TELL ME

w h y

M Y

C H I L D R E N

D I E D

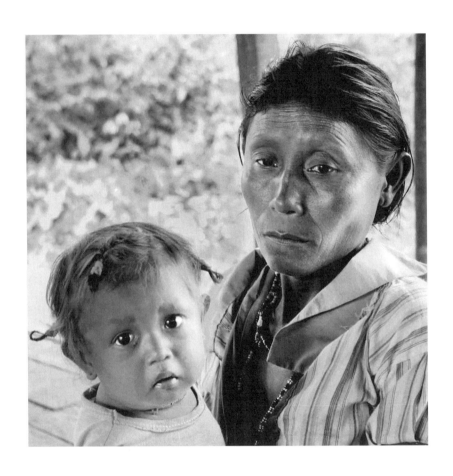

CRITICAL GLOBAL HEALTH *Evidence, Efficacy, Ethnography*
Edited by Vincanne Adams and João Biehl

TELL ME

w h y

MY

CHILDREN

DIED

———

RABIES, INDIGENOUS KNOWLEDGE,
and COMMUNICATIVE JUSTICE

Charles L. Briggs & Clara Mantini-Briggs

Duke University Press   Durham and London   2016

© 2016 Duke University Press
All rights reserved
Printed in the United States of America on acid-free paper ∞
Designed by Courtney Leigh Baker
Typeset in Garamond Premier Pro by Westchester Publishing Services

Library of Congress Cataloging-in-Publication Data
Names: Briggs, Charles L., [date] author. | Mantini-Briggs, Clara, [date] author.
Title: Tell me why my children died : rabies, indigenous knowledge, and
communicative justice / Charles L. Briggs and Clara Mantini-Briggs.
Other titles: Critical global health.
Description: Durham : Duke University Press, 2016. | Series: Critical global health:
evidence, efficacy, ethnography | Includes bibliographical references and index.
Identifiers: LCCN 2015038469
ISBN 9780822361053 (hardcover : alk. paper)
ISBN 9780822361244 (pbk. : alk. paper)
ISBN 9780822374398 (e-book)
Subjects: LCSH: Warao children—Diseases—Venezuela—Delta Amacuro—
History—21st century. | Epidemics—Venezuela—Delta Amacuro—History—21st century. |
Discrimination in medical care—Venezuela—Delta Amacuro—History—21st century. |
Communicable diseases in children—Venezuela—Delta Amacuro—History—21st century.
Classification: LCC RA650.55.V42 D458 2016 | DDC 362.196900987/62—dc23
LC record available at http://lccn.loc.gov/2015038469

COVER ART: Anita Rivas watches her husband's lament, Barranquitas, Venezuela, 2008.
Photograph by Charles L. Briggs.

FOR ELBIA AND MAMERTO
and the others who died in the mysterious epidemic

FOR LIBRADO

and

FOR FELICIANA, BILL, AND NANCY

and

FOR GUERINO, ESTRELLA, AND ALFREDO

CONTENTS

ILLUSTRATIONS

maps

figures

Inez Rivero Borges's one-room home in El Cocal has a green plastic roof and open walls on three sides, and is perched on stilts above the mud bordering a broad river. This is where she sits with her infant daughter to recount, over the span of forty-five minutes, the details of the mysterious deaths of her two sons, Jesús, age three, and Lizandro, age five (figure P.1). She is thirty-seven years old and has been married for a quarter century to Darío Garay Mata. She has given birth to twelve children, but only five are still alive. The infant girl she is now nursing will soon fall ill. She is one of scores of parents who moved frenetically from one caregiver to another in a desperate search to save their children, only to end up traveling to the cemetery—sometimes, as with Inez Rivero, over and over. They passed along their observations to anyone who would listen; they offered to collaborate in figuring out what was causing the mysterious epidemic. But even after the dying ended, their search for answers went on. They continue to demand, thinking both of their own children and many others, "Tell me why my children died."

First, Jesús "developed a fever out of the blue" in mid-March 2008. On the second day, when the fever grew intense, Inez said, "I went to my mother and told her, 'I just don't like it. Even though his fever is not high, I don't like the look of his eyes.' His eyes had changed color. His eyes weren't the same." When Jesús tried to swallow some acetaminophen in liquid form, "it didn't work for him; he felt like he was drowning." He swallowed a bit, "but then his eyes looked like they were crossed. His hands were stiff, like he was already going to die." By the third day, at times "he became immobile, as if he were asleep. When he was asleep, his legs kept moving." He was having trouble walking, and he fell a number of times. Soon, Jesús could no longer swallow food. Held tightly in his mother's hammock all night, he tossed and turned; whenever he started to fall asleep, he had strange dreams. "We didn't sleep at all that night."

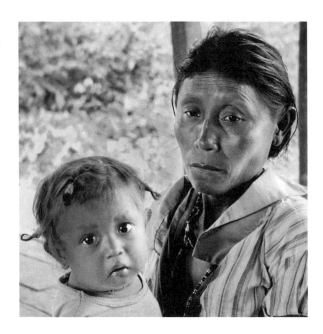

FIGURE P.I. Inez Rivero with her baby daughter, 2008. Photograph by Charles L. Briggs.

Strangely, "he would lose consciousness—but then seem just fine." Jesús also had frequent seizures.

Inez went to seek help from a healer who lived nearby. "I jumped out of the boat and went right up to him and stood before him: 'I came to you because my son is very, very sick and he couldn't sleep.'" He treated the boy and requested a return visit that evening. Back home, Jesús played actively with the family's dog and seemed fine, but later his legs were painful, and he seemed to be growing cold. His head hurt incredibly: "He wouldn't let anyone touch his head; he kept moving it from side to side, from side to side. He was dying. He was dying." Returning just as cooking fires marked the thatched-roofed homes in the waning light, the healer placed Jesús in a hammock and began to massage him, "but he died in the healer's arms." All that night and until noon the following day, Inez composed and sang *ona ribu*, laments for Jesús, while his father and other men fashioned a small coffin and built a small house-tomb for the child.

Two weeks after his death, five-year-old Lizandro "came down with a fever just like Jesús." At first, he continued to run about like a normal child, but "he had trouble sleeping; he would play by himself in the middle of the night." In the morning, he lingered in his hammock. On a visit to his grandmother, Lizandro ate taro and seemed fine, but, returning home, he got a bad case of hiccups and slumped into his hammock. Turning to the medicine that doctors and nurses could provide, Inez told the local nurse, "I came to ask for your help because my son is ending up just like his brother. He has a fever—give him an injection to bring down the fever." Lizandro got his injection and a hug from the nurse, which he returned. At home, Inez administered additional medication precisely as indicated, but it only seemed to make the child worse, and he began to have powerful seizures, falling down several times. The headache was so intense that he kept repeating, " 'My head, my head.' He was getting worse; it was just the way his little brother died."

Darío, Inez, and two of her sisters set out in a hired boat with Lizandro on an odyssey to find healers. Ready to go anywhere and stay as long as necessary, Inez said, "We took our hammocks with us." When the first healer failed, they traveled to a more distant settlement to consult another. When he failed, they went to a larger settlement closer to home, Arawabisi, where several healers joined forces on Lizandro's behalf. In España, farther down the Winikina River, they visited a healer who took out his sacred rattle and began to shake it, attempting to call *hebu* spirits/pathogens that might be lodged in Lizandro's body. But as soon as the spirit stones moved within the rattle, creating powerful sounds and visible sparks, Lizandro cried out, " 'That's terrible, no! That's scary, that's scary, Papa.' . . . The boy said that he was frightened, and so [the healer] stopped singing and using the rattle. Since Lizandro was older, he could express himself."

When the family returned to El Cocal, "He was near death—just like his brother." Desperate but not giving up, they called a healer from across the river. After touching Lizandro's body, feeling for the shape, hardness, and size of a pathogen and intoning a few words addressed to those areas of the spirit/medical world he commanded, he said, "No, that's not the kind that I know; another kind of illness has seized him." Healers had heard that a disease was afoot that neither they nor the nurses could stop. In all, Inez and Darío visited twelve healers, some more than once; the treatment sessions sometimes lasted most of the night. Still traumatized by Jesús's death, they did not sleep for days and were exhausted from restraining Lizandro during his many seizures. "Since he was big, he was strong."

But Lizandro's death, when it came, "took place very fast. . . . Toward the end, the saliva came; at that point his saliva just gushed." Inez, her sisters, and Lizandro's siblings combined their efforts, but they "could not wipe away the saliva before more came." Demonstrating, Inez's right hand moves rapidly some twenty times from her mouth outward. Lizandro was *amoni diana*, close to dying. His fever was high; he overreacted to sounds; and he couldn't perform simple bodily functions, such as swallowing or urinating. He lay in his hammock thrashing from side to side, thrusting his head and body backward as if his back would break. "His lungs were making sounds," and "he was having trouble breathing." Lizandro "loved everyone. . . . He hugged his father strongly around the neck and held on tightly; and his father hugged him too." Lizandro then asked for his brothers, calling their names, starting with his older brother, Armando. In Lizandro's voice Inez calls, " 'Come here, Armando, come here, Armando.' He wasn't around . . . but [Lizandro] called out to him." Then Lizandro named the names of "two *hotarao*," meaning nonindigenous persons, employees of a firm paid by the government to build cement bridges that would connect houses spread along the marshy ground, bridges that were never finished. "Now those drunken hotarao are gone. Back when there were many drunken hotarao here, they fell upon Lizandro, they hit him until he bled. . . .

"Then my son died."

This is a book we did not want to write, about a project that we did not want to undertake, about experiences that were not framed as research and that continue to create deep ambivalence within us. Nevertheless, there are times when the world calls you and you must either respond or face the realization that you have turned your back on it. This is our response to a call to "tell me why my children died."

The story we tell here looks into the depths of human misery, a nightmarish tale centered in a Venezuelan rain forest. It focuses on the death of children—sometimes one after another in the same family—from a disease that leaves no survivors, tortures bodies and minds, was never officially diagnosed, and, once symptoms appear, remains untreatable. Many of the words are not our own—they were spoken by parents who want the world to know about their children's deaths, parents who refused to let their children's deaths turn into memories deemed to be of significance only to them, only recalled as people lie in their hammocks in the darkness of rain forest nights. Other words are spoken by the nurses and doctors who tried to treat their young patients—only to watch them die in agony. Cuban and Venezuelan epidemiologists, in their turn, tried to solve the puzzle, which was as baffling and unprecedented as it was persistent. Healers were equally unsuccessful. Politicians and public health officials attempted to make the epidemic disappear—or turn it into more evidence of the supposed cultural inferiority of a population whose health they were charged with protecting. Journalists told readers and viewers around the world about the epidemic, only to drop the story after just two weeks, when the government claimed to have resolved the situation—without even providing the parents with a diagnosis or scientists with a scrap of evidence.

This book centers on a challenge that parents and local representatives continue to pose whenever doctors, officials, or journalists will listen: "Tell me

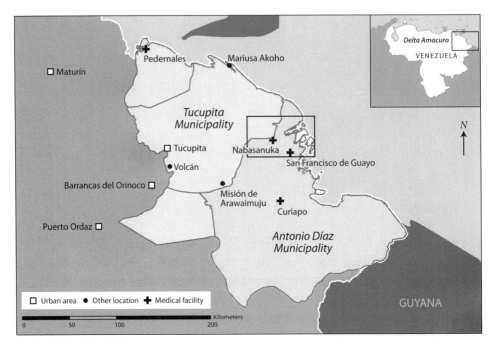

MAP P.1. Delta Amacuro State

why my children died." The epidemic occurred in 2007 and 2008. Nevertheless, their demand still reverberates in the mist that hovers above the vast delta that the Orinoco River creates as it enters the Caribbean Sea in eastern Venezuela (see map P.1). They demanded that doctors use their seemingly magical powers to turn suffering into a word, a diagnosis, the name of the disease that numbed their children's limbs and bedeviled their minds. Solving the medical mystery would, they hoped, enable doctors and nurses to tell them how to save the lives of their remaining children. The evidence we compiled as part of a team that included two local leaders, a healer, and a nurse suggested that the diagnosis was rabies, a disease that slowly and painfully takes control of the nervous system, and that vampire bats were the vector. Although rabies is almost 100 percent fatal, timely vaccination would have prevented infection and stopped the deaths; the vaccines, however, never reached the settlements where the children and young adults died. Bats still make their nocturnal visits, and the vaccines still have not arrived. Thus, the parents' demand actually goes far beyond just revealing a diagnostic category that would end the mystery— they want to know why, half a decade later, no one seems to care that they have grappled with some of the most acute health inequities in the world—and continue to do so.

The deaths led the parents, their neighbors, and leaders in the Delta Amacuro rain forest to identify lethal connections between disease and inequality. Activists noted bitterly that if the children who were dying were rich and white and lived in a nice part of the capital, Caracas, health officials would have mobilized armies of doctors and flown in international experts to solve the mystery. Why, the parents asked, did their children deserve only modest and fleeting attention? Why are their children's lives—and their own—deemed to be of so little value? Five years later, government officials still have not spoken the words that the parents demand to hear: "This is what killed your children, and we're sorry they died." So they refuse to be silent.

Our relationship to the delta and its residents has been long and intense. Charles began working there in 1986, learned the language (Warao), and studied healing, narratives, indigenous legal practices, gender relations, and interactions with government authorities. Given the precariousness of health conditions there, he witnessed numerous wakes and recorded the laments sung at several. Clara, a Venezuelan public health physician, began working for the Regional Health Service in April 1992, just months before a cholera epidemic killed some 500 delta residents. She served as the assistant regional epidemiologist and the state director of health education. After collaborating with residents in several areas to establish nursing stations and build cholera-prevention programs, we researched the underpinnings, bureaucratic as much as epidemiological, of such extensive death from a preventable and treatable bacterial infection. Afterward, we turned to other projects. One involved documenting how President Hugo Chávez Frías's socialist revolution had brought doctors, mainly Cubans, to live in most of the low-income urban neighborhoods in Venezuela.

After years of working elsewhere in Venezuela, it was our book documenting that epidemic, *Stories in the Time of Cholera*, that brought us back to the delta in 2008. Collaborating with healer Tirso Gómez and his daughter, nurse and paramedic Norbelys Gómez, and the residents of Siawani, we were using income derived from book royalties and prizes to explore new models for health programs. Upon our arrival in the delta, Conrado Moraleda, president of the local health committee, and his brother Enrique, a local political leader, approached us and asked us to join them and the Gómezes in trying to figure out what was causing yet another epidemic—this one ongoing and nameless. Chávez's frequent televised statements about constitutional guarantees to

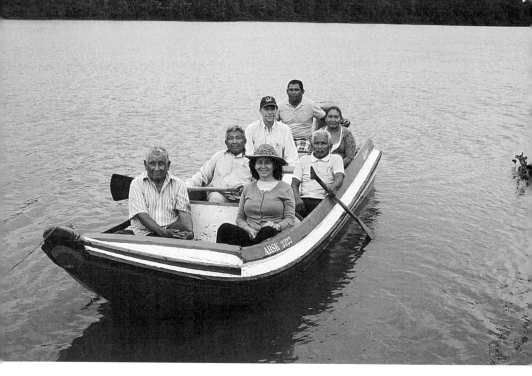

FIGURE P.2. The team in Enrique Moraleda's *balajú*, *Misluoy I*, 2012. Photograph by José Moraleda.

health as "a fundamental social right, [an] obligation of the State," in addition to his calls for an end to discrimination against indigenous peoples, struck a deep chord with Conrado and Enrique. They decided to unravel another mystery that the epidemic had revealed. If a revolution had brought doctors to and inspired residents in low-income neighborhoods elsewhere in Venezuela, why did health conditions remained abysmal in the lower delta? If the regional government lacked the will to bring the revolution in health to the delta, they resolved do so themselves, together with the parents who lost children in the epidemic.

This book is our response to the demands by parents and local leaders to make their words circulate, and it represents our participation in their efforts to solve the mystery and to help ensure that such a tragic scenario is not repeated. Centered on unknowns and mysteries, many of which have yet to be solved, it recounts how an unofficial epidemiological team of six people, traveling in a small wooden boat (figure P.2)and equipped with only a stethoscope, a sphygmomanometer for taking blood pressure, and a few medicines, and having no access to a diagnostic laboratory, tried to learn what was killing children and young adults so they could figure out how to stop it. In doing so, the team faced questions such as: what is causing these deaths? Why did it stump parents, healers, physicians, nurses, and Cuban and Venezuelan epidemiologists alike? Why did this disease arrive in 2007? Did ecological change prompt it? Why didn't Chávez's pro-poor, pro-indigenous government—which devoted massive resources to addressing health issues in other parts of the country— respond more forcefully and effectively to the outbreak? If the team encountered people dying from the disease, what help could we provide? Could we combine indigenous healing, clinical medicine, epidemiology, anthropology, and the impressive sophistication of Warao storytelling to more effectively investigate the epidemic? How could indigenous leaders, whose only experience with the press had been on the receiving end of stereotypes and discrimination, get reporters to take them and their story seriously?

Tell Me Why My Children Died is not simply a tale of suffering, and— emphatically—it is not about passive people who waited for others to speak and act on their behalf. Even before the epidemic began, leaders like Conrado and Enrique Moraleda had already placed health inequities at the top of the agenda of the indigenous social movement. Moreover, the situation we document is not unique. Nearly every year, bat-transmitted rabies causes outbreaks in some part of the Amazon basin. (It also periodically claims a life in the United States.) Thinking more broadly about these events, although the mysterious epidemic's toll in the delta is appalling, respiratory infections, diarrheal diseases, and malnutrition—which also kill some 26 percent of children under five in the delta—also take too many lives in too many other parts of the world. These sorts of unconscionable health problems have been widely documented, and drawing attention to them is not our primary goal here. Instead, our focus is on recounting the ways that, in the midst of a worst-case scenario, people came up with novel insights into how acute health inequities are produced and are made to seem "normal," and how they devised a creative vision of how we could all work together to end them.

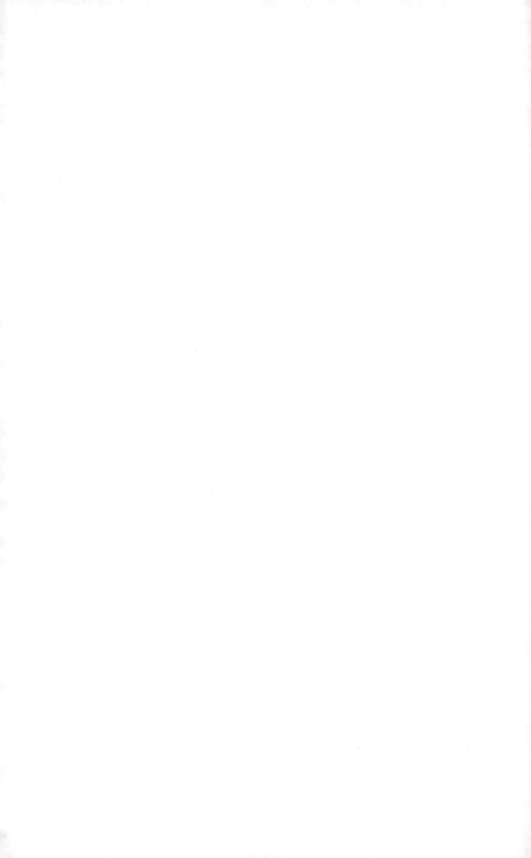

This book proposes a new way of thinking about health, from daily interactions with biomedical professionals and alternative practitioners to addressing some of the most pressing problems of global health. But the fundamental insights on which it draws did not emerge sitting at a desk or staring calmly at a computer screen, nor are we their originators. They were born in the middle of a terrifying and confusing epidemic in the Delta Amacuro rain forest of eastern Venezuela, forming part of parents' and caregivers' efforts to save the lives of their children. They also emerge from reflections on why the epidemic occurred and why it has never been officially diagnosed and on the unconscionable everyday health conditions that preceded and followed it. And, finally, they were born of a conviction on the part of people who face some of the worst health conditions on the planet that their ideas could play a crucial role in making a healthier and more just world. We accordingly need to introduce the book's contribution by placing it in the context in which it was forged.

The issue is global in scope. As we were finishing the manuscript, Ebola hemorrhagic fever was wrenching apart areas of West Africa. As of 6 May 2015, 26,593 cases and 11,005 deaths were reported in the region.[1] Some observers appealed to cultural logics—projecting West Africans as believing in "witchcraft" and "witch doctors" and impeding the efforts of physicians—in explaining the disease's wide dissemination and substantial case fatality rate.[2] Others rejected these sorts of cultural logics in favor of structural explanations, reading the epidemic as a symptom of the inadequacy of health infrastructures in the region,[3] exacerbated by rising global income inequalities and policies fostered by multilateral lending organizations and First World governments. When experimental drugs and multimillion-dollar treatment modes were used to save the lives of white health professionals from the Global North but not West Africans, perceptions that some lives were judged more valuable than others abounded. Ebola thus sharpened questions of access to health care, gaps within as well as between countries, as some people have access to organ transplants or drugs costing hundreds of thousands of dollars a year while the lack of cheap vaccines and treatments leaves others vulnerable to preventable and treatable infectious diseases.

Issues of access are indeed an important concern for global health. They were certainly key to incredibly high mortality from cholera in the 1992–1993 epidemic in Delta Amacuro. Caused by the bacteria *Vibrio cholerae*, the disease can be prevented by providing potable water and treated effectively with rehydration therapy, often supplemented with antibiotics. Nevertheless, if untreated, cholera can kill an adult through dehydration in as little as eight hours after the onset of symptoms. Given that reaching a clinic with a resident physician in an unmotorized canoe could take over a day, access to health care was crucial.[4] As commonly happens in epidemics (Rosenberg 1992), cholera X-rayed everyday inequalities in the region: nearly all deaths occurred in the population that is racialized as indigenous, specifically as the Warao ethnic group. These deaths came on top of what epidemiologists in the region refer to as the normal deaths from diarrheal and other diseases, including the staggering current figure of 26 percent child mortality (0–5 years).[5]

But when another epidemic began in July 2007, the deaths could not be as easily explained by questions of access to health care. This epidemic came in the midst of a socialist revolution. Starting in 2003, President Hugo Chávez Frías's Bolivarian revolution championed the health of low-income Venezuelans—the majority of the population—as a major priority. Ending decades in which access to public health eroded, most low-income neighborhoods in the country soon boasted a small health care facility, often staffed by a Cuban doctor. In the 2007–2008 epidemic in the delta, most of the patients were treated by a local nurse and taken to a clinic staffed by a resident physician. When he couldn't figure out what was killing his patients, the doctor sent them to the hospital in the state capital, Tucupita. Most were then transported to tertiary care facilities, where they were treated by specialists in the intensive care unit. Epidemiologists came to investigate, but they never determined the cause. No one was denied care, and no one was charged a dime. Nevertheless, the mysterious disease killed 10 percent of the population in one small settlement, Mukoboina. Some families lost two or three children. No one in the region had ever seen cases of the disease that caused this epidemic. Cholera was comparatively easy to diagnose, but the 2007 epidemic stumped doctors, nurses, epidemiologists, and healers. The underlying question thus shifts: despite significant improvements in access to care for Venezuelans, why did so many die in 2007–2008, and why did the disease elude diagnosis?

A crucial clue to unlocking the mystery—and to addressing key problems of global health more broadly—was provided by the parents' incessant demand, "Tell me why my children died." They still pose this challenge to doctors, nurses, health officials, healers, epidemiologists—just about anybody who will listen. It has, as they stressed, two components: First, they demand to tell their stories, to relate their efforts to save their children's lives. They were constantly observing symptoms and how patients responded to healers', nurses', and doctors' treatments. They thought insistently about what was going on and anything strange that might have preceded the illnesses. Their demand entails having their contributions taken seriously, sharing in solving the puzzle. Their insistence that people listen to what they have to say also involves recognition that their children's lives had value and that their deaths matter to more than just their relatives.

The second dimension of their challenge requires sharing: they asked doctors, epidemiologists, healers, and health officials to tell them what they had learned about the disease. The parents answered clinicians' questions and provided details requested by epidemiologists, but few health professionals deemed them worthy of a response, even to say, "We don't know, but this is what we are thinking." Or simply to say, "We're sorry your children died." "Tell me why my children died" thus constitutes a demand for dialogue, for a laterally organized and collaborative exchange of knowledge. What is at issue here is not a liberal, even paternal, gesture, an extension of empathy in the face of suffering. Given that the disease had never appeared before, pooling knowledge would seem to be a rather good idea. And, more generally, even when diagnoses are easy to come by but successful strategies for stopping preventable diseases and deaths are hard to find, breaking the monopoly held by "experts" who produce what they believe to be the only valid forms of evidence might open up exciting new possibilities for addressing global health problems.

When the children kept dying and health professionals did not respond to their overtures, the parents recruited two local leaders, brothers Conrado and Enrique Moraleda. Their deceased brother, Librado, had been one of the most respected indigenous leaders in Venezuela. Serving as the president of the health committee for the local clinic, Conrado listened to the parents' stories every time they brought their children for treatment. He realized how much knowledge they had to share and how their offers to share it had been rebuffed. They pressed him to approach the director of the Regional Health Service (RHS) in town, tell him about the epidemic, and request a more ambitious response. Conrado made the trip several times. After a second wave of deaths began in January 2008, the parents grew more anxious and angry; Conrado then bypassed health authorities, demanding a hearing with politicians and journalists. Health officials responded angrily; they discredited Conrado and the parents through rumors circulated in town, radio broadcasts, and articles in the local newspaper.

Try a thought experiment for a moment. You devote all of your resources—and place yourself deeply in debt—trying to save the life of your child. You go to every type of caregiver you can find, trying to figure out what he or she has to offer, and supply the requested information, in the language of the practitioner. Nevertheless, none have more than passing interest in what you have to say, and some denigrate what you have said and done. When one fails, you look for another. You end up in a strange city, your dying child surrounded by machines; you lack anywhere to sleep or resources to buy food. And then your child dies. Just as you return home to bury her, your parents tell you that another of your children has come down "with the same disease." Then you learn that doctors in the city are blaming you on the radio and in the newspaper for negligently killing your own children, by feeding them garbage or poisonous fruit or fish or intoxicating them with lead or mercury.

Reading these articles and listening to the parents' angry responses convinced Conrado and Enrique that the root of the problem, in the epidemic as much as in everyday death in the delta, did not lie with pathogens alone or the availability of health care but also fundamentally involved the production and circulation of knowledge about health. In 1992, health officials adopted a two-pronged strategy for dealing with the cholera epidemic. At the same time that they contained the spread of the bacteria, they countered political fallout generated by extensive national press coverage by claiming that the problem was not unhealthy health policies—the failure to provide potable water, sewage facilities, or adequate health care—but "the culture of the indigenous Warao ethnic group." As a result, the stereotype of "the Warao" that persisted right into 2007 was of a homogeneous population incapable of understanding what doctors say or participating adequately in caring for their own lives or those of family members, let alone contributing useful knowledge.

When a third wave of cases beginning in June 2008 was met with silence on the part of public health officials, the Moraledas decided that it was time to take action themselves against both the disease and the persistent lack of a response to the parents' demands. They began to connect the dots, perceiving how deeply the failure to value the voices of delta residents in clinical consultations, epidemiological investigations, and demeaning news stories lay at the center of both the failure to come up with a diagnosis and how the RHS was structured. If this pattern shaped the epidemic, the failure to diagnose it and the lack of concerted action on the part of public health officials required a bold effort to overturn public health business as usual. Deciding to form their own investigation, Enrique and Conrado recruited the two of us, healer Tirso Gómez, and nurse/EMT Norbelys Gómez. A novel type of collaborative work emerged, one that placed indigenous knowledge production at its core. Soon the parents' testimonies clearly revealed that the symptoms, not to mention the 100 percent case-fatality rate, lined up squarely with rabies and correlated with the incidence of nocturnal bites by vampire bats.

This book is not just an epidemiological thriller, a Sherlock Holmes–style narrative that reveals a viral killer. It rather explores other dimensions, ones that have implications that extend beyond the temporal contours of this particular epidemic and the delta's riverine geography. We are rather interested in how a socialist revolution, persistent ethnoracial inequities, relations between humans, viruses, bats, cats, chickens, trees, and other nonhumans, and interactions between parents, children, healers, physicians, nurses, epidemiologists, and journalists came together in producing an epidemic and impeding the collaborative knowledge exchange needed to diagnose it and stop it. Building on critical insights that emerged in the epidemic, our broader goals include diagnosing health and communicative inequities, analyzing their central role in creating health inequities, and reflecting on the call for justice pioneered by delta residents.

From Lay Labor in Health to Health/Communicative Labor

Two central features of the medicalization of health are the equation of clinical institutional sites with the labor of care and the identification of biomedicine as the locus of knowledge production in health. Even Annemarie Mol (2008), who envisions care as emerging collaboratively between patients and providers, identifies the clinic as the site where "the logic of care" unfolds. Argentine Mexican medical anthropologist Eduardo Menéndez (2009) rather explores ethnographically how clinical medicine depends on the labor of care performed by laypersons outside clinical settings. What scholars have missed is that the labor of care is coproduced with the labor of communicating about health, much of which is also performed by laypersons outside of clinical settings. Connections between care and communication have most commonly become visible to scholars and practitioners in the realms of "doctor-patient interaction" and health communication, but the epidemic and the way that the parents and the Moraledas responded to it revealed how other sites—such as epidemiological research, news coverage of health, and policy discussions—are involved and how deeply they are connected, if in precarious and shifting ways.

Who gets the credit for and who becomes invisible or gets blamed for the labor of care and communication follows the lines of professional hierarchy, but its distribution also parallels ethnoracial and class-based health inequities in complex and consequential ways. A landmark study by the esteemed Institute of Medicine hit upon this connection in seeking to explain why African American and Latino/a patients receive inferior treatment compared to Caucasians in the United States. It pointed to clinicians' perceptions that patients classified as members of these populations will be less capable of understanding diagnoses and treatment recommendations and less able or willing to turn this knowledge into behavioral changes as one factor that prompted clinicians to recommend less favorable treatments (Smedley, Stith, and Nelson 2002). By scrutinizing assumptions about the quality of the patient's labor of care and communication, this finding points to how health and communicative inequities are tied at the hip. Clinical medicine, once again, is not the only place where these inequities are coproduced: health/communicative inequities are inscribed deeply within health education and communication, epidemiology, public health policy, and news coverage. These health/communicative inequities reconfigure structural factors as the projected inadequacies of ethnoracial minorities in health communication.

Health infrastructures do not rely on cables, computers, CAT scans, record systems, software, and the Internet alone but also on the forms of communicative labor that situate people in relation to them. Health-related roles, including those of parent and child, physician and patient, are relationally defined, that is, constructed in relationship to one another on the basis of their difference. These positions are certainly constituted through care—who gets to touch whose body and use technologies like thermometers and stethoscopes in particular ways and administer or prescribe medications—but they are also defined through communicative labor. Learning to play the "sick role," in Talcott Parsons's (1951) terms, or that of the patient (Harvey 2008) involves learning when to call 911 and when to ask a receptionist for an appointment, how to talk about symptoms, how to answer receptionists', nurses', and physicians' questions, how to listen to diagnoses and treatment recommendations, and much more. The Institute of Medicine study suggests that medical outcomes depend not only on access to care or even how well individuals learn to play the patient role but whether clinicians give them credit for mastering these complex ways of performing biomedical literacies. A major focus of health journalism is providing advice regarding how to be an active patient who brings information to the doctor, asks questions, and helps shape decisions about treatment. Pharmaceutical ads teach television viewers to "ask your doctor if [a particular medication] is right for you." Parents are instructed in how to speak with their children about drugs, drinking, and sexually transmitted infections. Medical schools teach physicians not just how to talk with their patients but how to circulate medical information through notes, records, tests, and consultations with other health professionals (Cicourel 1992; Good and DelVecchio Good 2000). The complex forms of communication related to obtaining authorization and reimbursement from government agencies and insurance companies not only constitutes a great deal of the labor that professionals and patients alike devote to health in some countries but also fundamentally structures care—to the chagrin of many physicians and patients. Research suggests that ignorance and confusion are sometimes hardwired into such health services as Medicaid to cut costs by limiting how much people can overcome forms of "bureaucratic disentitlement" generated by "withholding information, providing misinformation, . . . and requiring extraordinary amounts of documentation" (Danz 2000: 1006; see also Horton 2014; López 2005). Looking closely at how the roles of caregiver and patient are relationally defined suggests to us that forms of health and communicative labor are deeply entangled and fundamentally out of sync, simultaneously crucial for enabling the work of care and constituting one of its fundamental obstacles.

A major reason that the importance of this nexus has been so seldom perceived is the commonsense opposition—largely reproduced by scholars— between media and communication versus the domains of science and medicine. Challenging this perspective, we follow Jesús Martín Barbero (1987) in suggesting that constructing "the media" or communication as a separate arena that exists apart from the spheres they seemingly represent should not be a presupposition that shapes our analytical framework; we should rather document ethnographically how, when, and why this category emerges and in opposition to what. This binary is particularly evident in news coverage of health issues, to which we return below. Scholars generally invoke health news only in extracting what seem to be transparent windows on popular perceptions; health professionals complain about how journalists sensationalize or distort medical issues, thereby relegating them to a sphere of "the media" that seems to exist apart from how these objects come into being and get imbued with value. Such treatments fail to take into account the pervasiveness of health news:

consuming health-related media forms, including direct-to-consumer advertisements, and ingesting pharmaceuticals and dietary supplements compete for being the most pervasive ways that health is woven into daily routines. Science-technology-society (STS) studies researchers almost never include journalists in the actor networks of scientists, politicians, microbes, technologies, and infrastructures they study. The epidemic revealed what scholars miss: that narratives circulate between news stories, clinical encounters, complementary and alternative medical practices, epidemiological investigations and reports, and health policy debates in complex and consequential ways. Again, sensing that health news can both reflect and extend health inequities, thereby buttressing unhealthy health policies, Conrado and Enrique turned their investigation of the epidemic into an alternative media strategy, one designed to produce medical and communicative justice.

The communication versus medicine binary also enters in other sites in which communicative and health inequities come together. Elliott Mishler (1984) and Howard Waitzkin (1991) argue that communicative inequities structure doctor-patient interaction in ways that thwart diagnosis and treatment; Brad Davidson (2001) details how medical translation can widen these gaps. Deborah Lupton (1994) and Mohan Dutta (2008) point to how fundamental inequities are built into dominant perspectives and practices of health communication, thereby turning efforts to overcome health inequities into key sites for extending social hierarchies. Clive Seale (2002) argues that health news similarly projects health communication as a hypodermic injection of knowledge into the minds of ignorant lay audiences. Herein lies the reason that we do not use the term "health communication" to frame our work here. What Dutta and others refer to as hegemonic perspectives in health communication imagine a linear, hierarchically structured process by which information produced by biomedical specialists—including scientists, clinicians, and epidemiologists—is transformed by health communication specialists into lay language and then transmitted to laypersons. Reproducing the media/medicine opposition thus excludes journalists, health promoters, and doctors and nurses—in their work of talking to patients—as well as laypersons as producers of knowledge. We accordingly introduce a new term, *health/communicative inequities*, to suggest how knowledge about health is coproduced by health and communication professionals and laypersons in a broad range of sites. We go beyond simply looking at both communicative inequities and health inequities to analyze how they emerge simultaneously, one powerfully shaping the other and often exacerbating its effects.

Even as researchers have explored how "neoliberal" or market-oriented restructurings of health and other institutions increase inequities by projecting normative models of rational, self-knowing, and self-interested subjects (Adams 2013b; Clarke et al. 2003; Rose 2006), João Biehl (2005) carefully documents how even progressive efforts to extend access to health care—mainly in the form of providing pharmaceuticals—can create "zones of abandonment." Critical epidemiologists (Breilh 2003) and social epidemiologists (Krieger 2011) scrutinize the way that epidemiology can turn assumptions and forms of social classification that reflect the position of dominant sectors into what seem to be objective, statistical measures of the distribution and causation of disease.

One of the central contributions of this book is to bring concerns that have largely been viewed in isolation into dialogue by ethnographically documenting how health/communicative inequities are coproduced in clinical encounters, epidemiological investigations, media coverage, and the development of health policies. By challenging the boundary-work (Gieryn 1983) that patrols borders between "health" and "communication," we demonstrate how health/communicative inequities structure care, epidemiology, journalism, and public health. We detail the different forms that these inequities take in each context, demonstrating how they form the social glue that connects sites as bodies, narratives, and reports accumulate, juxtaposing more and more extensive and complex assemblages. The parents' narratives that we highlight here focus as much on the health/communicative labor they performed as the work of care they undertook in trying to keep their children from dying. Breilh (2003) argues that documenting health inequities is not enough: we should go on, he suggests, to analyze how they are produced. We argue here that health/communicative dimensions play a central role in producing health inequities, as much in rich, industrialized countries as in those in which incomes and health services are more limited.

Failing to analyze health/communicative inequities limits research on the production of health inequities and bolsters the many ways that they come to feel like natural, inevitable features of contemporary life. In asserting demands for health/communicative justice, the parents and our fellow team members demonstrated that justice in health can only be achieved when efforts to challenge health inequities go hand in hand with more democratic health/communicative practices. Moreover, the labor of care and health/communicative labor are also often entangled and out of sync in situations that are not directly structured by marked inequalities. Thus, even as we are positioned in economies of the labor of care and health/communicative labor in different ways, this problem affects us all.

"Mystery Disease Kills Dozens in Venezuela":
An Overview of the Epidemic

A mystery disease has killed dozens of Warao Indians in recent months in a remote area of northeastern Venezuela, according to indigenous leaders and researchers from the University of California at Berkeley, who informed health officials of the outbreak on Wednesday.—*New York Times*, 6 August 2008

Given the complexity of the events that unfolded, a brief, chronological summary might help. The following overview encapsulates what happened, how people tried to diagnose the disease, and the work of the team that Conrado and Enrique organized. In July 2007, a strange disease appeared in Mukoboina, a settlement of some eighty persons located in the delta of the Orinoco River, the third largest in South America, near where the river enters the Caribbean next to Trinidad (see map I.1).[6] In Mukoboina, houses are open-air structures with thatched roofs built on stilts above the river and swampy land (see figure I.1). People call themselves Warao, claiming membership in a population that has lived in what is now Delta Amacuro State since before Columbus first stumbled onto the South American mainland in 1498. Residents speak an indigenous language, similarly called Warao; some also speak Spanish. There is no clinic, school, or other services. One by one, children developed fever, headache, and body aches. Parents took them to see Mukoboina's leader, Inocencio Torres, who is a healer. When he could not figure out what was wrong or stop the symptoms, they turned to a nurse practicing in a nearby settlement and other healers, but all failed. Strange symptoms appeared—a tingling sensation in the legs, followed by numbness and paralysis. The children stopped eating; then they couldn't drink. They sometimes had strange hallucinations and bouts of anxiety.

During this period, a team of nurses made a routine visit while vaccinating for childhood diseases. Ronaldo Domínguez, coordinator of the nursing program for the local Antonio Díaz Municipality, examined one of the Mukoboina patients shortly before he died. Seeing that something strange was going on, he returned several times in the following days while vaccinating nearby. When another child became ill, he, like the local healer and nurse, urged the parents to take the boy to the Nabasanuka clinic some forty minutes away by motorized canoe or several hours by paddle; it was staffed by bilingual nurses and a newly graduated doctor.[7] Hooking up IVs, the staff tried analgesics to stop the child's intense pain, antipyretics to lower the fever, antibiotics to treat

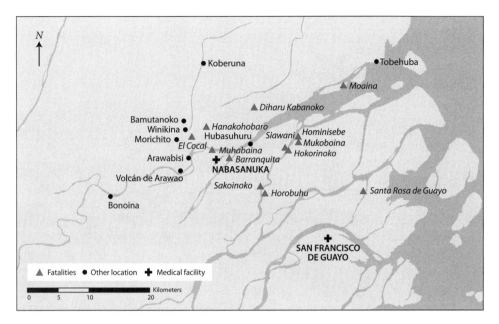

MAP 1.1. Area where cases were concentrated

a possible infection, and more. But nothing worked, and another child died. When the next patient appeared, an eleven-year-old boy, the doctor sent him to the maternal-pediatric wing of the hospital in Tucupita. Physicians there could not figure out what was wrong, and soon the symptoms worsened. They transported the boy by ambulance to Maturín, a larger city several hours away, which boasted more advanced care, where he was placed in the intensive care unit. The results, however, were the same—death without diagnosis.

All in all, seven Mukoboina children between three and eleven years of age died in July–September 2007 and one more the following January—some 10 percent of the population. Four children died in nearby settlements in September and October and four more in January and February 2008, all with similar symptoms. Taking their children to town imposed new forms of anguish on parents—once there, they had no place to stay and little or no food or money, and generally felt ignored and mistreated by the hospital staff. Back in the delta, many parents stopped taking their children to the clinic, even for easily treated diseases.

As president of the local health committee in Nabasanuka, Conrado Moraleda visited the clinic each time a new patient arrived and kept an eye on his or her progress. Like the nurses, he first heard about the initial deaths through

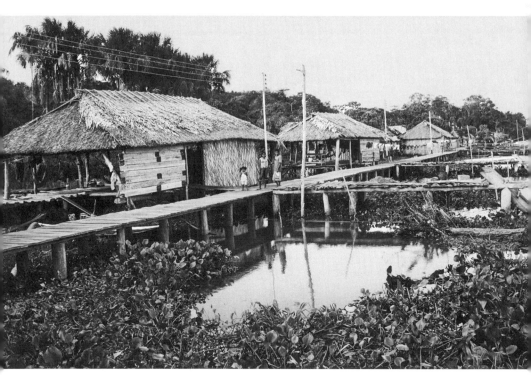

FIGURE 1.1. Houses in Mukoboina, 2010. Photograph by Charles L. Briggs.

what is jokingly called Warao Radio, the passing of news from mouth to mouth, settlement to settlement. Conrado then saw what happened when patients reached the clinic; he listened to the doctor and nurses tell how the disease baffled and worried them. Starting just after the first cases reached the Nabasanuka clinic, Conrado repeatedly visited the director of the RHS and the regional epidemiologist in Tucupita; he expressed concern about the situation, related that residents were terrified, and asked for action. The regional epidemiologist and a Cuban epidemiologist affiliated with the Mission Barrio Adentro program visited Mukoboina in September 2007. They obtained detailed data on the children who had died and the households in which they lived. They filed reports that presented several hypotheses but reached no conclusion as to the cause of the disease. After one more child died in October 2007, the strange disease seemed to go away, and nothing further was done.

Then five more children died in January and February 2008. Parents, nurses, and local leaders believed that the regional government in Tucupita was indifferent. Conrado joined parents of the dead children and nurses in trying to press the regional government to act. Traveling to Tucupita, they asked sympathetic members of the Legislative Council to hold a public hearing, resulting in embarrassment and anger on the part of RHS, which then conducted a large epidemiological investigation. Jesús and Lizandro died in El Cocal in March and April, but then the disease seemed to disappear again.

June 2008 ushered in a new wave of deaths over an even wider area, including eight in Santa Rosa de Guayo to the southeast, three in Muaina, a settlement near the coast, and one around the corner from Nabasanuka in Barranquita—seventeen deaths in three months (see map I.1). Local leaders were frightened and furious, and their anger focused on Conrado and other activists, blaming them for failing to force the government to act. Conrado and Enrique hatched a bold plan—they would compile their own data and then bypass the state government and go straight to Caracas. But without documentation or a diagnosis, it would be hard to get a hearing. That's why Conrado and Enrique almost literally pounced on us when we arrived in Nabasanuka on 24 July. They weren't looking for outsiders to tell them what to do—they had had enough of that. Rather, they thought that a physician and an anthropologist with whom they had worked for decades might be of some value. They also recruited an indigenous nurse, Norbelys Gómez, and a healer, Tirso Gómez.

Our six-person team traveled in a small wooden boat throughout the entire region, visiting thirty settlements (figure P.2). We located fourteen places in which someone had died from the disease. In each, we set up meetings in which parents who had lost children, local representatives, nurses, and other people could tell us their versions of what had happened. Many located the deaths within the broader context of hunger, social conflict, exploitation by businesses operating in the area, ecological change—whatever they felt was important. Our goals were twofold: first, because we had no idea what disease was afoot or exactly when it had started, we wanted to cast a wide epidemiological net—to collect any potentially relevant detail. Learning, as we did, that all of the chickens had died a year earlier or that many people had adopted cats might be irrelevant—or might be crucial to solving the mystery.

We sought, second, to provide a more substantive response to the parents' demand, "Tell me why my children died." Anger, pain, and fear were rampant. Even when epidemiologists and public health officials had visited, as in Mukoboina, people did not feel heard, never gaining the sense that their questions and observations had been taken seriously or their grief acknowledged. They wanted answers, but they also wanted public recognition of their loss and their struggles to keep their children alive. Listening to their stories, recording their

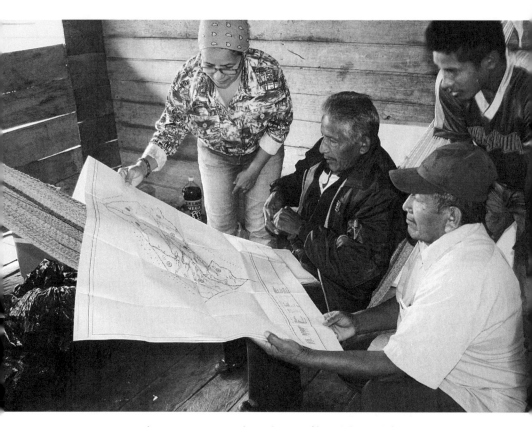

FIGURE I.2. Clara, Enrique, Conrado, and Eumar (from left to right) view map of Manuel Renault Parish while planning the team's investigation, 2008. Photograph by Charles L. Briggs.

perceptions, thinking with them about what could be happening, and just plain saying that we were sorry that their children had died was important. Enrique asked Charles to photograph each parent, resulting in the images that emerge in these pages, and to videotape as much of the work as possible.

When relatives asked Clara and Norbelys to examine Elbia Torres, whose husband had just died, we came face to face with the disease. Now there was clinical information to complement the "verbal autopsies," the parents' accounts of their children's illnesses. This enabled Clara to reach a presumptive diagnosis, which would have to be confirmed by laboratory tests: clinically, the disease seemed to be rabies. And if rabies was the disease, there was no cure, so all Clara and Norbelys could provide was palliative care; visiting Elbia twice a day, they eased her pain as we supported her relatives.

By the time Elbia died on 2 August, the team had compiled detailed information on thirty-eight cases. Using a laptop computer in a house deep within the rain forest, we pulled data from handwritten notebooks and fashioned them into a spreadsheet and a report. Conrado, Enrique, Norbelys, and Tirso wanted to stop the epidemic, but they also wanted to fundamentally change the way Delta Amacuro State's government treated the people they classified as indigenous. The report and photographs would demonstrate that delta parents care deeply about their children, that indigenous people had important knowledge about health to share, and that residents had the right to participate fully in the design, implementation, and evaluation of health programs. Our work was interrupted several times as we returned to participate in Elbia's wake and funeral; the sounds of her parents' laments and the hammer nailing her coffin shut rang in our ears each time we returned to the task of writing.

The team showed up on 6 August in the lobby of the national headquarters of the Ministry of Popular Power for Health in downtown Caracas. We made it clear that we were not trying to embarrass the government but were all supporters of President Chávez who were looking to present high ministry officials with a report that would assist them in addressing a health crisis. It was a fiasco. We were greeted by security guards, not the minister. They told us to go back to the delta—that we should never have left. Officials refused to meet with us or even accept a copy of our report. Reporters for the *New York Times* and *El Nacional*, a national newspaper aligned with the anti-Chávez opposition, witnessed the standoff. Finally, Conrado, Enrique, Norbelys, and Tirso were allowed to meet with the national epidemiologist. The six of us became a cause célèbre, appearing in newspapers around the world and on the government's two television stations, applauded as heroes by many Chávez supporters and members of the opposition alike. At the same time, however, national and regional government officials were pulling out all the stops in attempting to discredit us. They declared variously that there was no epidemic, that it was smaller than we stated, that we had confused the disease with "normal" diarrheal infections, that the real problem was "Warao culture," and even that it was all dreamed up "by an agent of the Empire" (referring to Charles's status as a U.S. citizen). We were harassed and threatened with incarceration. Commissions were sent to the delta, but their major goal was to prove us wrong; they never publicly presented an alternative diagnosis or took significant steps to address the underlying health issues.

In the end, officials simply erased the entire affair: Chávez's socialist government defended a regional administration affiliated with the United Socialist Party of Venezuela (PSUV) rather than standing by its commitment to provide health care to low-income Venezuelans and countering discrimination against indigenous people. The parents were forgotten. Officials forbade nurses to talk about health conditions or strange diseases with anyone other than RHS supervisors—and particularly not with reporters or researchers. Conrado, Enrique, Norbelys, and Tirso were threatened, warned to keep quiet and stay out of sight. They expressed deep discouragement and some bitterness that their leadership and aspirations for a better world had sparked only official contempt and denial. Meanwhile, to this day the parents continue to demand, "Tell me why my children died," and to press the six team members to keep the memory of their children's lives and deaths circulating—"We want lots of people to know!" Conrado, Enrique, Norbelys, and Tirso keep insisting that what we did involved more than the epidemic itself, that our efforts demonstrated that people who face acute health inequities can lead the way to a healthier and more just world. We collaboratively produced a memoir in Spanish, *Una efermedad monstruo: Indígenas derribando el cerco de la discriminación racial en salud* (A monster disease: Indigenous peoples breaking down barriers of health-based racial discrimination), aimed at readers who face similar health problems and policymakers. The present book rethinks the epidemic from a variety of participants' perspectives and focuses on the relationship between health and health/communicative inequities, bringing a range of analytical tools to the task of sorting out what happened and reflecting on its broader implication.

Narratives, Knowledge, Mourning, and Biomediatization: Forging New Points of Departure

Such a simple, linear, straightforward narrative of the epidemic was never told in the delta from start to finish, with all participants and places woven together and without the narrative being interrupted by fear, anger, and uncertainty or by accusations and recriminations. If this book simply retold the story in this manner, it would place us in the position of omniscient narrators and clairvoyant analysts, turning patients, parents, local leaders, doctors, nurses, healers, and epidemiologists into characters in need of our assistance in order to render their thoughts and actions transparent. Such a book would simply reproduce the health/communicative inequities that helped give rise to the epidemic and amplified its destructive effects. Our approach is rather to unsettle established ways that scholars, practitioners, activists, and others think about health inequities and open up new possibilities.

Our efforts to slow down conventional approaches takes several forms, two of which are primary.[8] In part I—which focuses on the participants' lenses—we complicate and fragment this story, bringing out the uncertainties and contradictions, the links and gaps between ways that different participants tell the story. We start with the perspectives of parents who lost children in the epidemic, following their efforts to save them, their observations, and their views of the healers, nurses, and doctors with whom they collaborated. Their stories reveal how intimately their labor of care was woven together with that of health/communicative labor, as well as the obstacles they faced in attempting to foster exchanges of knowledge that could have yielded a diagnosis and a way to save their children. As the stories build on one another, they can feel relentless, unnerving. Our writing here is deliberate. During each of the three waves of cases, the epidemic produced a feverish, chaotic, frightening avalanche of stories, bodies, and encounters with healers, nurses, doctors, hospitals, and coffins. For parents who lost more than one child, their own stories seem to haunt them at each step as they started to be repeated even as the principal character shifted to a second—or third—child.

We then consider the perspectives of doctors, nurses, and healers. Some physicians and nurses may initially be taken aback at having their stories placed in dialogue with those of vernacular healers. We mean no disrespect; indeed, Clara herself is a physician, even as Charles was trained as a healer in the delta. In juxtaposing healers, nurses, and physicians, our point is not to suggest that they share a common lens. Rather, we explore the differences and similarities in how they faced the enormous challenge of diagnosing the mysterious disease and trying to save patients. One common thread between them is that none succeeded in diagnosing the disease or saving patients, and we explore the diverse affective trajectories that shaped their responses.

We then join the individuals—mostly physicians but also nurses and other professionals—who looked at the disease epidemiologically, trying to find forms of evidence and patterns that would help them figure out what the heck was going on. Listening to their stories also entails reading the reports that they drafted. We listen to them as they try to balance their drive to find a diagnosis with public health officials' efforts to limit potential political fallout from the epidemic. Eventually, the disease rose to prominence in the regional, national, and international news media, and the last lens we follow is that of journalists. We focus in particular on the two individuals who were most involved in reporting on the epidemic, one who worked for the local newspaper and the other a leading health reporter for a national, opposition newspaper and a national radio network. Rather than singling out the work of journalists, we look closely at how their professional ideology and practices were woven into the fabric of public health, electoral battles, and social movements.

In part I, our writing takes on an experimental edge. Beyond disrupting a single, linear, definitive account of the epidemic, we place readers in the middle of the work of care (and epidemiology and journalism) and of health/communicative labor as they unfolded during the epidemic. We have tried to avoid presenting any perspective as being more exotic, rational, commonsensical, or authoritative than any other. We do not project the members of any class of practitioners as sharing a homogeneous perspective: no two parents, physicians, nurses, healers, or epidemiologists reacted identically. Nor were individuals themselves always consistent. In the case of the resident physician in the local clinic, for example, there seemed to be two Dr. Cáceres, two voices in one body, and we tried to let both of them emerge.

Entering someone else's head and revealing what transpired there is tricky, particularly when we must rely on memories and interpretations that themselves change over time as controversies emerge, stories circulate, and conversations unfold. Indeed, we could not claim to be able to reveal transparently the contents of even our own hearts and minds during the epidemic; these events were challenging and confusing for us too, as much emotionally as conceptually. We cannot offer clairvoyance, only honesty and a certain depth of familiarity that follows from having worked in Delta Amacuro and having known many of these individuals for decades and from tracing the resonances and the discrepancies between their accounts.

After engaging the frenetic pace of the epidemic in part I, we focus on slowing it down, analytically, in part II, on disrupting and reconfiguring the frameworks that scholars, practitioners, and laypersons bring to thinking about these issues. Unraveling the many mysteries that unfolded and exploring what they can teach us requires a complex work of unwriting the story even as we write it, of challenging the commonsense categories—notions that are widely accepted, without reflection, as being just the way things are—that shape these issues. Each chapter in part II unravels a particular set of prevailing frameworks in order to open up new possibilities.

Chapter 5 breaks new ground by rethinking the relationship between care and narration. Scholars often position narratives in their accounts as providing a window on how the narrator—such as a patient, relative, or practitioner—thinks about a disease or treatment. The rich social scientific and medical literature on doctor-patient interaction views patients' efforts to tell a story about their illness as aiding the diagnostic process and establishing a supportive clinical relationship. Arthur Kleinman (1988) argues that a physician's willingness to grasp patients' lifeworlds and understandings of illness through the narratives they tell lies at the center of patient-centered medicine. Good and DelVecchio

Good (2000) note that becoming "competent" as a physician is intimately caught up with learning to tell particular types of stories about patients, one-self, and other doctors; medical students are thus taught to overlook details that are not deemed medically relevant and to position the particulars they do use within medical narrative structures.

Even approaches that celebrate such stories generally place narration out-side the realm of care; like Linda Garro and Cheryl Mattingly (2000a), we rather focus on how the two are intimately entangled. Drawing on Menéndez's attention to forms of care that are provided outside the clinic, we examine how care was entangled with the work of narration in complex and consequential ways in each site where it unfolded, including the anticipation of how that particular moment would be carried forward narratively. For the parents, narrating and the work of care emerged simultaneously with each touch, ob-servation, treatment, and trip. Except for the parents of the first child to be infected, their stories—and their perceptions of symptoms—started with other stories of children taken by the strange disease; narratives thus tied their children's bodies to other diseased bodies and the forms of care they received. The parents' labor of storytelling thus did not simply report on their labor of care but formed a crucial part of it. In clinics, hospitals, and encounters with epidemiologists, however, health professionals reduced their narratives to an-swers posed to their own questions; they excluded this rich archive of observa-tions and the forms of care provided by the parents and other caregivers they had recruited from entering clinical spaces.

In this book, we point out how placing narration at the center of care requires a rather different work of documentation. These stories did not emerge exclusively in clinical spaces; epidemiologists, journalists, and local leaders told stories about the epidemic. Moreover, stories were not confined to particular contexts but rather circulated broadly through Delta Amacuro State. Public health officials spent at least as much time trying to stem, channel, and transform the circulation of other people's stories about the epidemic in clinical settings, epidemiological investigations, and newspapers as in telling their own or undertaking other types of interventions. By deciding when the story began and when it ended, the places in which it unfolded, who constituted characters, and what types of actions and perspectives were included, narrators tried to shape what would count as evi-dence and what types of explanatory logics could be used.

Our goal is not to add to the body of research that celebrates the place of nar-ratives in medicine and healing. Having professionals interrupt and discredit their stories and hearing stories told by health authorities that turned them into inadvertent murderers of their own children greatly deepened the parents' pain and anger and augmented its persistence, right through the present. The problem was not a shortage of stories any more than it was a shortage of access to health care. The challenge here is to broaden the analytic lens beyond the usual attention to how narratives circulate in one site, generally a clinical one, to think about why this hypercirculation of narratives impeded diagnosis and more productive modes of collaboration. When the team created a context in which everyone could speak, different types of stories and other genres could be brought into dialogue, thereby expanding evidentiary frames and juxtaposing perspectives in ways that facilitated collaboration in producing a diagnosis. This experience thus opens up possibilities for thinking about new types of relations between narration and care.

We did not find this project—it found us after we returned to the delta to collaborate on a health project. After we acceded to Conrado's and Enrique's insistence that we join their project, the team's work did not begin with interviews or clinical examinations. Invited to participate in a meeting, Tirso, Norbelys, and the two of us showed up shortly after dawn one morning in a small coastal settlement to find a group of mourners gathered around the body of a young man, Mamerto Pizarro. They were singing laments, acoustically and affectively charged songs in which mourners collaboratively remember the dead and decry the loss. Our work thus began not with epidemiological reports, clinical narratives, and the stories about the epidemic that circulated through the lower delta but with a very different genre. As Enrique put it later, "We wanted each word spoken about the epidemic to connect with the sounds of [Mamerto's] relatives' wailing." The lamenters framed the investigation that was beginning that morning as part of their work of mourning.

This phrase comes from Sigmund Freud's classic essay "Mourning and Melancholia." In chapter 7, we build a dialogue between ways that psychoanalysts and the lamenters have thought through the complexities of mourning. Collectively composed and performed songs asked tough questions about not only the physical death of a young man but also the social deaths of the people who died in the epidemic: the apparent lack of acknowledgment by government officials that their lives were of sufficient value to require public recognition and more concerned action particularly troubled lamenters. Even as we use psychoanalysis, anthropology, and public health to think about how relatives mourned the individuals who died in the epidemic, we ask how these fields might be transformed by reconfiguring them as part of the work of mourning, meaning not just responses to physical death but to demands for collaborative knowledge production and epistemological openness. In a number of fields, researchers have stretched beyond the borders of academic research to think about how their work can respond to critical situations that emerge in contemporary life; these include Latin American social medicine and critical epidemiology, popular epidemiology, community-based participatory research in public health, and public or engaged anthropology, to name just a few. We ask how this call to join the work of mourning—not just in response to physical death but to demands for acknowledgment that all lives and deaths matter—might enable scholars and practitioners to sharpen analytical frameworks, broaden modes of investigation, and increase the impact of their work.

All parties wanted to stop the deaths, and everyone agreed that knowledge was needed to identify the disease and figure out how to end the epidemic. Parents, their neighbors, local leaders, nurses, doctors, healers, epidemiologists, and others all actively sought to produce knowledge while the children were dying; some persisted when new cases were not appearing and even after Elbia Torres Rivas—the epidemic's last fatality—died on 2 August 2008. But why did so much knowledge fail to produce a diagnosis? Why is the epidemic still officially undiagnosed? This problem raises issues faced by researchers in a number of disciplines. The STS scholar Bruno Latour analyzed how scientific practices, technologies, and forms of writing enable knowledge to circulate (Latour 1999), as quintessentially embodied in "immutable mobiles," objects of knowledge ideally capable of traveling anywhere without shifting reference or losing significance (Latour 1988). Nevertheless, a great deal of health officials' efforts went into trying to produce *immobility*, to prevent scientific knowledge regarding the epidemic from spreading. They invested substantial energy in ensuring that even the most scientifically authoritative accounts—as compiled by their own epidemiologists—would circulate only in very particular ways and end up in administrative dead files. We also need to account for ways that producing knowledge was intimately entangled in producing nonknowledge, in relegating other perspectives on the disease to the categories of ignorance, superstition, error, or political interference.[9]

In chapter 6 we draw on STS and linguistic anthropology to think in new ways about the nitty-gritty, the mechanics of the production of knowledge and nonknowledge and of circulation and immobility. All parties based their claims to produce knowledge on their relationship to the same dying and dead bodies, providing a powerful common focus. The types of relationships that people claimed to those bodies, those of kinship, care, statistics, laboratory analysis, clinical examination, and journalism, turned them, however, into what STS scholars refer to as boundary objects, held in common by actors occupying distinct social spheres but defined and used in different ways by each (Star and Griesemer 1989). We reflect on how participants sought to position the bodies in relationship to space, time, medical technologies, and forms of care in such a way as to define the points at which they might yield the knowledge needed to produce a diagnosis. We look at the role of genres in invisibly shaping dividing lines between knowledge and nonknowledge: epidemiologists elevated laboratory results and epidemiological statistics as most accurately and transparently representing knowledge; clinicians favored clinical histories; and healers privileged myths and dreams. Nevertheless, people who are not versed in these specialized genres were cast outside the sphere of knowledge production and circulation. The stakes here for understanding health inequities are huge, given that these mechanisms ensure noncollaboration and miscommunication between people who want to figure out what leads to negative health outcomes and to address skewed distributions of health and illness. The sort of zero-sum game in which I have to cast your observations as ignorance or error in order to elevate my own as knowledge turns out to rest less on self-interest or ill will than on complex interactions between these sorts of generally unstated ways of configuring knowledge production and circulation.

Trying to figure out why the epidemic occurred, why it went on so long, and what thwarted diagnosis also entailed considering nonhuman actors as integral to knowledge production. The epidemic brought together not only patients, parents, physicians, healers, and other human participants but also viruses, bats, chickens, cats, and tigers, as we detail below. Clinical and epidemiological accounts of the epidemic cast humans exclusively as knowledge producers, while nonhumans became natural phenomena that had to be known and controlled by humans. Tirso Gómez, a healer as well as team member, disrupted this projection of a gulf between nature and culture, human and nonhuman actors by challenging the relegation of the vampire bat—who played a crucial role in the epidemic—to the status of a natural phenomenon lacking in knowledge-making capacity or any relationship to the social world until it became a disease vector. Other healers invoked the power of water spirits and magical candles, as unleashed by people classified as nonindigenous who were bent on adding supernatural violence to the forms of political and economic power they wield.

Here our story leaps to the heart of issues connected with what has been called "the ontological turn" in anthropology and other disciplines. Eduardo Viveiros de Castro (1998, 2004) argues that Amerindians view persons, animals, and objects relationally through the way they "apprehend reality from distinct points of view." Isabelle Stengers (2005) suggests that recognizing multiple ontologies engenders a "cosmopolitics," that is, political recognition of the coexistence of different ontological worlds and their divergent and often competing epistemological and ethical claims. Marisol de la Cadena (2010) points to the inclusion in the Bolivian and Ecuadorian constitutions of the Quechua phrase *sumak kawsay* (translated as "good living") at the center of relationships to other humans, animals, the environment, and material objects. Eduardo Kohn (2013) developed a semiotic analysis, based on fieldwork with an Amazonian people, to think about particular ways that humans and animals communicate, thereby shaping ongoing definitions of the human in response to nonhuman perspectives and actions. Mel Chen (2012) examined how representations of nonhumans, including animals and seemingly inanimate things like lead and mercury, are used in casting some humans as fully sentient, alive, and agentive and, at the same time, relegating other humans—racialized, queer, or disabled—along with nonhumans to a lower status, one that lacks full animacy.

Bringing nonhuman actors and forms of knowledge to the fore helps us think through a continuing puzzle: if the epidemic was caused by bat-transmitted rabies, why did the vampire bats suddenly increase their nocturnal attacks? A partial answer lies in a preceding sudden die-off of chickens, which form a major part of their blood supply. Why did the chickens die? Why did the rabies virus proliferate in the bats' saliva? Why did one to three individuals die in some households, leaving as many as a dozen family members untouched? Why did dying patients speak in sometimes horrifying, sometimes endearing ways that seemed to lie beyond "normal" human powers of articulation? When a nine-year-old's last words generate a new understanding of the meaning of life and death, even as he attempts to provide his mother with words that will soften her mourning, who is speaking? We dare to ask if viruses speak through human bodies and if animals—including chickens and bats—might have been providing the clues to discover not just the name of the disease but shifting ecologies of human, nonhuman, and environmental interactions. At the same time that these sources provide us with ideas for thinking beyond biomedical and other frameworks that reserve knowledge-making capacity to humans, how our delta interlocutors juxtaposed myths, laments, healing, political critique, and science points to ways that proponents of multiple ontologies and natureculture (nonbinary) perspectives might underestimate how contemporary afflictions (Das 2015) require complex and sometimes fatal ontological balancing acts.

Another focus of these conceptual reworkings centers on the issues of health and media that we raised earlier. One of the largest and most pervasive dimensions of communicative infrastructures of health now lies in media, the constant circulation of health information through television, radio, newspapers, the Internet, and social media. For example, epidemiologists track disease outbreaks by monitoring Internet traffic, social media, and health news. Scholars generally cast such "media representations" as immaterial, secondary features that come after the primary facts of research, diagnosis, and treatment have already emerged. Research on the pharmaceutical industry suggests, however, that media and public relations professionals collaborate with scientists all the way through the process of producing a new drug, from the creation of a new disease or risk factor to laboratory research, the design of clinical trials, publications in medical journals, approval by federal regulators, advertising, media coverage, and efforts to convince clinicians to accord it a central place in their pharmakon.[10] In short, biological and media components are coproduced, but we know relatively little about how they are made and circulated in widely dispersed sites by media and health professionals, marketers, and laypersons.

Understandings of health news reflect commonsense cultural models of the production, circulation, and reception of health knowledge. The most prevalent construction envisions this process as reflecting the production of knowledge about diseases and treatments as enacted by health professionals in such specialized sites as hospitals, laboratories, and epidemiologists' offices. This knowledge is projected as then being translated into popular representations by "the media" and health communicators for reception by lay audiences. Health news stories thus both teach audiences a given body of biomedical content and impart ideas about what counts as health knowledge, who makes it, and how laypersons are required to assimilate it. The types of health subjects who are projected in this process are hierarchically ordered in terms of knowledge, authority, and agency; ethnoracial differences often project minority populations as simply being out of the loop, too ignorant, inattentive, or irrational to learn how to save their own lives and those of their children.

Looking ethnographically at how news about the epidemic was produced and received—rather than relying on content analysis alone—enabled us to see that it resulted from complex collaborations between health officials and journalists. Rather than coming after the medical facts had been determined, the news coverage sometimes structured subsequent epidemiological investigations and shaped their policy implications. Indeed, as we document in chapters 3 and 8, news coverage sparked the two largest epidemiological investigations carried out in the delta during this period, both of which were geared toward producing particular sorts of stories and precluding others, toward casting some actors as producing knowledge and others as reproducing superstition and ignorance.

Looking closely at the epidemic thus pushed us to document what we call *biomediatization*,[11] the coproduction of medical objects and subjects through collaborations between health and media professionals, laypersons, and others, as unfolding in a wide range of sites. We trace how news coverage informed what took place in homes, clinics, hospitals, and public health offices as well as the complex and shifting alignments of health officials, journalists, politicians, and activists that shaped what figured in coverage, how it was framed, what did not get covered, the roles assigned participants in stories, and the complex, heterogeneous political effects of coverage. News stories about the epidemic were consequential even for people who violently challenged their veracity. Conrado and Enrique grasped the powerful role of biomediatization in shaping public health policies and practices in the 1992–1993 cholera epidemic. They accordingly insisted on mediatizing knowledge about the epidemic even as we were producing it; recording stories, producing statistics, and asking Clara to come up with a diagnosis and Charles to take photographs were all designed to infuse delta residents' accounts of the epidemic with mobility, to enable them to reach Caracas. By telling the story themselves to national and international journalists, Conrado, Enrique, Norbelys, and Tirso were determined to disrupt biomediatization-as-usual and how it reproduces fatal stereotypes. At the same time that this discussion opens up a new line of inquiry, it suggests that no attempt to locate health/communicative inequities and no effort to achieve health/communicative justice will be adequate if they fail to address biomediatization.

A Note on Names and Images

A few final words about names and photographs. Our narrative practices follow the guidance we received from the parents and our fellow team members. The demand, "Tell me why my children died" goes hand in hand with a challenge to circulate the parents' stories about their children and how they died. In their continuing efforts to counter the social deaths that followed their children's physical demise, the parents want their children's names spoken and demand recognition for their labor of care and communication. The nurses and healers also asked to be recognized for their efforts to save their patients. On the other hand, many were concerned that naming doctors, epidemiologists, health officials, and journalists would engender retaliation; some of these professionals requested anonymity, expressing similar concerns. We have honored these requests.

The parents expressed particular interest in photographs. They asked that "people everywhere" learn about their children, how they lived, how they died, and what the parents did in trying to keep them alive. Given the uneven distribution of money and photographic technologies, few of them had pictures of the children who died. Enrique asked Charles to photograph and film the parents' testimonies; the photographs became a crucial part of the act of witnessing, of hearing these stories. They were also designed to help increase the mobility of the parents' accounts, to equip them to engage national health officials and journalists and, simultaneously, to keep our work from turning into disembodied numbers and clinical descriptions. In Caracas, Enrique took these photographs out in each meeting with officials and journalists. Having been asked to participate in the work of mourning, these photographs signal our recognition of this role. When we return to the delta, the parents proudly treasure the copies of the photographs we bring them, despite the pain.

We have thus included a great number of photographs of the parents and, in several cases, of their children. They are presented as images, not ethnographic supplements, standing beside the text, not subsumed under it (Stevenson 2014). We present them for three reasons. First, they are of and for the parents. We want them to see themselves, literally, in the pages of this book. The images signal that the parents, nurses, healers, and others are crucial members of the audience for this book. Second, the photographs invite readers to construct their own relationships with these individuals and use their own experience and imaginations to enter into these stories. Finally, they are for us, interpellating the book's authors as part of its audience. As we suggest in chapter 7, the parents charged the six members of the team with participating in their work of mourning. Every time we look at them, these images keep us focused on this responsibility at the same time that they enable us to imagine new ways of undertaking it, new types of relationships with the parents, their lost children, and the world around us. They remind us that this book is just part of a larger project, one that is not linear, not finished, and not of our own making.

part I

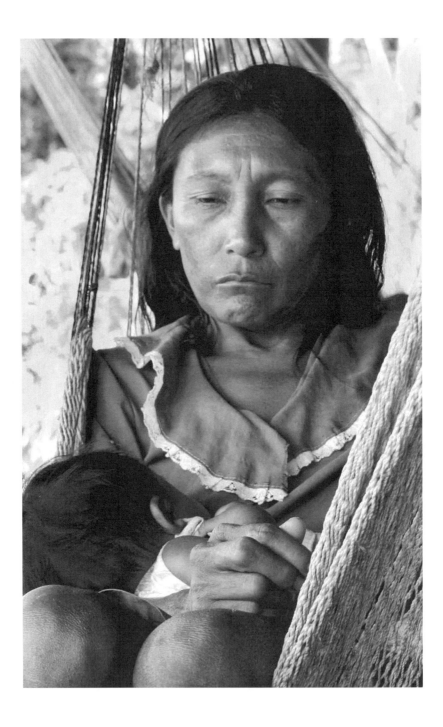

1

———

R E L I V I N G

T H E

E P I D E M I C

Parents' Perspectives

For three months, all we did was cry. Another would get
sick, another would get sick, and another would get sick; it was
impossible. . . . They were finished off, one by one.
—Alfonso Torres

My relatives, you must narrate exactly how all of this began.
—Enrique Moraleda

Mukoboina: Revisiting Ground Zero

Mukoboina, the first place hit by the mysterious epidemic, could have won an
award for being the most nondescript among hundreds of other small settlements in the lower delta—until it became in July 2007 the lead story on Warao
Radio, the popular designation for word-of-mouth transmission within the
area. That was when the first Mukoboinian child died of a strange and terrifying new disease. Mukoboina has around eighty residents and just a dozen
thatch-roofed houses perched on stilts above the mud and water of a midsized
tributary of the Orinoco River. It was literally sliced out of the surrounding

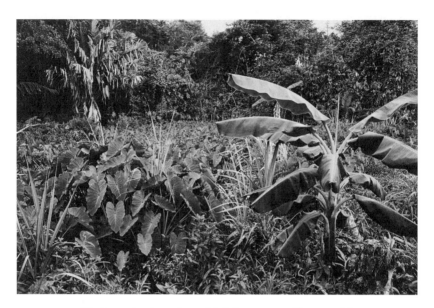

FIGURE 1.1. The Baeza family garden in Mukoboina, 2010. Photograph by Charles L. Briggs.

jungle.[1] Relatively new, it was settled around 1990 by José Manuel Florín and Alejandrina Morales. They liked the area: there was a good beach and catfish were abundant, prompting the name, which means "the place where catfish are plentiful."[2]

There is no store, mission, school, or nursing station, although the Institute of Nutrition did fund a small "community hearth" to provide nutritional assistance for a short while. Mukoboinans live primarily off their gardens, where they grow taro, bananas, plantains, yucca tubers, pineapples, sugar cane, and other crops (figure 1.1). Most houses have a few mango and coconut trees next to them. When fish are scarce, Mukoboinan men travel by canoe to the coast, where catches are more plentiful. Residents visit the clinic and stores in Nabasanuka and make occasional trips to Tucupita, some six hours away by motorized canoe, to sell hammocks and baskets, buy consumer goods, and petition government bureaucrats. With minor variations, Mukoboina is the delta's "everytown."

Mukoboina is a primary destination on the team's itinerary in July 2008 as it begins its investigation into the cause of the deaths. Our boat pulls up at the last house, looking for Mukoboina's local representative and *wisidatu* healer, Inocencio Torres. Rosaura Romero, a woman of about thirty, recognizes Tirso in the boat and, accompanied by half a dozen children, welcomes us. A boy of about four, clad only in white briefs, jumps up and down shouting, "*Pollo, pollo!*" "He does that every time a boat arrives with criollo [nonindigenous] passengers," Romero explains. "He thinks you're *bongueros* [itinerant fluvial merchants] selling chickens. He loves chicken!"

Inocencio, Rosaura's brother-in-law, emerges wearing a smile that makes you feel like you have known him for years; he climbs into the boat. Taller and thinner than most Mukoboina men, he is in his midfifties. His father was a criollo fisherman who returned to his "legitimate," nonindigenous wife in Barrancas after impregnating Inocencio's mother. Although he grew up in the delta, Inocencio spent a year as a teenager on the mainland with his father; he can understand Spanish, even though he seldom speaks it. The lines on his forehead appear to map the anxieties wrought by the way his ordinarily nondescript settlement has become a focal point of death and controversy. He is a charismatic and capable leader who listens intently when people speak. The Mukoboinans know all the team members, particularly Norbelys and Tirso, one of whose daughters-in-law hails from Mukoboina.

Accompanied by Charles, Inocencio gathers residents, stopping at each family's dock to announce, "The leaders have arrived; come and tell your story!" Except for one father, all the parents are at home; they crowd into the boat, often with several children in tow. Fearing it would capsize, the last family opts to skip from log to log over the mud to Inocencio's house, which has already begun to fill up. It is divided into two sections. The one on the right features a bench-desk combination rescued from a school modernization program, where Enrique sits surrounded by fascinated children and takes notes. Conrado settles into a plastic chair near the outside edge of the room. Some fifteen other people have already gathered. The left side of the room, where the family sleeps, contains four hammocks, shielded from the sun and rain by sheets of black plastic and *temiche* palms. Several parents sit nearby, cuddling their surviving children, while others listen from the dock and adjacent kitchen that jut out above the river. While taking their turn as narrator, parents stand in the middle of the room, simultaneously embraced by every eye in the house and isolated in unseen worlds of pain.

Mukoboina is regarded by all parties as the ground zero of the mysterious epidemic, the first place it tortured bodies and shattered lives. Nearly every story of the strange epidemic begins with Mukoboina, so ours does as well. In July 2008, parents seemed still to be living in mourning, terrified, and furious that other visitors had come before us but had not expressed interest in hearing their stories; they just asked questions and left without sharing their observations and hypotheses. More than anyone else, Mukoboinans had been demanding for over a year, "Tell me why my children died." Now, one parent after another rises to give testimony about the deaths of one, two, or three of their children.

WILMER TORRES AND ZOILA TORRES:
THE FIRST COUPLE TO FACE THE DISEASE

We had no idea what was going on. . . . His little sister developed an identical fever. It was the same sickness.—Wilmer Torres

Zoila Torres and Wilmer Torres are in their late twenties (figure 1.2). Social and outgoing, they enjoyed their trips to Tucupita, where Zoila sold the beautiful *moriche* palm fiber hammocks she made. They had four children. Gabriel was a bouncy eight-year-old who particularly loved to imitate the roar of an outboard motor as he played in the water, racing tiny boats around on a string. Six-year-old Graciela was a charmer whose frequent smile revealed wonderful dimples. Yuri, only two, had an oval face and the same large dark eyes as her siblings.[3] With newly arrived Maricelia, Zoila and Wilmer could not have dreamed of a happier beginning for their family.

Wilmer comes to the middle of the room, grabbing the roof beam so firmly that his strong biceps bulge. Zoila sits silently against the wall holding Maricelia, who clings tightly. She appears prematurely aged and lost in an inner realm. Although Wilmer's face never loses its seemingly stoic quality, his head turns, his arms flutter, and his whole body seems to dance as he recounts the couple's efforts to save their children.

"Gabriel suddenly developed a fever in July 2007," Wilmer begins. The symptoms appeared on 18 July during a quick trip to Tucupita. The fever was not high, and the boy was in good spirits. As the return trip in the hot sun wore on, however, his fever climbed, and he grew weak. Once home, his parents took Gabriel to the nearby house of their uncle Inocencio, a wisidatu healer. Unfortunately, he could not locate the source of the disease, nor was he able to reduce the symptoms. It was well past midnight when the family departed. "Afterwards," Wilmer continues, "he was just the same. The illness remained." They sought out another type of specialist, a *hoarotu* who could look for *hoa* pathogens. But "it was impossible, impossible. He treated and treated him, but, just like before, nothing happened. Then heavy saliva appeared. I said, 'Let's take him to Nabasanuka, to the clinic.'" On the way, they stopped to see a third healer, but he could not locate the source of the illness either. Just as they reached Hubasuhuru, over halfway to Nabasanuka and with night falling, Gabriel died in his father's arms.

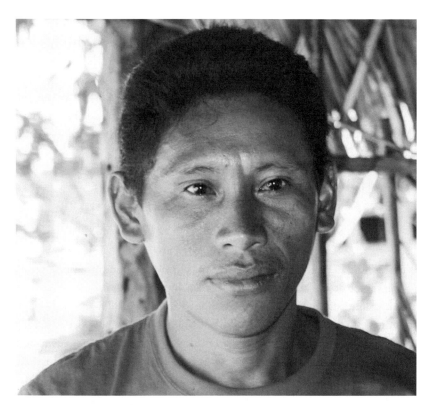

FIGURE 1.2. Wilmer Torres, 2008. Photograph by Charles L. Briggs.

That was on 24 July 2007, the first case to appear in Mukoboina—and possibly in the delta. "We had no idea what was going on," Wilmer reported. On 8 August, "just the same way, his little sister developed an identical fever. It was the same sickness." They took two-year-old Yuri to see Uncle Inocencio, who again worked much of the night, but the results were no different. The next day, the parents visited Nurse José Pérez in Siawani, telling him, "We took her last night to the wisidatu, but she was just the same in the morning." The nurse placed her in a hammock to treat her, but his medicines failed too. Next they headed for the clinic at Nabasanuka. During the trip, "Yuri just kept getting sicker." She cried out continually and she couldn't even walk by the time they arrived. Yuri was the first case of the strange disease to reach Dr. Ricardo Cáceres's clinic. Wilmer could provide few details about the visit, except that it didn't help. The parents then took Yuri to another wisidatu but brought her back to the clinic the next day. She was terribly ill and died on 11 August before Dr. Ricardo could send her to the hospital in Tucupita. "We didn't know what had happened," Wilmer practically whispers. "We were very sad. Her mother, when she touched her little body, became very sad."

A year later, Zoila is still too numb with grief to tell her story at Inocencio's house. Moreover, it is now the same time of year the children's deaths occurred. "We're scared," Wilmer reports. "If this disease comes again, it will be really dangerous." Zoila holds Maricelia even tighter.

GRACIANO FLORÍN AND MATILSE CARRASQUERO CONFRONT THE THIRD AND FOURTH CASES

[The hospital] just gave us the boy['s body] and we came back here.

—Graciano Florín

The second parent to talk about the strange disease, Graciano Florín, walks to the center of the house. Heavier-set than most Mukoboinans, he has just a hint of moustache and a face that appears unwilling to yield its childlike roundness. Like Wilmer, he grabs the beam above him for support to tell his story (figure 1.3). His wife, Matilse Carrasquero, has a serious, quiet demeanor. Comparatively well off, they live in a large home complete with exterior walls and built with commercial rather than hand-hewed lumber. In their early thirties, Graciano and Matilse had three children in July 2007: Ángel Gabriel, age eleven, Adalia, six, and Mary, who was only a few months old.

On 23 August, Ángel Gabriel was the next child to develop the strange fever. His national identity card, the parents' only image of their son, shows a boy with short black hair, deep and serious eyes, an arrow-straight nose, and slightly prominent ears (figure 1.4). Though ordinarily his parents would have just watched carefully to see if the fever got worse, the first two deaths had changed that pattern: a mild fever had become a parent's worst nightmare.

As he recounts the way the disease claimed Ángel Gabriel's body, Graciano traces its effects on his own powerful torso, creating a moving and somewhat surreal juxtaposition of bodies. The course of the disease was already familiar: fever, sore throat, headache, and body aches that were followed, on day three, by profuse salivation. Ángel Gabriel asked for food, but he grew frightened and rejected it when it was offered, just as with water. The parents consulted Inocencio, as both wisidatu and local leader, who again tried to treat this disease. He urged them to visit Nurse José Pérez, and they rushed Ángel Gabriel to Siawani. Again the nurse used his medicines, but the fever did not diminish. Nurse José took the child and parents in his

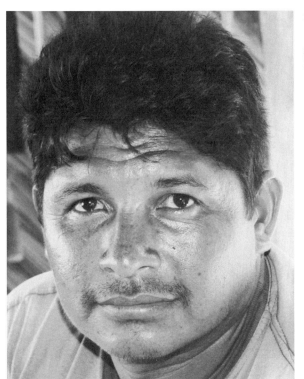

FIGURE 1.3. Graciano Florín, 2008. Photograph by Charles L. Briggs.

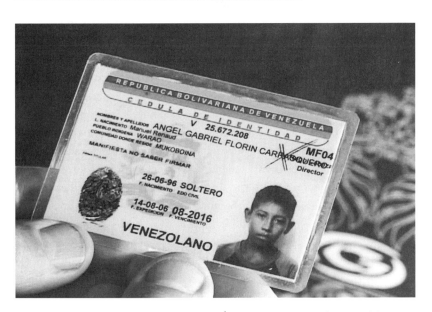

FIGURE 1.4. The national identity card for Ángel Gabriel Florín. Photograph by Charles L. Briggs.

little boat to Nabasanuka, and Dr. Ricardo quickly referred Ángel Gabriel to Tucupita.

Graciano and Matilse knew very well what had happened when Wilmer and Zoila refused to let Dr. Ricardo send Yuri to Tucupita, taking her first to a wisidatu. They accordingly accepted the physician's recommendation immediately. "Early the next day we took him to Tucupita." Alerted to Ángel Gabriel's imminent arrival, an ambulance met the family at the port at Volcán, made the twenty-minute journey to Tucupita, and continued to the Maternal-Pediatric Dr. Oswaldo Ismael Brito wing of the Tucupita Hospital. After spending a day and night there, doctors sent Ángel Gabriel to Maturín, the capital of neighboring Monagas State. Maturín boasts more sophisticated medical centers, but expertise and technology did not help Ángel Gabriel. He died there on 31 August, a week after he developed a fever.[4] Graciano recalled that medical personnel only told them, "Your son is dead." Regarding what killed Ángel Gabriel, his father said, "I don't know. They didn't tell us. I have no idea." The couple did exactly what physicians ask of delta parents—they recognized the seriousness of their son's condition, went to the local nursing station and then the clinic for help, and trusted his life to nurses and doctors. When Ángel Gabriel died, "They just gave us the boy and we came back here."

Arriving in Mukoboina with Ángel Gabriel's remains, Graciano and Matilse learned that their daughter Adalia, who had been in her grandmother's care, had come down with "the same fever." Despite their misgivings about the care Ángel Gabriel received, on 5 September they took six-year-old Adalia to Nabasanuka, where Dr. Ricardo hospitalized her and administered antibiotics. When she failed to improve, Dr. Ricardo proposed sending her to Tucupita, but after their recent experience, her parents refused.[5] They trusted the kind young physician in Nabasanuka and the bilingual nurses, but their experience with hospitals in the city gave them the shudders. Graciano doesn't say it in front of everyone at this meeting, which includes a doctor and a nurse, but they had come to share a growing sentiment that, in view of intubation and other procedures—particularly given the lack of any effort to explain them to the parents—hospital personnel were torturing their children.

Several healers attempted, unsuccessfully, to treat Adalia before the parents accepted Dr. Ricardo's recommendation the following morning. Adalia was rushed by fluvial ambulance to the Luis Razetti Hospital in Tucupita, and the next day she followed in Ángel Gabriel's footsteps to Dr. Manuel Núñez Tovar Hospital in Maturín. She died the next day. Graciano speaks only briefly about Adalia's death; losing a second child just seems to be too much for him.

My daughter said to me before leaving for Tucupita [Hospital], "Mama, I'm dying. I'm leaving you. I'm dying. I'm dying."—Santa Morales

The only mother to speak at this assembly, Santa Morales has small, deep-set eyes that are surrounded by circles of fatigue. She is fifty years old, and ten of her eleven children (ages five to twenty-nine) are alive (figure 1.5). Her husband, Alfonso Torres, fifty-nine, a local leader, is away. Santa smiles warmly as Conrado gets up and offers her the plastic chair he had been using. At first her voice waivers, seeding doubts about her ability to press on. She ties a palm fiber string into knots as she speaks about the disease that took her second youngest child, six-year-old Yanilka, as if she is trying to keep herself anchored in the here and now rather than slip into a world of pain. She musters a force that transfixes her audience.

Yanilka was a happy and charming child who loved to play with her sisters and nephews, nieces, and cousins. That night Yanilka told Santa, " 'Mom, I'm not going to eat. It hurts.' The fever started then and lasted for three days." Three Mukoboinan children had already died, and Adalia was ill. When healers had failed to save them, a collective decision had been made to take them to the Nabasanuka clinic. Why did Yanilka's family wait for three days before seeking treatment? Yanilka came to her parents late in life and was *muy consentida* (meaning both "spoiled" and "treasured"). She brought out her father's tender side, and he was deeply attached to her. A serious man and deep thinker who reflects on issues carefully before speaking, Alfonso had a different strategy to save her life (figure 1.6). The delay was caused by the time it took him to secure loans from relatives and friends and hire a boat; these preparations in place, he left Mukoboina before dawn with Yanilka in his lap, wrapped in a blanket to protect her first from the chilly dawn and later from the sun's rays. Alfonso bypassed Nabasanuka and took Yanilka directly to the Tucupita Hospital; he wanted to stack the deck. He wanted Yanilka's case to turn out differently.

Having circumvented the Nabasanuka clinic, Alfonso reports, no ambulance was waiting at the dock. Carrying his daughter, he got into a small, dilapidated taxi that blared salsa music during the trip to the emergency room entrance in Tucupita. Although indigenous patients are often kept waiting for hours, a nurse had a good medical eye and a good heart. When Alfonso gave Yanilka's name, age, and particularly her place of residence—Mukoboina—

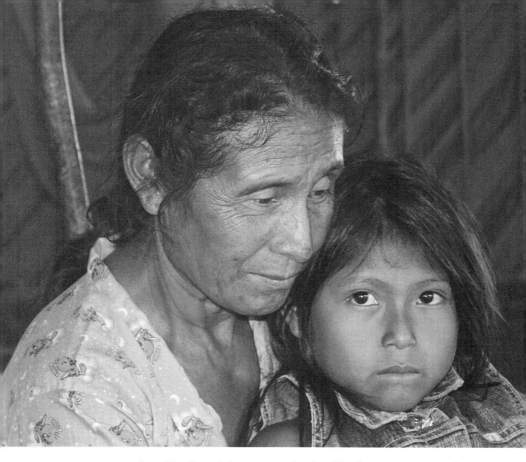

FIGURE 1.5. Santa Morales with her youngest daughter, Yamileta, 2010. Photograph by Charles L. Briggs.

and the thermometer registered a fever, the nurse gasped and immediately fetched a physician, who ordered Yanilka hospitalized. The nurse inserted an IV, and father and daughter were ushered into a room where they spent three days.

Alfonso could not tell doctors what had happened in Mukoboina; the staff did not summon the Warao patient advocate to translate. Having spent nearly all of his money to get her to the hospital, he could buy nothing to eat, and hospital food was for patients only. Yanilka grew worse. Only at the end of his stay did doctors call in the patient advocate, who informed him that Yanilka was being referred to Maturín. The advocate reassured Alfonso, who was worried that no one there would understand him, that there were Warao speakers at the hospital. The ambulance took over an hour to reach Dr. Manuel Núñez Tovar Hospital, where Alfonso saw "only criollos."

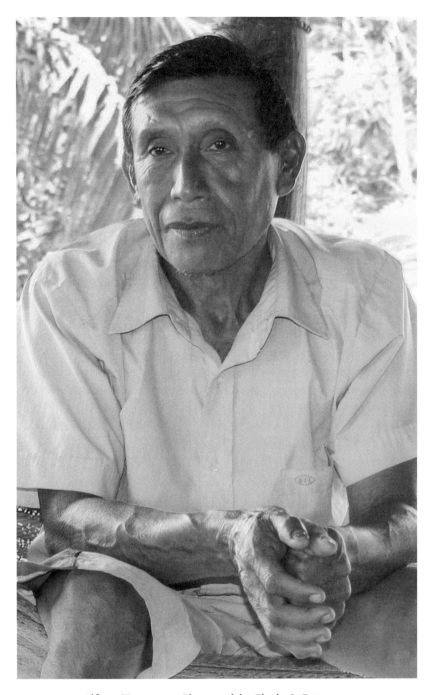

FIGURE 1.6. Alfonso Torres, 2010. Photograph by Charles L. Briggs.

Yanilka was immediately hooked up to a host of machines. Alfonso, who had not eaten for over three days, refused the food he was offered, saying he could not eat with his child gravely ill. And then Yanilka died on 10 September. When Alfonso asked about his daughter, they pointed to a closed door marked Morgue. He languished in Maturín for three more days. Finally, Santa related, he confronted the medical authorities, using as much Spanish as he could remember in order to say, "My daughter is dead. I want to go home with my daughter. I can't stay here. Her mother and all of our relatives are in Mukoboina—I want to take her to them." The criollos told him, "We're finished now." They donated a coffin and sent father and daughter to the port in Volcán, where they arrived at night. When dawn came, their boat left.

Santa confides to her audience that until Alfonso returned, "I waited and waited. 'What is happening to my daughter there, so far away?' I kept saying that over and over. Then the news came: they've taken her to Maturín, that's where she is." A boat arrived as darkness fell; Alfonso appeared with her corpse. "I was just sitting there. Her father is not a woman, but although he is a man, he was screaming and crying, 'My daughter is dead!' Since I was her mother, my world faded away. I began to wail. When we see our children die, it causes us intense pain, so we wail. When something like this happens, words come to us: 'Our loved one has died.' My daughter said to me before leaving for Tucupita [Hospital], 'Mama, I'm dying. I'm leaving you. I'm dying. I'm dying.' 'You're dying?' 'I'm dying.' "

ODILIA TORRES AND ROMER TORRES LOSE THREE CHILDREN

They had split her head open from front to back!—Romer Torres

Walking to the center of the house, thirty-year-old Romer Torres clings to the roof beam with both hands as if he would collapse (figure 1.7). His first words are "Tai monika hase" (It was just the same), suggesting how closely his own experiences are interwoven with those that have just been told. He married Odilia Torres (figure 1.8), twenty-nine, Inocencio Torres's half sister. In July 2007, Odilia was seven months pregnant and they had three healthy children—Yordi, who was seven, Yomelis, four, and a one-year-old boy, Henry.[6]

Odilia sits behind Romer as he narrates, holding an infant daughter, Yuneli, and occasionally adding to the story. As he begins speaking, she interjects, "All my children died." Romer relates, "The same fever infected" Yordi on 28 August. He had a sore throat and a cough, even though Odilia could not recognize any signs of a cold or any other disease. Well aware of the previous deaths, they

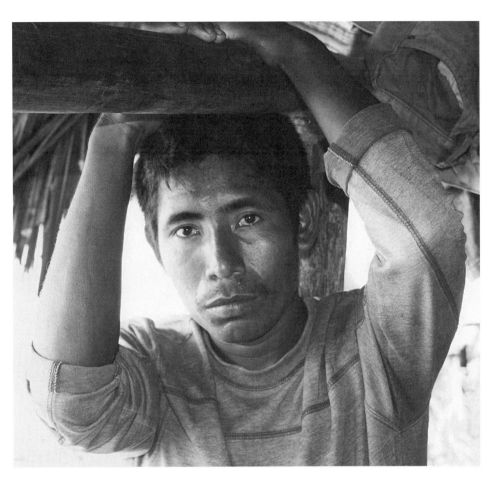

FIGURE 1.7. Romer Torres, 2008. Photograph by Charles L. Briggs.

knew that seeing "the same fever" meant anticipating their worst nightmare. What to do? Zoila and Wilmer had trusted their children to healers; both died. Graciano and Matilse took the biomedical route, and Ángel Gabriel died in Maturín. Though all avenues had failed, doing nothing was unthinkable. And because the sick children were being given nothing more than acetaminophen at the clinic, parents could see that care there was inadequate.

Odilia immediately crossed the bridge over the swampy space that separates her house from her parents' residents to consult with her mother, a *yarokotarotu* trained in herbal therapies. After her mother prepared an herbal treatment, they watched and waited. When Yordi's condition had not improved in a couple

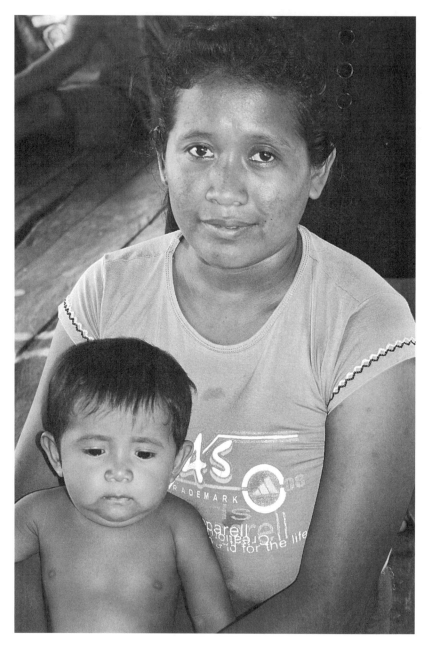

FIGURE 1.8. Odilia Torres with her daughter, Yuneli, 2008. Photograph by Charles L. Briggs.

of hours, Odilia and Romer inaugurated a process of moving hurriedly from healer to healer, starting with Inocencio. Yordi just got worse. The family went to Nabasanuka, where clinic personnel hospitalized him. Dr. Ricardo wanted to send him to Tucupita immediately, but Yordi said, "Mommy, I don't want to go. If I go, I'll die." He had heard about Ángel Gabriel's death in Maturín, and he was now afraid of doctors; ailing Mukoboinan children had begun voicing their own perceptions of what was happening and what should be done for them. Odilia did not want her own child to be taken away from her, only to return in a coffin.

When they respected Yordi's wishes, refusing the trip to Tucupita and taking him out of the clinic, they could tell that the doctor was unhappy. They took him to a nearby healer for treatments that lasted all night. At dawn, Yordi was worse. The healer gave up, and they went home. Yordi, Odilia reported, "didn't get better. He was getting much worse. His head hurt. His fever was worse." Odilia's mother was helping with his care. He was "turning from side to side. 'Grandma,' that's what he said, 'my head really hurts.'" Yordi wouldn't eat, and wouldn't drink. "When he saw a glass of water, he couldn't look at it. He was afraid. And saliva kept coming."

Yordi declared, "I'm going to die very soon," but his parents refused to accept that verdict; they rushed him to the Nabasanuka clinic. Yordi died there on 7 September. Romer worked with relatives to clean a space in the cemetery, built a house-tomb, and buried his son, while Odilia was the lead singer in the wake for her firstborn child.

"Two days later," Romer tells the gathered listeners, "the disease embraced his younger brother, just the same." Henry had a fever and he stopped eating, drinking, urinating, and defecating—he was getting very sick very quickly. The parents took him to Nabasanuka right away; the staff gave them medicines and released him. After three days he was in very bad shape. A healer worked on the child all night, but he was sicker by dawn. As with his brother, heavy saliva started to pour from his mouth. Just approaching two years of age, Henry could not articulate the experience of his illness like his brother Yordi. "He said, 'Mama, Mama,' that's all he said, because he was still so little." Romer was unable to muster more than a fragmentary account of Henry's illness and death, concluding simply that the same disease had taken him. He died on 14 September.

In November 2007, Odilia gave birth in the *neihimanoko* or menstrual house behind the family's house to a daughter, Yuneli. Still reeling from losing two children, it seemed as if death was moving slowly away like the Orinoco's currents. But, Romer continues softly, "this past January, Yomelis . . . got a fever, just the same way." Then four years old, she appeared fairly normal during the day. She bathed in the river in front of the house, but at night the fever got stronger, and at dawn it was worse. The family began another round of frenetic trips among practitioners, hoping to save her life. They took Yomelis at once to Nabasanuka, borrowing a motorboat and racking up debt to pay for oil and gasoline—they had not lost faith in doctors. Arriving on 11 January, Yomelis was treated for an ear infection but did not improve. Dr. Ricardo recommended hospitalizing her, but Odilia and Romer took Yomelis to two different healers. Though the parents asked themselves, "What fever could this be?" they knew it was the same one; they thought, "Our children are being finished off!" After healers failed, the family returned to Nabasanuka; the clinic arranged their transport to Tucupita. "It was Sunday," Romer recalled. "They immediately put her in the boat and hooked up an IV. It was getting dark, around 6:30, when we arrived at Volcán. In the hospital in Tucupita, she was a bit better at dawn, but she was really sick by the afternoon." The parents recall that it was really hard on them in the hospital. They were penniless and hungry, and Yomelis was restless and in pain, turning from side to side in the strange bed.

Romer concludes, "It was two o'clock. The doctor called us into the hallway. Yomelis was holding my arm tightly. I was watching her closely, sitting right next to her. The doctor called to us again: 'Your daughter is not going to recover. Your daughter is dying. Sit down out here, next to me [indicating chairs outside].' We sat down next to her. 'You can't go near her right now.' I didn't say anything. We went back inside." Odilia adds, barely whispering, "She died there. She died." Romer continued, "She was already dead. The criollo doctor called us again: 'Come here, sit down next to me.' We sat next to her. 'Your daughter has died. Do you want to leave [for Mukoboina]? There is a Warao representative here, María Fernández. If you speak with her, she will help you.' We went to her. 'What do you want? Are you the dead girl's father?' 'I am.' 'Is your name Romer?' 'My name is Romer.' 'Very well.' She sat down. She took out papers. She went in and out. She gave me a document. 'Will you be leaving tomorrow?' 'Yes.' 'Okay, come back tomorrow.'"

Romer left the hospital with Odilia, who carried Yuneli secured to her torso in a cloth sling; they looked for acquaintances in the shantytown by the river where delta refugees build shelters from discarded lumber and large sheets of plastic. The city evicts them periodically and bulldozes their dwellings. Lacking hammocks, they sat by the Manamo River in an illegal encampment of refugees from other areas of the delta—waiting sleeplessly for morning, waiting to take their dead child home.

Finding their way back to the hospital, they greeted María. "Have you come?" "We've come," Romer responded, observing proper Warao etiquette. "She took a paper, wrote everything down, and gave it to me. So we left; it was about 10:00." At Volcán, they waited. And waited. In the late afternoon, a boat and the coffin bearing Yomelis's body arrived, but no gasoline. " 'Tomorrow you can leave for sure. We'll give you oil and gasoline,' that's what he said. We spent the night there. They put our daughter's coffin into the boat, and we slept there, next to her." The next day their departure was delayed again and again. The throng of people waiting to return to the delta told and retold the Torreses' story. The boat left as night fell, not a propitious time to traverse waters frequented by pirates. "We finally arrived here in the middle of the night."

Romer ends his narrative with a chilling description: "And when we arrived here and opened the casket, it looked as if they had split her head open from front to back, and she was cut from her neck down." He slides his finger down to his navel. Seeing the incision on their daughter's body led Odilia and Romer to surmise why the doctor had taken them out of the room when Yomelis was dying, why the Warao advocate had told them to come back in the morning: they wanted to perform an autopsy. The liaison told Romer that the documents she assembled were needed in order to release the body, but they may have included mention of an autopsy. Odilia and Romer do not know Spanish and could not read the documents; the advocate did not translate or explain.[7]

Odilia and Romer's experience is not unique: several of the parents remark that their children were "mistreated." When Yanilka died, Alfonso, too, wondered why he had to wait so long at the doors of the hospital in Maturín. When he opened Yanilka's coffin during that sleepless night in Volcán, he saw that "they also cut her all the way around here. There were stitches all over. Damn, that was inexcusable." The most intense anger and pain expressed in Mukoboina concerned the autopsies. When Conrado and Enrique came for several of the wakes and funerals, the parents angrily demanded that they ask Dr. Ricardo about the autopsies. They were initially satisfied with the physician's response, that authorities performed autopsies in order to "figure out what is killing their children" and "we [doctors] are still waiting for the answer." But nearly a year later, as they surround us in Mukoboina, the parents still have not received any response, and they are still angry. The autopsies have become the last straw heaped on a burden of mistrust.

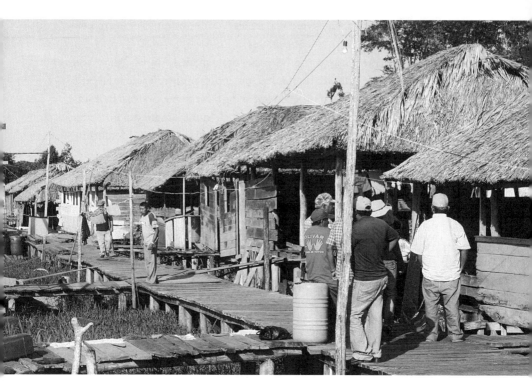

FIGURE 1.9. Muaina, 2008. Photograph by Charles L. Briggs.

Muaina July 2008: A Meeting and a Wake—Searching for Causes

Muaina, which means Land of Many Ants, rises like an impressionist paint-ing composed of brushstrokes of blue-brown water, blue sky, and green forest (figure 1.9). It lies on a medium-sized island in the mangrove swamps where the delta rain forest meets the coast. In a matter of minutes, one can be out in the Caribbean, looking back at densely forested islands.

Muaina is a product of the utopian activism of Librado Moraleda, one of Venezuela's most important indigenous leaders, the brother of Enrique and Conrado Moraleda. His goal was to create a Warao social movement that could challenge the colonial legacy of nineteenth-century plantations and rubber tap-pers that survived in the form of cattle ranches, palm heart factories, lumber mills, and the *caudillo* political system itself. It was largely through Librado's activism that the government closed the palm heart factories and lumber mills. He helped establish the Union of Indigenous Warao Communities and served as its president. Teaching in the Nabasanuka school, he authored several bilin-gual texts.[8]

After his father-in-law, Victor Pizarro, established a fishing operation in Muaina in 1988, Librado retired from teaching and moved there. He brought with him new residents and a utopian vision for combining socialism, the indigenous social movement, Warao cultural practices, and access to formal education and agronomy. Librado's revolutionary vision caught the attention of Chávez's pro-indigenous socialist government; by 2001, Muaina boasted an elementary school, nursing station, small-scale agricultural and fishing projects, and seventy-seven residents, most of them descended from the Pizarro family. When Librado died in 2006, Muaina pushed ahead under the leadership of his wife, Olga Pizarro.

The meeting we attend in Muaina takes place at Olga's house. Enrique and Conrado arrive with eleven men in their sixties, representing the male political and spiritual leadership of a wide swath of the lower delta (figure 1.10). They have concrete reasons for participating. Some treated patients with the strange disease; they hope participants can figure out why they failed. Others have lost people in their settlement and want to keep more from dying.

Why assemble so much patriarchal firepower? Central to both political leadership and health in the lower delta is a process for sorting out disputes that threaten to become collective conflicts. Known as *monikata nome nakakitane* (roughly, making a problem "straight"), it requires each party to a conflict "to speak everything in their heart," taking as long as necessary. Once all parties testify, elders take turns reflecting on what gave rise to the conflict and what should be done. Then elders make the crucial pronouncement: all of the angry words have now been spoken and the conflict is over—no one may do anything to reignite it.[9] Here, the deaths over a large area from a strange disease suggest that a broader, unprecedented problem is afoot. Enrique has scaled up the process with a powerful cast of players.

Opening the meeting with the oratorical style required for monikata nome nakakitane, Enrique gestures next door, saying, "Here we have an adult, still quite young, who was just beginning his life.... We have his corpse here in the house. That's why I ask the people of Muaina, with all my respect and consideration, we want to record from beginning to end. This record can provide a base, a support, a force to enable us to convey this painful situation that is taking place" (figure 1.11). In addition to working collectively for a diagnosis, Enrique has organized the meeting to ensure that knowledge about the disease would be mobile—that it would reach officials and journalists in Caracas. His introduction indicates that he is just as interested in figuring out how to ensure that journalists and national health officials will pay attention to the epidemic

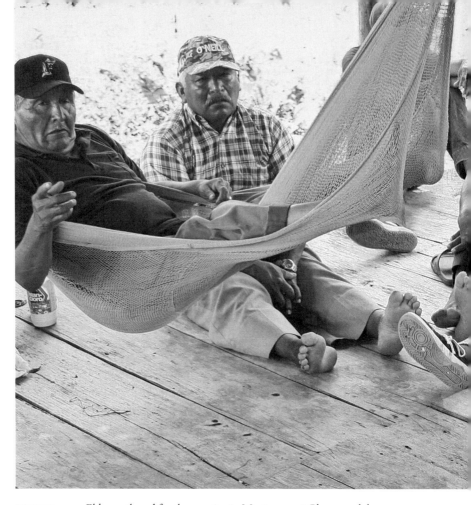

FIGURE 1.10. Elders gathered for the meeting in Muaina, 2008. Photograph by Charles L. Briggs.

and health conditions in the delta in general as in responding to the parents' demand to tell the story of their children's deaths and to participate in the process of solving the mystery. Then he calls out names of people who had asked to speak, defining their task: "My relatives, you must narrate exactly how all of this began."

Throughout the presentations and accusations regarding the suspected causes of the disease—ranging from irresponsible school boat drivers to vindictive healers to foreign companies to ecological disruption—the wailing next door serves as a constant reminder that the epidemic is inflicting intense pain on four Muainan parents.

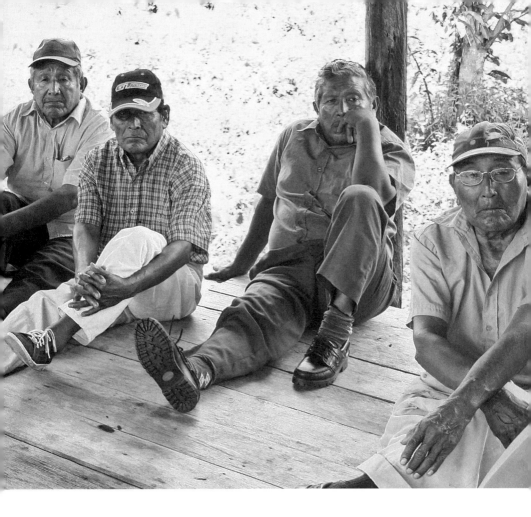

FLORENCIA MACOTERA AND INDALESIO PIZARRO:
MUAINA AND THE DELTA LOSE A FUTURE LEADER

*I can see that you will not recover. Your brother Dalvi has been dead a week,
and you have the same disease.—Florencia Macotera*

Florencia Macotera and Indalesio Pizarro are in their early forties (figure 1.12).
Indalesio has a powerful build and radiates boyish enthusiasm. Born in Guayo,
one of the largest delta towns with a sizeable Catholic mission, he reacted against
his parents' "abandonment of Warao ways"—they had embraced Catholicism,
emphasized individual achievement, and rejected Warao healing. He became
a wisidatu healer. Florencia Macotera stayed firmly rooted in the small settlement of Siawani until she traveled with her parents to Tucupita, where she met
Indalesio. They married and lived in Nabasanuka for eleven years; he was em-

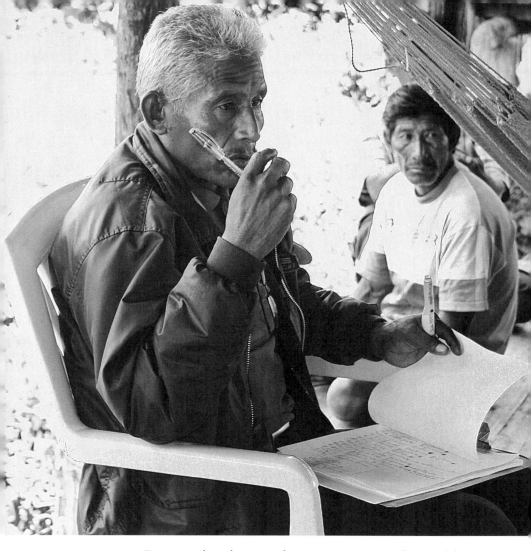

FIGURE I.II. Enrique speaks as the meeting begins in Muaina, 2008. Photograph by Charles L. Briggs.

ployed as a school boat operator. Edgar Mamerto was the couple's first child. He was followed by two girls who died as infants, then by Melvi, now fifteen, then Wilme, Argelio, and Dalvi, and finally two girls, Imelda and Melisa. Melisa was just three years old in 2008.[10] When Librado obtained a grant to expand horticultural and fishing operations in Muaina, he chose Indalesio as coordinator.

When Enrique calls on Mamerto's parents to speak, Indalesio has already left for the cemetery to build Mamerto's tomb. Florencia leaves the other wailers

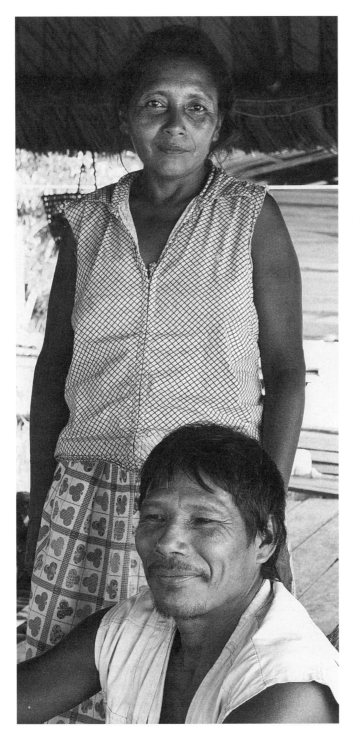

FIGURE 1.12.
Florencia
Macotera
and Indalesio
Pizarro, 2010.
Photograph
by Charles L.
Briggs.

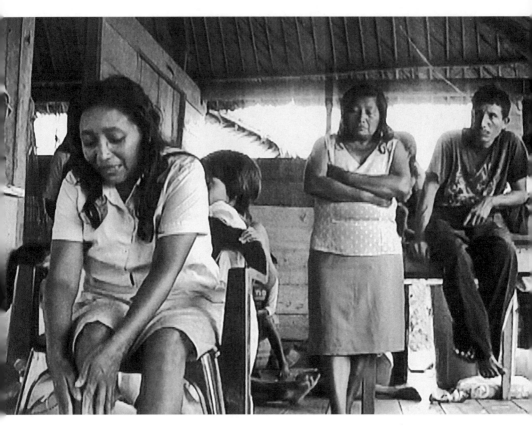

FIGURE 1.13. Florencia Macotera narrates Dalvi's death in the Muaina meeting, 2008. Olga Pizarro and Eduardo Pizarro listen. Photograph by Charles L. Briggs.

and walks slowly, as if in a trance, across the bridge. All eyes shift from the previous witness, who wraps up swiftly, as Florencia enters the area. Everyone steps aside, allowing her to go directly to the white plastic narrator's chair. Florencia's uncombed hair hangs around her face and she seems exhausted to the point of delirium. The sound of the ritual wailing moves toward a crescendo as she begins her story, not with Mamerto's death but with that of his little brother, Dalvi.

She speaks rapidly, her voice raspy from days of crying and punctuated by sobs (figure 1.13). Her youngest, Melisa, hovers near her. The ordeal began, Florencia reports, when nine-year-old Dalvi said weakly one day, "Mama, I'm cold. I think I have a fever," and went to lie down. His illness emerged even as a wake had begun for Muaina's first fatality from the strange disease, Florencia's nephew, Eduardito Pizarro.

Florencia's nephew, Eduardito Pizarro, was already sick with a fever and had been taken to Guayo. She didn't know how severe the disease was until his mother came back at 2:00 AM and called out loudly, "My son is dead!" Indalesio rushed to his brother's house to learn what had happened, then helped with funeral preparations while Florencia wailed over the body. While Dalvi was gazing at his cousin's corpse, Florencia noticed that he was not well and said, "Let's go home." She asked Nurse Mirna Pizarro for assistance, receiving a bottle of liquid acetaminophen. It did not help; by dawn Dalvi was worse and said that his head hurt a lot. Given more liquid acetaminophen, he "vomited and vomited."

Indalesio, being a wisidatu, tried to diagnose his son. After smoking a *wina* cigar to activate his helper spirits, he touched Dalvi's head, which felt like it was on fire, then rubbed his chest and abdomen, lightly intoning healing songs bearing the names of *hebu* associated with Dalvi's symptoms while moving his sacred rattle rhythmically in circles. He hoped to force the pathogen to reveal itself, but he felt no mass or movement.

When the nurse saw Dalvi shortly after dawn, his temperature was high. Florencia bathed him in infusions she prepared of mango and soursop (*Annona muricata*) leaves. She is a yarokotarotu, trained in the use of herbal medicine; Nurse Mirna used her medicines, too. Dalvi felt an intense itching sensation in his feet, which he scratched so hard they started bleeding. Florencia reaches down to demonstrate on her own bare legs how intense Dalvi's scratching had become.

The following day, the itching turned into numbness. Touching his hips, Dalvi said, "Dad, it's up to here!" Dalvi developed insomnia and had strange dreams. He said repeatedly, "Mama, I can't close my eyes because when I do, Eduardito comes up to me and says, 'Let's go, let's go. There are movies up there. There are cartoons.'" A decision was made to make the thirty-minute trip to Guayo, which must have been excruciating for Dalvi. They finally arrived at the home of a much more experienced wisidatu, Basilio Estrella, whose grandson, Eduardito, had just died in his care. He felt around for hebu—but his hands and rattle failed him and he turned away, leaving Dalvi with his parents.

As death drew near, Dalvi appeared to be fighting the cartoon villains that are regularly beamed into Muaina via DirecTV satellite dishes. He declared, "Mama, the monsters have killed me. They have taken my heart." His voice began to fade: "Mama, I am leaving without you now. I'm going now. My dead cousin Eduardito has come to get me. He's with me. I'm going now. We're going now." Attempting to hang onto Dalvi, Florencia pleaded, "Don't die yet son. Wait a little longer for me." He comforted her: "Okay, I'll stay. I won't die. I'm not going to die, Mama." But she could see that his eyes were closed, his body growing cold, his voice fading away. "Mama, Mama, I won't die. I won't die. I won't die, Mama, for you I won't die. My body will grow cold, but I won't die. I'm going to come for you, Mama. Wait for me, Mama. When I die, don't cry for me. Don't cry for me." "And then," Florencia concludes, "he grew silent. My son Dalvi died." On the way home from placing Dalvi in his tomb, Florencia's firstborn, twenty-two-year-old Mamerto, complained that he was not feeling well.

Mamerto attended first through fourth grades in Muaina. Because he was a good student, his parents then sent him to live in Nabasanuka with his uncle, nurse Jesús Moraleda. Jesús counseled Mamerto to press ahead with his studies. His uncle Librado had helped establish the Indigenous University of Venezuela (IUV) in 2004. An ambitious, innovative attempt to train a new generation of indigenous leaders, the IUV is based on an intercultural model that attempts to deepen rather than displace the students' foundation in what are considered indigenous knowledge systems. Sensing Mamerto's potential even as he felt the cancer grow inside him, Librado recruited him for IUV, announcing, "When I die, we will need a well-trained leader." Fellow students and professors alike realized that Mamerto—known there by his Warao name, Naku (Monkey)—had talent; he excelled academically (figure 1.14). Everyone said that Mamerto had a dream.

While studying in Nabasanuka, Mamerto met Elbia Torres Rivas, from nearby Barranquita. Elbia was beautiful, and Mamerto found her shyness and soft laughter beguiling. He missed her when he went to study in Tauca; when illness forced him to return to the lower delta temporarily, they were married.

Florencia begins her story of Mamerto's illness by gesturing toward his corpse and saying, "This other son of mine complained that he was not feeling well." After returning from Dalvi's burial, Mamerto went alone to visit his cousin, Mirna, complaining of a headache. The nurse gave him some acetaminophen tablets and sent him home, but the headache did not go away. Then Mamerto's feet starting itching "just the same" as his brother Dalvi's, and after a while he said, "Mama, I feel as if my legs are getting numb." Feeling worse the next day, he returned to Mirna, who gave him more acetaminophen. By morning, "his legs hurt, and he was just dragging his feet along as he walked," Florencia reports. These sensations of numbness reached his hips; he told his mother, "My legs have died!"

When medication did not help, his father concluded, "Look, this isn't a fever. We Warao always think like that. It could be hoa sickness." Indalesio's

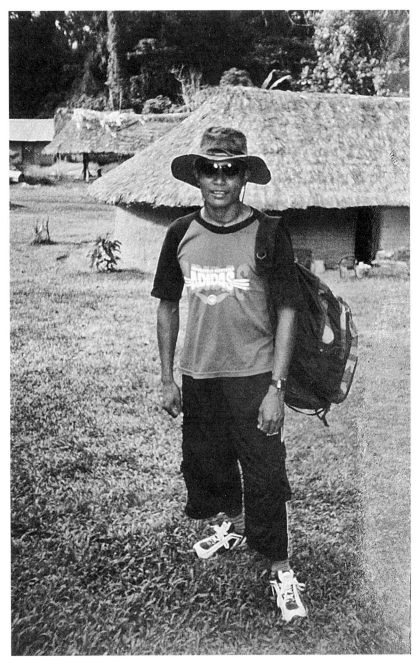

FIGURE 1.14. Mamerto Pizarro at the Indigenous University of Venezuela. Photographer unknown.

efforts to find hebu had already failed. So he brought in a highly experienced hoarotu, a specialist in hoa sickness, from Guayo. The hoarotu thought that he had found something: "He sang and sang, but nothing happened, absolutely nothing."

Two days later Mamerto appeared at Mirna's clinic-kitchen complaining that on top of everything else, he could barely urinate, resulting in acute pain. This had been going on for some days, but he had not told his parents. Florencia says she then noted that her son had acute abdominal pain. Mamerto went to the Nabasanuka clinic.

"He began to talk exactly like his little brother," Florencia reports. "Mama, I'm going away without you now. When I die, the television set is going to be yours. The DVD is going to be yours. Everything I have is going to be yours." Then Mamerto closed his eyes, saying, "Mama, I see lots and lots of houses, lots and lots of people. 'How are you?' [Mamerto greets the people in his vision.] 'We're fine. How are you?' 'I'm just fine. What have you brought?' 'Nothing, we're just looking around.' 'Well, go ahead and look around, the settlement is very large.' " Mamerto "was delirious," which alarmed Florencia. Then he fell asleep but awoke suddenly and jumped out of his hammock. "I was fighting with the bad guys," he told his mother. "They were pursuing me. I fought with them, punching and kicking them and throwing them to the ground. But they surrounded me." She concluded that he had entered a cinematic world. "I'm in bad shape. I can't sleep, Mother. What's happening to me? Every time I try, these things appear. I don't know what's happening, Mother." Each episode awoke Elbia, sleeping in the adjacent hammock, with a start; her soothing words did little to ease her husband's terror.

Florencia's voice grows quiet. A young adult died with similar symptoms in Siawani in February, followed by a mother who had given birth only two weeks before, but these deaths had not led clinicians to realize that the strange disease was now killing young adults. Florencia made the connection. She recounts her words to her son: "I can see that you will not recover. Your brother Dalvi has been dead a week, and you have the same disease." She then breaks off in midsentence and rises to leave, overwhelmed by grief: "That's the end of my story; I just can't say anything else." At this point, Clara asks two short diagnostic questions, knowing that more would be inappropriate. "How did they react to water?" "They asked for water," Florencia replies, "but then said that it frightened them, and they refused it." "Were they bitten by any animal?" "Yes, Mamerto was bitten by a bat about a month before he died." Dalvi and Eduardito also received nocturnal bat bites just over a month before they became ill.

Returning to her seat at the head of Mamerto's coffin, Florencia's voice again rises above the others as the wailing reaches a new intensity.

Florencia's sudden departure leaves us in suspense. In March 2010, Charles spent a day with Florencia and Indalesio and heard the father's account of accompanying Mamerto to urban hospitals, thus filling in the missing details. Indalesio says, "Once both hebu and hoa treatments failed, I realized that I could do nothing more." He found this very painful, but remembers thinking, "We should take him elsewhere." Indalesio, Elbia, and Mirna accompanied Mamerto to Nabasanuka; Florencia stayed behind to care for her other children. Mamerto told the nurse, "I have a really bad headache, and I pass out sometimes. My whole body hurts, and it really hurts when someone touches me." Elbia and Indalesio spent the night alternating between standing next to his bed and sitting on the uncomfortable plastic chairs on the porch outside. Neither slept. When he could not control the fever—or explain why Mamerto was dying—Dr. Ricardo referred him to the Tucupita Hospital.

An ambulance took Mamerto from the port to the emergency room of the Luis Razetti Hospital in Tucupita, where Indalesio implored the staff members, "We've just arrived from the delta, and my son is in really bad shape. Help us!" His command of Spanish and the history of patients coming from Nabasanuka with the strange disease secured a more positive response than the one afforded most patients classified as Warao. Attendants found a stretcher and wheeled Mamerto right in. His wife and father sat in plastic chairs near the entrance, so exhausted that they hardly noticed the stares, some hostile, from passersby. After a few hours, a physician emerged: "The doctor just said, 'Well, there's nothing we can do for him here,'" adding that Mamerto needed another referral, this time to the Uyapar Hospital in Puerto Ordaz, a city in Bolívar State, that could provide a higher level of care.

Within minutes, Mamerto was wheeled out on a stretcher and put into a waiting ambulance that raced along the only road leading out of Tucupita. The siren's scream and the flashing lights contributed to Elbia's and Indalesio's sense of desperation. When they finally turned onto Caroní Avenue, which leads to the hospital, everything seemed strange: either out of scale, such as a huge tire store and looming apartment buildings, or adorned with peculiar colors and lights, like the Burger King and McDonald's fast-food outlets. The journey partially retraced Mamerto's trip from Muaina to the IUV.

The fortress-like Uyapar Hospital loomed just ahead. The large parking lot in front was cluttered with debris from the massive remodeling afforded by President Chávez's revolution in health. They stopped at a huge sign marked

EMERGENCIA; within seconds, a guard pulled back the large gray gate protecting access to the emergency room, and two uniformed workers emerged with a gurney for Mamerto's seemingly lifeless body. Elbia and Indalesio followed them into the emergency room, through double doors, and down a corridor to an elevator. Elbia and her father-in-law were immediately struck by how much cleaner and better maintained this facility was than the Tucupita Hospital. Big digital clocks popped up everywhere, the colon between the hour and minutes flashing at them unnervingly.

On the fifth floor, attendants pushing Mamerto knocked at a closed steel door marked Intensive Care Unit A; a man opened the door slightly, took the papers, and then allowed them to wheel Mamerto in. His wife and father caught a glimpse of a couple of other patients, each surrounded by a host of machines, tubes, and personnel before the doors swung closed and a guard suddenly appeared. She wore a white uniform with black seams and a stern expression and said gruffly, "Come this way!" She led them past the elevator and across a strangely depopulated waiting room to the stairwell. Here the hour portion of the ubiquitous clock was strangely blank; to the right of the flashing colon it read ":82," as if time stood still there or had been erased.

The guard motioned them into the stairwell where the vacant waiting area gave way to a mass of anxious bodies. On the landing, perhaps 2 by 2.5 meters, some fifteen people stood, sat on portable chairs or the floor, or leaned against a mound of coolers, thermoses, pillows, backpacks, and satchels stacked against the wall. Another two dozen people claimed the stairwell leading down to the fourth floor. Their beleaguered, anguished faces suggested that they were relatives of patients in the two intensive care units or the nearby surgical pavilion, waiting for news about their critically ill relatives. Rather than welcoming Elbia and Indalesio as two more relatives of poor patients in a public hospital, people reacted as if they might contaminate the already chaotic atmosphere of the stairwell. A young boy pointed at them and said, "Look, Mama, Indians!" Gradually, the crowd maneuvered the two of them down the stairs. Elbia and Indalesio already felt that each step of their arduous journey from Nabasanuka had progressively dislodged them from all that was safe and familiar—and from Mamerto. Being unwelcome in this disorderly space in a modern, orderly hospital was just too much.

After about an hour, the guard reappeared and shouted, "Indalesio Pizarro!" She escorted him and Elbia through the intensive care unit door where a man in light blue scrubs—from surgical cap to shoe covers—ushered them to Mamerto's side. He was connected to numerous machines, but the physician said only, "He's in critical condition; we don't know what's wrong." Recalling that moment, Indalesio says, "Then everything fell on top of Mamerto. . . . The machine failed him there—everything failed him."

Soon the nurse ordered them back into the stairwell. Elbia, exhausted, sat back in a corner and slept. Indalesio mostly stood but sometimes sat on the steps; he could not sleep. At 5:00 AM, a nurse appeared, called out, "Indalesio Pizarro," and led him to a physician standing outside the intensive care unit. "Your son is dead," he said matter-of-factly. Indalesio continues, "In about an hour they let me see him. The machine [respirator] had stopped." He was told, "Go downstairs and wait." Awakening Elbia on the landing, he echoed the doctor's curt, unfeeling words: "My son is dead." "What are we going to do?" she asked. "We have to wait."

The sun was rising as they descended from the hell of the stairway to the spacious waiting area by the main entrance. Indalesio longed to call Florencia from one of the three pay phones on the wall, but Muaina was clearly beyond their reach. Shortly after 9:00 AM, a secretary called out, "Indalesio Pizarro," then moved to stand behind a large glass panel. Speaking through a circular opening, she pushed a document at Indalesio through a slot. "We've alerted Tucupita, and they will send an ambulance for your son in the afternoon. Sign here." He signed the paper and returned it. The secretary disappeared into an inner office, where an official signed and stamped the forms; she then reappeared and shoved a copy through the slot before turning away to sip from a tiny plastic cup of coffee.

They waited. At midmorning, Elbia walked over to a glass-enclosed bulletin board where she found a typewritten notice with the heading Patient Rights. She read: "TO BE treated equally, with consideration, and without discrimination. . . . TO KNOW everything about your illness, laboratory results, procedures, and success or failure of treatments. TO MAKE decisions regarding your treatment, among them, to accept or reject proposed procedures or treatments. . . ." Who, she wondered, enjoys these rights? Who receives this kind of care?

Shortly after 1:30, "Indalesio Pizarro" rang out one last time. The secretary escorted them to an entrance near the ER where the ambulance was waiting. They watched as Mamerto—now a corpse in a coffin—emerged through a set of doors marked Anatomical Pathology and was placed in what looked like a large icebox in the back, much like the ones used to bring delta fish to mainland markets. They retraced their steps toward home. Neither slept, and Elbia appeared distant and unresponsive. At the Tucupita Hospital, employees took Mamerto's body and sent Elbia and Indalesio away, telling them to come back in the morning. "Where will we sleep?" Elbia asked her father-in-law. "On the street?" With no other place to go, they retraced Odilia's and Romer's route to the shantytown next to the river. There Indalesio asked, "Friend, do you have an extra hammock? My daughter-in-law wants to sleep." Exhausted, Elbia slept, but Indalesio embraced Warao practices of mourning and refrained from sleeping or eating, despite already having missed three nights of sleep. Hearing that Enrique Moraleda was in town for his daughter's graduation, Indalesio asked him to help navigate the maze of paperwork needed to take Mamerto back to Muaina. Elbia awakened, dazed and feverish, with no idea where to find her father-in-law.

Our arrival at Muaina coincided with the end of Mamerto's wake and burial, infusing the beginning of our investigation with marked intensity and edginess.

Elbia Torres and Her Family

My Daughter, tomorrow you will be in the forest, and weeds will grow over your tomb.—Anita Rivas

Elbia's birthplace, Barranquita, is right around the corner from Nabasanuka (figure 1.15). Her mother, Anita Rivas, is a vibrant woman in her early forties (figure 1.16). After she married Arsenio Torres, forty-six, they took up residence in the Rivas household in Barranquita. Anita gave birth to nine children. Elbia was the eldest; two of her siblings did not survive childhood.

Anita and Arsenio doted on Elbia (figure 1.17). Like Mamerto, she liked to accompany her parents on annual trips to make palm starch deep in the forest. Nevertheless, her life did not match any romantic vision of a timeless traditional Warao childhood. The family bought a television and VHS, later a DVD player. Elbia particularly liked to imitate the singers of Mexican *rancheras* and watch Arnold Schwarzenegger action movies. In school, she always did her homework and learned quickly. After they married, the couple split their time between Barranquita and Muaina—"They gave me a garden," Anita said with a smile. Though most people described Elbia and Mamerto as a happy couple, Anita believed that there was a sad, dark side to Mamerto's personality.

When news reached Mamerto that his cousin Eduardito had died suddenly in Muaina and that the strange symptoms had jumped into his little brother, Mamerto and Elbia caught a ride to Muaina.[11] When the mysterious disease started to claim his body, Mamerto confided details of his symptoms to her that he withheld from his worried parents, but no one ever asked Elbia for her observations, discussed possible courses of treatment, or explained what was taking place, and she was too timid to speak up.

When the nurse and her father-in-law announced that they were taking Mamerto to Nabasanuka, she said nothing and quickly untied their hammocks,

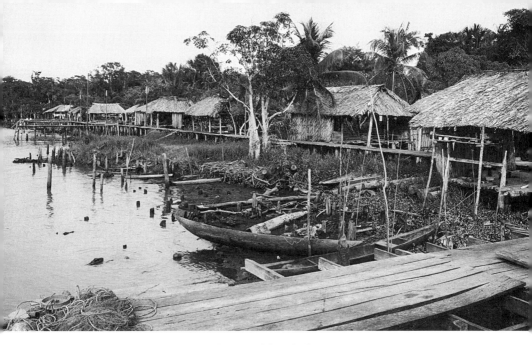

FIGURE 1.15.   Barranquita, 2010. Photograph by Charles L. Briggs.

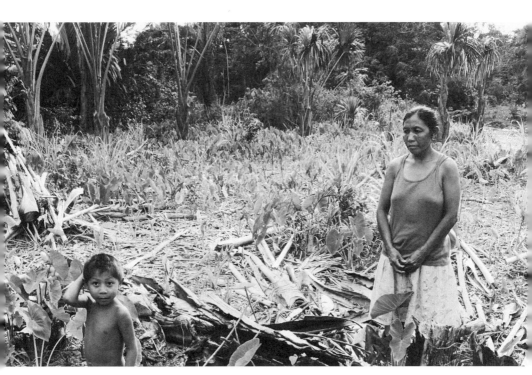

FIGURE 1.16.   Anita Rivas and her son, Romeliano, in her garden, 2010. Photograph by Charles L. Briggs.

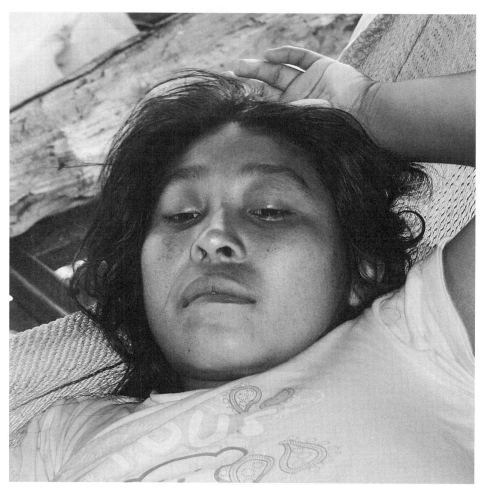

FIGURE 1.17. Elbia Torres Rivas, 2008. Photograph by Charles L. Briggs.

grabbed their few possessions, and climbed into the canoe next to Mamerto. In the clinic, Indalesio spoke with the nurses and Elbia sat by her husband's dilapidated, rusty bed and whispered to him about the garden they had planted. Sleepless, she spent the night on a blue plastic chair on the porch replaying in her head her mother-in-law's words to Mamerto: "I can see that you will not recover. Your brother Dalvi has been dead for a week, and you have the same disease." During the six-hour boat ride to Tucupita, she spoke softly to Mamerto about building their own house in Barranquita and about the children they would raise. He appeared to see and feel nothing. She begged him not to leave her. She wanted to cry but focused on the noise of the motor and cleaned the saliva that poured from Mamerto's mouth.

In the Tucupita Hospital, the attendants didn't even look at Elbia when they admitted Mamerto. It was Indalesio the physician called aside to announce the transfer; Indalesio who said, "We're going to Puerto Ordaz." Although Indalesio's Spanish was much better than the other parents' he was treated similarly: asked little, no explanations offered. Elbia spoke Spanish fairly well, but—young, female, and classified as indigenous—she was rendered mute. In the ambulance she felt as queasy as she had on the boat from Nabasanuka; she attributed it to exhaustion and emotional upheaval and said nothing.

At Uyapar Hospital, the sight of Mamerto connected to so many machines both frightened Elbia and offered a ray of hope—the machines and doctors might bring her Mamerto back. She wanted to stay awake but felt weak, had a splitting headache, and was asleep when her father-in-law received the doctor's brusque announcement. When he awakened her and said bluntly, "My son is dead," she wished she were back in Barranquita. She began to compose the verses that she would wail alongside Mamerto's mother. Exhaustion gave way to a flood of silent tears, but she did not dare to give verbal, let alone musical, form to her thoughts and feelings there on the hospital landing.

Elbia felt worse and worse during the return trip down the bumpy, two-lane highway to Tucupita. Some men take it for granted that indigenous women are always interested in the sexual advances of criollo strangers, so she was grateful to fall asleep in a borrowed hammock in the Warao squatters' camp. But when she awoke a couple of hours after daybreak, Mamerto's death hit her as if for the first time. Terrified, she called out for Indalesio, but the lean-to's other occupants replied, "*Naruae*" (He left).

Anxious, feverish, and weak, she arose like a zombie and left the shantytown. Cars honked at her as she crossed the street, traversed the plaza, and looked dazedly at face after face, panicked that her father-in-law might have taken Mamerto's body and left for Muaina. Her whole body hurt; her feet felt heavy, slightly unresponsive. She remembered Mamerto describing the strange sensations that came from nowhere; she grew even more terrified. "Is Mamerto taking me with him?" She determined there and then that if she had to die, it would not be in a clinic or hospital.

Trying to retrace the once-familiar way to Tucupita Hospital, she kept getting inexplicably lost. In the central plaza she heard someone speaking Warao and asked if they knew Indalesio Pizarro and where to find him. "His son died," an old man replied, "and he is at Volcán with his body, waiting for the boat."

Indalesio had given her a fifty-Bolívar note and, desperate, she stopped the first taxi that came along. The loud bass of reggaeton music pounded at her head, and the twenty-minute drive seemed to take hours. Fleeing the taxi and moving as quickly as she could manage down the cement ramp, her sense of relief at seeing Indalesio vanished as he scolded her in front of the crowd at the landing for failing to wait for him in the Paseo Manamo, for disappearing. She just stared at the ground, not saying that on top of her grief she also had symptoms just like Mamerto described, that getting lost paled in comparison with feeling as if she, too, was on the way to the graveyard. Silently, she climbed aboard the boat and sat down next to the shiny coffin, imagining herself inside it with Mamerto.

In Muaina, Florencia began to wail as soon as the boat arrived. Elbia listened for a few minutes, then added her voice, weaving in her own twists on the images constructed by other lamenters. She was wailing for Mamerto's death and her own simultaneously. For Elbia, lamentation gave musical form to an interior world that she had entered the previous day, one that was claiming her body as much as her mind and larynx. Her parents arrived shortly, and Elbia collapsed in their arms. No longer mute and invisible, she unleashed a torrent of words and tears that left them frightened and confused.

After singing again briefly, Elbia grew so weak and feverish that she and her parents spent most of that day and the next morning in the house next to that of community representative Olga Pizarro, where they could hear the wailing. Learning that Indalesio's support for Elbia had turned into a rebuke at Volcán, her parents declared angrily that they would have nothing to do with Indalesio and Florencia after Mamerto's funeral. Between a family in grief and one in panic there was no space for negotiation. But Elbia's parents received their greatest shock when they offered to take her to the doctor in Nabasanuka. "No," she replied, shaking her head both resolutely and anxiously, "I'm not going to any clinic. I'm going to die in my home." "Die?" they gasped.

The meeting at Olga's house took place the morning of Elbia's second day back in Muaina. Before returning to Barranquita, Anita and Arsenio requested that the team, particularly Clara and Norbelys, visit their daughter. Like the other parents, they were recruiting all possible help from healers and medical practitioners. If Elbia wouldn't go to the clinic, the clinic would come to Elbia. Anita's parents' house had been converted into a sort of hospital, with brightly colored sheets hanging vertically in one corner to shield Elbia from the sun reflected off the river and provide a measure of privacy.

As Elbia's grandmother, Jacinta Gómez, pulled aside a sheet, Clara and Norbelys came face to face with the disease and a human being it was claiming.

Anita squatted at the head of her daughter's hammock, her face filled with exhaustion and worry. Elbia lacked signs of acute illness, but she had descended into a state of depressed resignation. As doctor and nurse knelt near her, Clara asking questions and Norbelys and Charles translating, Elbia replied succinctly. Gasping slightly for breath, she noted that her symptoms had begun three days earlier. She was in a lot of pain, weak, and feverish, and she felt as if her legs were paralyzed. Asked if she were thirsty, Elbia said yes, but when Clara offered her a glass of water she cried out, "Obononaha!" (I don't want it!) in an agitated voice and looked away. "Masaba aisda" ("It's bad for me," or "I don't like it"). Asked if she had been bitten by an animal, Elbia said, "No, but Mamerto was bitten by a bat on the head and feet while we were visiting Muaina. . . . A little over a month before he got sick. I'm really scared." We visited Elbia each morning and evening, and these encounters punctuated our investigation. Clara and Norbelys provided palliative care. They obtained the best medications that the Nabasanuka staff could offer—intravenous analgesics and rehydration solution—and administered them during each visit. They noted the progressive worsening of Elbia's symptoms, interrupted only by one remarkable morning after her visit to healer Avelino Campero, when she felt much better.

We visited Elbia for the last time on the morning of 2 August. In keeping with the family's wishes, Charles took photographs. She lay in her hammock, conscious but unable to move; the drugs helped ease her intense pain. "I'm dying now," she said softly. "I'm really scared." The face of Elbia's grandfather, Tito Rivas, was a study in grief and anguish (figure 1.18). Her lips were parched. Clara fetched swabs of cotton from our medical supplies and showed Anita how to dip them in a bowl of water that Elbia could not see, then moisten her lips. It was the last time Anita was able to care for her daughter (figure 1.19).

Upon our return that night we found ourselves in the midst of an equally distressing but visually and acoustically contrasting scene, one in which Anita, Arsenio, and other relatives stood wailing over Elbia's corpse; we return to this moment in chapter 7.

The next day the men sealed Elbia's coffin, placed it in a canoe, paddled it across the river, and placed it in the small opening that provides access to Barranquita's cemetery (figure 1.20). Then the men cleared away overgrown forest, fashioned boards to construct the house that would become Elbia's new dwelling, and built a wooden structure within it to hold her coffin securely. Tirso, a relative, supervised the work. They carried the coffin to the tomb-house, lifted it up, and placed it in its niche as the women watched in silence: the

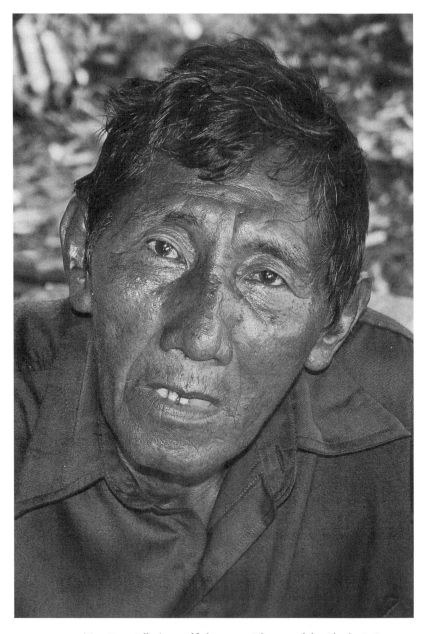

FIGURE 1.18. Tito Rivas, Elbia's grandfather, 2008. Photograph by Charles L. Briggs.

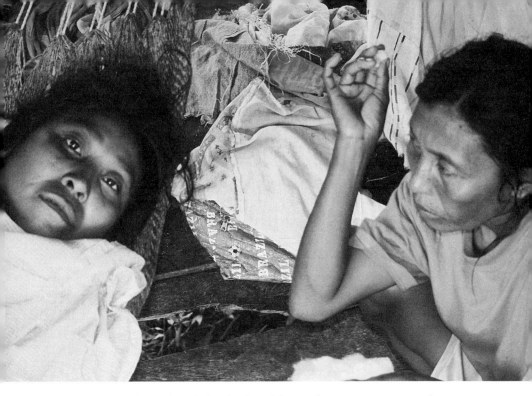

FIGURE 1.19. Elbia, an hour before death, with her mother, Anita Rivas, 2008. Photograph by Charles L. Briggs.

laments had ended (figure 1.21). In the final phase of the ritual, a canoe full of oozing mud arrived at the landing. A double line of women and men formed and passed big gobs of mud from the canoe to the grave site. As the participants became more and more caked with mud, a transformation occurred. Laughter and joking replaced wailing and crying (figures 1.22, 1.23). Soon even Elbia's relatives began to smile as they watched this phase of the work of burial transform pain into mirth. Anita left her mother's side to join relatives filling Elbia's new house with mud until it lay some fifteen centimeters deep over the coffin. Everyone then crossed back across the river, ritually washed off the mud and overt signs of grief, and found a way to get on with their lives.

The Parents' Testimonies Suggest a Presumptive Diagnosis

Given the time to tell their stories, the parents provided detailed accounts of their children's symptoms that were remarkably consistent. Soon it added up: headache, fever, generalized aches, malaise, itching or tingling in the extremities

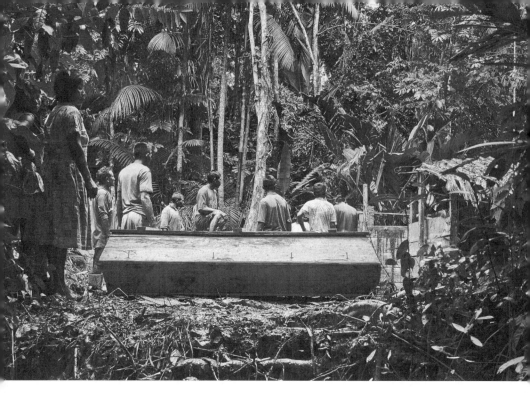

FIGURE 1.20. Elbia's coffin has just been placed at the entrance to the Barranquita cemetery, 2008. Photograph by Charles L. Briggs.

(paresthesia) that progressively changed into feelings of numbness and paralysis, hypersensitivity to touch, difficulty swallowing (dysphagia), first of food then of liquids, and excessive salivation. Some patients presented vomiting, stomach upset, and diarrhea, but not all. Most telling was hydrophobia, fear of water. All persons who exhibited symptoms died within seven days. Then came the series of clinical encounters with a patient—Elbia Torres Rivas. She felt pain when touched lightly and had a 39.5°C (103.1°F) fever. Stethoscopic examination revealed hoarseness, crackling sounds in the lungs, and abdominal sounds. Neurological examination suggested a partial loss of sensitivity in the lower extremities and great difficulty walking. A test for the Babinski response, repeated on both feet, was positive, indicating a significant neurological abnormality.[12] Salivation was excessive. Elbia had a cup on the floor to expel the saliva; when she looked in its direction, her mother would retrieve it.

Over the course of our investigation, the team had entertained a number of hypotheses, none of which were borne out by the parents' testimonies: Could it be intoxication from a substance derived from the landfill at Cambalache? No: in many of the places where people had died, residents had not visited a landfill

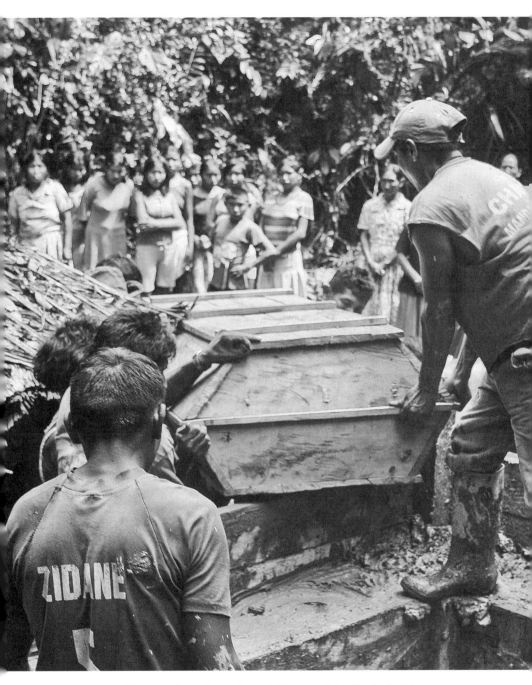

FIGURE 1.21. Placing coffin in the tomb, 2008. Photograph by Charles L. Briggs.

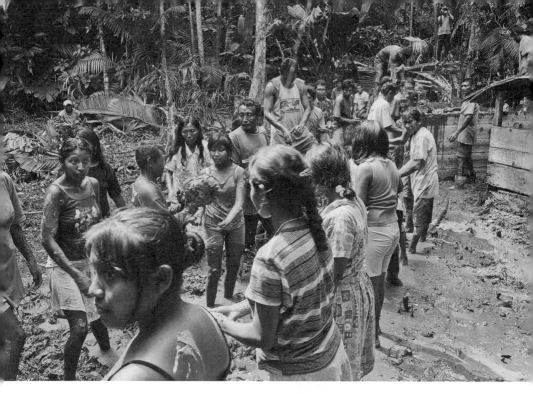

FIGURE 1.22. Passing large gobs of mud, 2008. Photograph by Charles L. Briggs.

FIGURE 1.23.
Muddied and laughing,
2008. Photograph by
Charles L. Briggs.

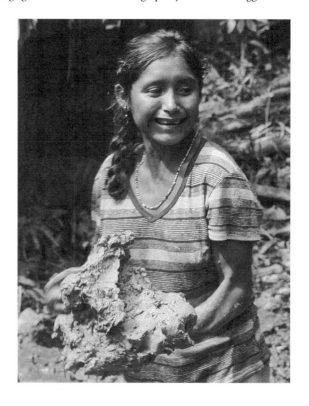

or received objects taken from it during the previous twelve months. Could it be a food or other product sold by bongueros, itinerant merchants? No: several communities had deaths but had not received visits from bongueros during the preceding months. From the start, the parents' testimonies pointed to some sort of neurological connection due to the tingling in the feet and ascendant paralysis, along with the strange visions and sensations, perhaps due to some form of encephalitis (inflammation of the brain). Some symptoms of mercury and lead poisoning, such as difficulty sleeping, headaches, low appetite, difficulty breathing, numbness, and difficulty walking, correspond to those reported by the parents, but we found no evidence of exposure to lead or mercury. It similarly did not make sense that only one or two individuals in a house would die as a result of drinking the same fluids, bathing in the same water, and eating the same foods as everyone else, or that the same pattern would be evident in Mukoboina or Muaina and settlements located kilometers away. Rather, the parents' accounts and the clinical evidence pointed strongly toward rabies.

Rabies is an acute viral infection of the central nervous system caused by the rabies virus, generally transmitted in the saliva of a rabid animal who bites the victim. The virus infects muscle fibers at the site of the bite, then slowly—some 50–100 mm per day—travels from neuron to neuron along the central nervous system toward the brain, initially producing no symptoms. Once the brain is infected, however, neurological symptoms begin, resulting in the strange visions and other sensorial abnormalities reported by patients. Nevertheless, consciousness can be present even late in the course of the disease, resulting in patients who can bounce back from strange dreams and seizures to articulate moving and poetic last words; others, like Mamerto, slipped into coma. The disease is commonly spread through bites from mammals such as dogs, skunks, and raccoons through the injection of infected saliva; different species can transmit different strains of the rabies virus, a single-stranded negative-sense RNA virus of the genus *Lyssavirus*. Hydrophobia results from selective infection of neurons that control the swallow reflex, resulting in an exaggerated response that feels like gagging. After repeated attempts to deglutinate (swallow) fluids results in a drowning sensation, even seeing a glass of water can stimulate this response. Eventually, multiple organ failure results in death.[13]

Obviously, a rabid dog was not wandering from place to place, biting people, so what was the vector? Because people sleep in hammocks in houses that generally lack walls on at least two sides, the occasional nocturnal bat bite is common. From the day we arrived in Hubasuhuru, however, people reported an unusual number of vampire bats, as signaled by the new presence of cats, which

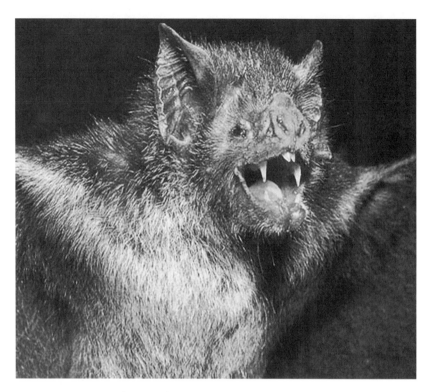

FIGURE 1.24. *Desmodus rotundus.*

people had adopted due to their ability to kill bats when they fly into houses. The team added animal bites to the list of questions it had compiled as soon as the rabies hypothesis emerged. The parents reported that many of the children who died had been bitten nocturnally by vampire bats approximately four to six weeks prior to developing symptoms, which falls within the interval between exposure and the onset of symptoms for most patients (World Health Organization 2014). The species of vampire bat that is common in the delta, as in many other parts of Venezuela (Linares 1986), is *Desmodus rotundus* (figure 1.24). In keeping with the age of the people who died in the epidemic, detailed research in the Peruvian Amazon suggests that persons twenty-five years of age or younger are most likely to be bitten by these bats (Gilbert et al. 2012, 208). As cases of rabies transmitted by dogs become less common in the Americas, the Pan American Health Organization reports that similar outbreaks of bat-transmitted rabies have occurred in recent years in Brazil, Colombia, Ecuador, Peru, and other Latin American countries (Schneider et al. 2009). Although bat-transmitted rabies cases in the United States are commonly attributed to insectivorous bat species, human cases in Latin America are most commonly transmitted by *D. rotundus* bats (Gilbert et al. 2010, 206).

Rabies has the highest case fatality rate of any conventional disease, nearly 100 percent fatal once symptoms emerge. At the same time, rabies vaccines are remarkably effective in preventing the disease. According to WHO (2010), anyone bitten by a bat should receive antirabies vaccine and immunoglobin as soon as possible—whether or not cases of rabies have been reported in the area. A study by leading specialists of rabies and *D. rotundus* in the Peruvian Amazon suggested that rabies prophylaxis (vaccination) should be provided for all persons living in communities in which bies are common (Gilbert et al. 2012). Despite the rapid increase in the incidence of nocturnal bat bites, no one was being vaccinated in Delta Amacuro. Once we suspected rabies, we began health education in the affected areas, suggesting that people take precautions to prevent bat bites, wash all bites with soap and water as soon as possible,[14] and request vaccination immediately. Our goal was to prompt authorities to vaccinate residents as well as to further investigate the epidemic. This step has been undertaken in Ecuador and Peru where bat-transmitted rabies has been reported.

We did not have access to a laboratory, and we did not perform autopsies. The clinical evidence was sufficiently strong, however, that Clara could present a presumptive diagnosis of rabies. Knowing that people were being bitten nocturnally by vampire bats cried out for a rabies vaccination program, a need further underlined by the finding that the cause of the deaths seemed to be rabies. The stress of listening to the parents tell such horrific tales of their children's deaths and watching Elbia die was deepened by the specter of rabies. It is clearly not just a nosological category, not just another an entry in the *International Classification of Diseases*; rabies has been a horrific figure in popular culture for centuries (see Wasik and Murphy 2012).

Welcome to the New Wing of the Mukoboina Cemetery

The clearing across the river from Barranquita was not the only cemetery we visited while investigating the epidemic. On 11 August 2009, we traveled with Alfonso and Inocencio Torres three kilometers upriver from Mukoboina. As we entered a *hana* (a smaller river that connects two tributaries), an opening suddenly emerged in the dense forest. A muddy bank, brown water below, an upper edge of temiche palms, then a glimpse of low houses in a circular clearing some 100 meters in diameter. On the right, three diminutive houses were eroding back into the forest. On the left, a line of new, five-foot-tall houses (figure 1.25).

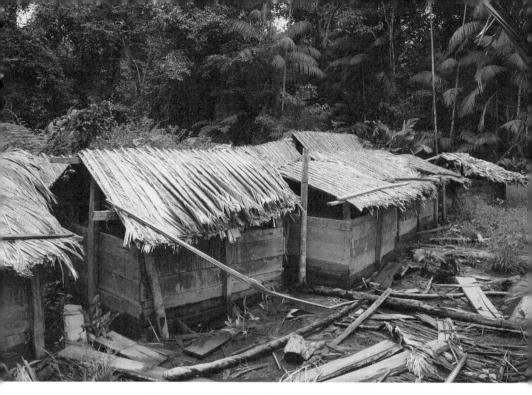

FIGURE 1.25. The new section of the Mukoboina cemetery, 2008. Photograph by Charles L. Briggs.

"This was the first," Alfonso explains. "This next one is for Romer's children. There are two here in a single house. This one is for Wilmer's children—there are two here as well." His tone is so matter-of-fact this could have been a tour of Mukoboina proper. At the next he says simply, "Ine, isaka" (mine, one). His voice deepens. "She [Yanilka] died in Maturín. . . . I cried, I was so sad. After it happened, I was in really bad shape. When I saw [this house], I felt so badly, I couldn't do anything but cry. I lost consciousness, my will to live. When we don't think about it so much, we feel a little better. But when we see it, when we come here, our minds go blank, we just cry. We think about her. Our minds fail us." He continues, "For three months, all we did was cry. Another would get sick, another would get sick, and another would get sick; it was impossible. By the time we finished here [burying one child], another died. That is how they were finished off, one by one."

The mysterious epidemic had split Mukoboina into the land of the living and, slightly upriver, the land of the dead. After two waves of death washed over Mukoboina, residents petitioned the government for a nursing station with medicines and a primary health care worker. Nothing happened. Between

July 2007 and January 2008, eight of their children died, plus one from Hokorinoko across the river, three in Sakoinoko, and three more in Horobuhu, both just a few kilometers upriver. Not to mention the four in nearby Siawani and eight in Santa Rosa de Guayo, both of them places of origin for Mukoboina families. Healers had failed them. Doctors and nurses let them down. They felt they and their children had been mistreated in urban hospitals. In spite of it all, Mukoboinans had not renounced what they understood to be their "fundamental social right" to health care, as guaranteed by the Venezuelan Constitution. Alfonso continues, "We don't want this to happen anymore. That's why when diseases come, we want a nursing station in Mukoboina, so we won't die." Alfonso remembers that in her lament, his wife, Santa, had cried, "Because we have no nurse or doctor here, my daughter died. Although the politicians have resources, they didn't help us. They only come and see us when it is time for elections. Now that they have ended, politicians don't bring medicines for our children. They bring nothing. Our children have died now. They have died."

Alfonso turns away from the houses and says in a measured, calm voice that betrays an edge of anger, "This is not a lie. I'm telling the truth." Then, pointing at Yanilka's house, "She died."

2

———

WHEN

CAREGIVERS

FAIL

Doctors, Nurses, and Healers Facing an Intractable Disease

When the first patients were admitted,
we thought it was a simple virus.
—Alonzo Moraleda

Even as they faced a common dilemma—trying to save their children from a 100 percent fatal disease that guarded its secrets carefully—the parents' approaches to it varied widely. Some went straight to the doctor; others bounced between healers; most asked anyone and everyone they could find to help. The people on the other side of this equation, the caregivers who were entrusted with sick and dying children, were also all over the map in what they said to the parents, how they attempted to figure out what was going on, and which forms of treatment they tried. By placing these caregivers in dialogue in this chapter, our goal is not to put them in a relationship of equivalence—a magical reversal of social hierarchies that none would accept—but to explore the different ways they all faced what was perhaps the greatest challenge of their careers. We use ethnography, interviews, and years of our own engagement in the delta as physician (Clara) and anthropologist and healer (Charles) in trying to move among complex, shifting, and heterogeneous perspectives. In the end, these practitioners held three things in common. First, all of them did their best to save the patients who were brought to them with strange symptoms. Second, they all failed—no one could achieve a satisfactory diagnosis or save the life of a single patient. Third, for all of them, the failure hurt. Particularly as the deaths multiplied and some parents lost more than one child, their inability to figure it out troubled them profoundly, prompting them to search deeper for clues. Each specialty afforded insights into what was taking place and each imposed barriers to communicating with the parents—or even sometimes with their fellow practitioners. Here is what we have been able to reconstruct about their diverse experiences.

Dr. Ricardo Cáceres and the Medical Interns at the Nabasanuka Clinic

If Mukoboina provides a snapshot of the hundreds of small delta settlements— each consisting of one or two dozen houses surrounded by gardens—then Nabasanuka functions as an urban center, with its clinic, school, stores, mission, and visibility to the world beyond the rain forest. Nabasanuka was founded in 1932 by Capuchin missionaries for students leaving their boarding schools. Like San Francisco de Guayo, it was designed to radiate "civilization"— Catholicism, education, and market-oriented horticulture, fishing, and craft production—to the surrounding area. With some 500 residents,[1] Nabasanuka boasts wooden, fully enclosed houses linked by a cement sidewalk, contrasting, in settlements like Mukoboina, with palm-thatched houses largely devoid of walls and connected—if at all—by bridges built over a swampy surface.[2] Stores offer such items as flour, rice, sugar, soda pop, oil, soap, batteries, fishhooks, gasoline, and oil at prices three to five times greater than in Tucupita. The mission is now staffed by Kenyan priests and Italian nuns of the Consolata order.

Beside the mission stands a principal destination of visitors to Nabasanuka, a Type II Rural Clinic. It was founded in 1975 by German-born physician Egon Herbig: he fled the Nazis, built the clinic, and periodically came in his small plane, fitted with pontoons. After a crash killed him and most of his family in 1977, the Regional Health Service (RHS) provided a resident physician and nurses,[3] medicines, and a boat to transport critically ill patients to Tucupita.

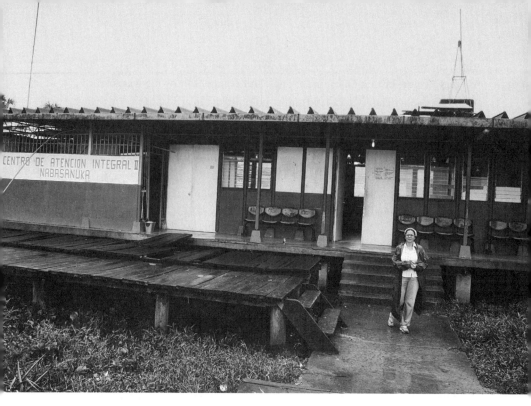

FIGURE 2.1. The Nabasanuka clinic, with Dr. Clara Mantini-Briggs in the foreground, 2008. Photograph by Charles L. Briggs.

The clinic is now a somewhat dilapidated rectangular structure painted bright blue on the bottom and white on top (figure 2.1). As boats pass along the river in front, it stands out sharply from the mission and nearby houses. Cement steps lead from the dock to a porch with a row of aging blue chairs used by relatives to pass the long days and nights. The middle door opens onto an area with a rusting metal desk that serves physicians and nurses as a place to conduct initial interviews with patients and relatives and record basic information in the daily log. Each week, the case information is transferred to Tucupita. Behind the desk is a two-way radio, used to communicate with administrative offices in Tucupita and the other four Type II clinics in the lower delta. A screen divides this area from one graced by a table used for examinations and short-term treatment. To the left is a small room with the stock of medicines, brought by physicians or nurses during trips to Tucupita and provided free of charge to patients. Sometimes patients must be turned away by exasperated physicians and nurses with the words, "We don't have anything, not even aspirin!" or given prescriptions to be filled in Tucupita. On the far left is a room formerly dedicated to the tuberculosis screening program administered by the Malarial Institute.

On the other side of the examining/reception area is the pediatric clinic, with a desk and a small examining table with a scale, used for routine pediatric examinations and less serious cases. The walls are adorned with Ministry of Popular Power for Health (MPPS) posters, drawings, and photographs taken from magazines featuring children and pregnant or lactating women, often with texts emphasizing vaccination, breast-feeding, and rehydration. Many drawings picture mothers and babies with skin so white that they look more like the tourists who occasionally appear than patients or staff. Next door is a small room with two beds for hospitalized patients. Last is the obstetrics clinic, with an obstetrical bed and a small metal table for instruments. This area served as the physician's residence—sometimes a family or two physicians shared this cramped space—until a new structure was built next door with a living room, kitchen/dining room, and several bedrooms. A boathouse in front houses the fluvial ambulance and stores gasoline and oil. Behind is an electrical generator. By the time it was replaced in 2012 by the adjacent Dr. Luís Beltrán Zabaleta Hospital, the clinic had conjoined generations of newly minted doctors and advanced medical students, generations of bilingual nurses, and a steady stream of patients.

The life of the rural doctor embodies both the utopian vision and the discouraging constraints confronting physicians in public practice. Upon graduation, physicians in Venezuela are required to work their first year in an underserved area, either rural or urban. Each year in Nabasanuka, a young, newly graduated physician, working for the first time without immediate supervision, collaborates with nurses in overseeing disease treatment and prevention for a large swath of the lower delta, diagnosing a succession of cases of diarrheal diseases, respiratory infections, tuberculosis, cancer, skin diseases, HIV/AIDS, and other illnesses. The doctor can solicit advice from more experienced physicians over the two-way radio and in person during monthly visits to Tucupita, but these efforts generally yield little counsel or support. Charged with supervising the nursing staff, some physicians acknowledge that bilingual nurses assist the monolingual Spanish-speaking physicians with more than translation and drug administration. These nurses are, in any case, the only staff members on hand when the doctor is in Tucupita for a week or on vacation or a new doctor has not yet been appointed. Even under "normal" circumstances, the job of addressing abysmal health conditions is challenging. And in 2007–2008 things were anything but normal.

The parents were very nervous because they could see that this child was
going to die. . . . I had never seen any disease like that.
—Ricardo Cáceres

Dr. Ricardo Cáceres is a generally relaxed and friendly, if somewhat reserved
man in his late twenties. He came to Nabasanuka in June 2007, shortly after
receiving his medical degree from the Central University of Venezuela and just
before the initial outbreak of the mysterious disease.[4] Of medium stature, with
short black hair, brown eyes, and an aquiline nose, Dr. Ricardo thinks cautiously
before speaking. There was a quite sense of energy and intensity in his reflections about the epidemic, but they were carefully modulated by a voice that exuded restraint. We sought him out the day we learned about a series of strange
deaths from a Siawani man who had lost his young wife. Dr. Ricardo generously ushered us into the residence next to the Nabasanuka clinic and told us
of his extraordinarily challenging first year of medical practice.

After arriving at the clinic, Dr. Ricardo initially treated diseases that had
become familiar in the course of his training. Then he began to see children
with a disease that he could not diagnose and that stubbornly refused to respond to treatment, even to antipyretics to control the fever. Once the strange
cases started to appear, the children just kept coming. Yuri Torres was the first
patient to reach the clinic in Nabasanuka. Nurse José Pérez of Siawani brought
her in when his medicine could not bring down the fever. Dr. Ricardo did not,
however, remember her case as part of the epidemic. Reflecting on these events
a year later, without consulting any records, Dr. Ricardo told us that "the first
case was an eleven-year-old Mukoboina boy." He recalls that the child had a
very high fever, 41 degrees Celsius, an intense headache, chest pain, and great
difficulty breathing. In this case, Dr. Ricardo also detected a number of unusual symptoms, including seizures and excessive salivation. When the child
grew delirious, he reported that he was fighting a monster. Already a conscientious physician who was struggling to relate what he had learned in medical
school to what was seeing, Dr. Ricardo paused poignantly, then continued, "I
had never seen any disease like that." He reported, "I administered rehydration
solution and an antipyretic to control the fever." A stethoscope revealed "severe
hoarseness and a crackling sound, so I also nebulized him," that is, administered
an inhaler. Dr. Ricardo paused, inhaled deeply, and then related that three
more Mukoboina children, between six and eight years of age, soon arrived
with the same symptoms; given the gravity of the situation, he referred them
immediately to Tucupita. Then the disease mysteriously disappeared, but

there was a second and then a third wave of cases. He again sent patient after patient upriver, only to have them all return in caskets, causing him frustration and deep anguish.

When he was speaking about his work at the clinic and efforts to figure out the strange epidemic, we sensed his subdued but detectable intensity and excitement. When asked what sort of guidance he had received from his superiors, however, that was replaced with an equally muted sense of anxiety, even despondency. When he sent patients to Tucupita, they were always accompanied by a one-page sheet in which Dr. Ricardo carefully listed his clinical observations. He never received in response a report summarizing clinical data or the results of laboratory tests and autopsies. Thus, when another patient with similar symptoms appeared, he had no diagnosis to suggest, no revised treatment plan to recommend. The doctor used the radio to ask about the status of his patients and to request guidance, but no answers were forthcoming. Pressing officials in person during trips to Tucupita was fruitless. When Dr. Ricardo could not diagnose the disease and his treatments did not help, when children returned from urban hospitals in coffins, the parents and residents of Mukoboina and beyond wanted answers; the tone in which they questioned Dr. Ricardo grew increasingly worried, then insistent, then, eventually, angry. Dr. Ricardo was caught between unresponsive specialists and health authorities and the imperative to render effective treatment and answer the parents' questions. When parents catalyzed Conrado and others to organize a trip to Tucupita to demand action, he assisted them, attending the meeting they organized and writing yet another letter to his superiors. These efforts earned him a rebuke on the part of RHS officials, who were working to keep the mysterious disease quiet even as he was trying to draw attention to it.

Dr. Ricardo had been very well received as a physician in Nabasanuka—he was acknowledged to be hard working and conscientious, with good medical judgment, good working relations with nurses, and a respectful attitude toward patients and their relatives and neighbors. Being unable to diagnose or treat one patient after another began to undermine his developing sense of competence as a physician. When the only way he could respond to the growing chorus of questions was to repeat ad nauseam that he was still waiting for word from Tucupita, Dr. Ricardo felt that people were losing faith in him. The autopsies proved to be the tipping point. When Conrado and Enrique confronted him with the Mukoboinan parents' demand for answers, he sensed their anger and defended his profession by saying that the autopsies were performed in order to aid diagnosis. Dr. Ricardo repeatedly requested but never received the results. Time passed. The answers never came. Trust in him and his medicine suffered.

We should have a team here . . . so that we could reach a conclusion as to
what it is!—Leoncio D'Ambrosio

In May 2008, Dr. Ricardo was joined by four medical students in their final
year in the School of Medicine of the Central University of Venezuela. They
were full of enthusiasm, already highly professional and committed to their
patients. When only one physician is in residence, it is hard to leave the clinic;
having the medical students on board made it easier to follow up with patients
in their homes, survey health conditions, give health education talks, and address prevention issues. Two students were at the residence when we first met
with Dr. Ricardo, and they participated actively in the conversation; the other
two were on duty in the clinic.

Medical students Leoncio D'Ambrosio and Roselia Narváez did not mince
words, even as they spoke in front of their supervisor.[5] Dr. Roselia is a slender
woman in her twenties with black hair, large black eyes, and an expressive face.
Even at this early stage of her career, she exuded a sense of confidence and
authority, an assurance that permitted her to speak critically yet professionally
about what she saw as shortcomings in RHS and how it treated rural physicians,
pointing as well to structural factors that undermined the health of people in
the lower delta. Dr. Leoncio cuts a tall, athletic figure with dark brown hair and
a slightly roundish face. More cautious in how he positioned himself within
medical hierarchies and given to a more analytic bent, he nonetheless joined
Dr. Roselia in criticizing how RHS had handled the epidemic, and he went
on to question RHS's acceptance of "normal" health conditions, including
the persistently high infant morality rate. Both were strongly supportive of
Dr. Ricardo, sympathetic to the problems he had faced, and distressed with the
way his superiors had responded to his work on the epidemic. Having arrived
in May 2008 for the most extended clinical practice of their training, and just
months away from graduation, they treated numerous patients during the third
wave of cases of the strange disease.

Dr. Roselia reported that she examined Mamerto several times. "The first
time he was walking by himself. He had a fever; that was the symptom he
presented." Nabasanuka nurses treated him as an ambulatory patient and prescribed an analgesic and an antipyretic. Mamerto returned two days later and
was reexamined. Dr. Roselia remembered, "Against medical advice, he left with
his family. . . . They took him to a wisidatu. The next day he was back and in
generally bad condition. His relative said that the wisidatu took out a spirit that
was supposedly affecting him." Returning with acute urinary retention and in

great pain, Mamerto told Dr. Roselia about the strange headache, itching, and numbness. She continued, "They brought him to the clinic again because he 'couldn't go pee'—those were the colloquial words of his relative." Dr. Roselia and the nurses hooked up a catheter. Because he fitted a different demographic than the children—although similar to a patient from Siawani—Dr. Roselia relegated the case to a more familiar diagnostic category: she suspected a sexually transmitted infection and prescribed antibiotics. She noted neurological abnormalities—paralysis, excessive salivation, and seizures—but they didn't fit. They sent him to Muaina with an antibiotic and instructions for nurse Mirna Pizarro to inject it every six hours.

The interns were clearly moved by their experience in the epidemic. As Dr. Roselia put it, "We have felt the worry of the mother who knows that her child is going to die." She filled in Dr. Ricardo's blanks: "I believe that [RHS] should have taken this situation more seriously; it should have attacked it in depth in order to end these deaths." Her frustration was evident in keen observations regarding how problems persist in the delta, where doctors come and go: "This is alarming, because we are leaving. . . . Each of us is going home, and the problem remains hidden here." Dr. Leoncio jumped in at this point, arguing that cases of the strange disease had been undercounted: "We haven't treated many cases precisely because people don't dare to bring the patients to our clinic anymore, because they know that they will just die. We can see that they know. The symptoms are so similar that the Warao can see that a patient has the same thing that the other one had and that he will die." Dr. Leoncio discerned how the situation was undermining health care as parents refused to bring their children for any disease. For him, the proper response was clear: "This is an epidemic." Accordingly, he asserted, "We should have a team here," including epidemiologists, pathologists, and lab technicians, "working with residents, so that we could reach a conclusion as to what it is!"

Probably reflecting both their self-confidence as students of the preeminent medical school in Venezuela and their lost faith in RHS, they hoped to recruit their professor at the Central University of Venezuela to take charge. The hierarchical structure of public health institutions dictates that medical students should report to the local physician who then reports to RHS officials; going over all of their heads to Caracas would have constituted a serious breach. We were moved by their spirit and conviction and imagined they were destined to become excellent physicians. We were also aware that they had a great deal less on the line than Dr. Ricardo. We continued to exchange observations and words of encouragement with Dr. Ricardo and the four interns until they left the lower delta on 4 August 2008.

The Delta's Bilingual Nurses

NURSE JOSÉ PÉREZ: SIAWANI

Patients come here with a fever all the time . . . and usually they recover
in a couple of days. But with this fever, I use medicines and it's just the same,
just the same—it even gets worse!

—José Pérez

Dr. Ricardo was not the first biomedical health professional to encounter the strange disease. Mukoboina lies near Siawani and falls within the jurisdiction of its nurse, José Pérez.[6] The space in which José sees patients does not resemble the octagonal structures that became the trademark of socialist medicine in urban centers; despite repeated requests, he does not even have a simple wooden nursing station but sees patients in the palm-thatched house he shares with his wife and two young children (figure 2.2). Although he has a desk and chair, his examining table and observation area consist of a hammock strung close to the living area where his children sleep. A thin man with short, unruly dark hair and a shadow of moustache, José has a calm voice that inspires confidence (figure 2.3). His experience speaks eloquently to how nurses in the lower delta endeavor to serve their profession and their neighbors—and how the health bureaucracy appears to do its best to thwart their success, if not to drive them away from nursing altogether.

José graduated from high school in the Capuchin boarding school in Arawaimuhu, subsequently studying simplified medicine in Tucupita. "I received both theoretical and practical training; I learned a lot." Returning home to Siawani in 1997 to practice, he was determined to succeed where five predecessors had failed. He reflected modestly, "I am just a nurse. I received training so that I could help my Warao brothers and sisters. I am not a doctor, but I have gained some knowledge." He showed us the manual he uses to refresh his memory if and when an unfamiliar set of symptoms emerges. After eleven years in a house without walls, insects had nibbled many pages.

José needs to be on hand as much as possible to receive patients and, if necessary, transport them to Nabasanuka, but the only way to stock his medicine cabinet and collect his salary is by traveling to Tucupita. Until he was granted use of a small motorboat in 2007, he had to pay for a ride to town. Once there, José reported, he meticulously provided RHS with a list of patients, including date of service, diagnosis, and treatment, along with information on pregnancies and births. Reporting to the Nursing Division, he waits for an order for medicines; he is sometimes delayed another day if the proper officials are not in their offices. Particularly because provisioning the lower delta is a lower priority for

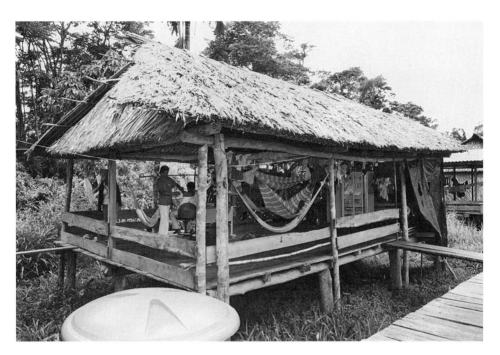

FIGURE 2.2. Home of Siawani's nurse, 2008. Photograph by Charles L. Briggs.

warehouse workers, he often has to wait until the next day or—when supplies are low—several days. Meanwhile, José has to use his own meager salary to eat. He can either pay for a hotel room, find a friend or relative who will let him set up his hammock in their home, or sleep in a boat in the port. He has to leave his patients and family for at least three days a month, but the trip often takes a week. Then he must pay the cost of transporting the medicines. By the time he returns home, a good portion of his salary has disappeared. Under such circumstances, many nurses burn out, deciding that fishing and keeping a garden is an easier way to make a living, or they stay on the payroll but devote most of their time to other pursuits. By 2008, José had served Siawani for eleven years.

Keeping a stock of medicines on hand, being available to receive patients, traveling to the surrounding localities for prevention-oriented work and to see patients, and transporting more serious patients to Nabasanuka is challenging. But in July 2007, José's work became much more complicated. "The first case I saw was a child from Mukoboina," he recalled. This was Yuri, daughter of Wilmer and Zoila Torres. "She arrived in the afternoon. I could see right away that she had a high, a very high fever." The parents told José, "Last night the wisidatu treated her; he worked all night long, but she was just the same at

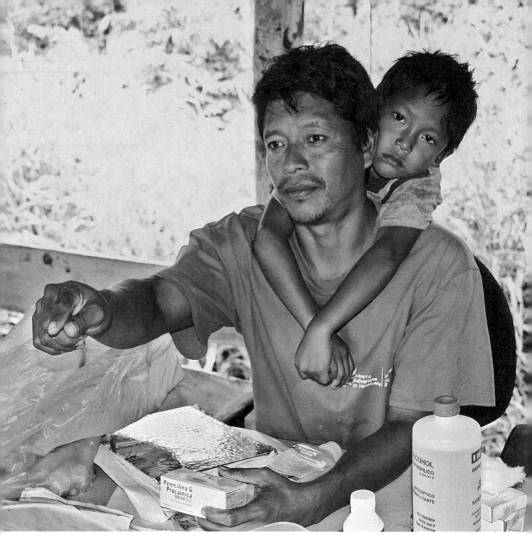

FIGURE 2.3. Nurse José Pérez with his son, 2008. Photograph by Charles L. Briggs.

dawn." José continued, "I gave her acetaminophen to bring down the fever." He was running low on medicines, but he had a supply of acetaminophen. "But the fever wouldn't come down. It just wouldn't come down. And foam was coming from her mouth. The child was in critical condition." After treating her for less than an hour, he told Wilmer and Zoila that they should take her to Nabasa-nuka, providing a note for Dr. Ricardo.

Two weeks later, another Mukoboina child, this one an eleven-year-old boy, arrived in José's home; this was Ángel Gabriel Florín. José had not received any word back about Yuri, so he had no better idea about how to treat Ángel Gabriel. The fever was similarly high. He administered an analgesic and an antipyretic, but the fever did not come down. "I thought, darn, what could it be? Patients come here with a fever all the time. I bring it down with an analgesic, antipyretic, or some other medication, and usually they recover in a couple of days. But with this fever, I use medicines and it's just the same, just the same—it even gets worse!" This time he decided to transport the child to Nabasanuka himself. He wanted to see how Dr. Ricardo and the nursing staff would treat Ángel Gabriel and if Dr. Ricardo could provide him with advice for treating patients with these symptoms. "Unfortunately," José reported, "the only words he said to me were, 'When you get this kind of case, bring the patient to me immediately. We don't know what disease it is either.'"

The epidemic began to create problems for José's practice. His neighbors "thought that they were going to get infected," he explained. "They said that they had never seen a disease like that. 'We have children, we have grandchildren: isn't it possible that they will come down with it too?'" He went to Mukoboina and spoke with Inocencio, asking him to send word but not patients if more cases appeared; José would then go to Mukoboina and transport the child to Nabasanuka. He tried to reason with his neighbors, to say that diseases don't spread in this fashion, but "they were afraid."

NURSE MIRNA PIZARRO: MUAINA

I began to think that it wasn't a disease, but that it was something else, some kind of bad medicine.—Mirna Pizarro

In some ways, the work of thirty-one-year-old Mirna Pizarro in Muaina was similar (figure 2.4). She also was born in the settlement she serves and is its only nurse. She likewise trained for a year in simplified medicine, half in Tucupita and half in Nabasanuka; she had nine years' experience. Librado Moraleda convinced the government to build a nice structure and furnished it with a desk, filing cabinet, pediatric and adult scales, and a tank and water filtration system. After his death, the building fell into disrepair; like José, Mirna now sees patients in her home.

A large difference emerges, however, in the populations they serve. José's jurisdiction includes six settlements; he must navigate carefully among alliances and fissures. Muaina, on the other hand, is populated by the Pizarro family. When Mirna gives prevention-oriented talks or apologizes for a shortage of medicine, she noted, "I speak with my family," meaning Muainans as a whole, "and they say, 'thanks.'" Although they both faced patients with strange symptoms, José was confronted with the first cases and Mirna with the last. She had heard about the strange disease for a year, but for her the epidemic began when her cousin Eduardo said, "My son has a fever." She did what she was taught

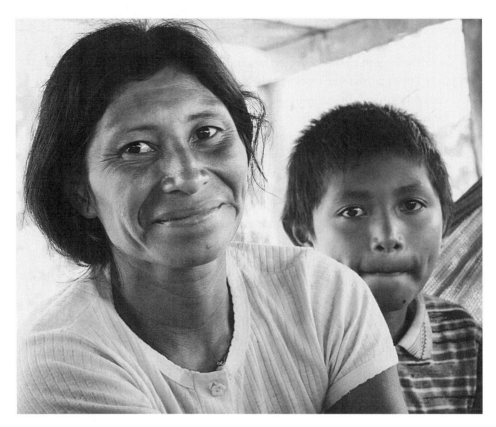

FIGURE 2.4. Muaina nurse Mirna Pizarro with her son Roberto, 2010. Photograph by Charles L. Briggs.

to do for fevers, giving Eduardito acetaminophen. Two days later, "he was just the same, with fever and diarrhea; his father told me, 'He's in really bad shape.'" Mirna injected him with a more powerful analgesic and antipyretic, "but the fever never diminished." She then injected him with a nonsteroidal anti-inflammatory used for pain or fever. In short, Mirna used everything in the toolkit she learned in Nabasanuka and Tucupita. She considered other ways of explaining the cases and the failure of her medicines: "I began to think that it wasn't a disease, but that it was something else, some kind of bad medicine."

Then Florencia Macotera found Mirna at Eduardito's wake and told her that Dalvi had a fever. The nurse gave Florencia a bottle of liquid acetaminophen, administering a spoonful. Mirna came to see Dalvi shortly after dawn. She took his temperature; it was just below 40°C (approximately 103.5° F). Her medicine complemented Florencia's herbal treatments. Mirna then injected him with an antipyretic, just as she had tried with Eduardito; these treatments only lowered his fever briefly. Mirna lost another young patient.

Dalvi's older brother Mamerto went to visit Mirna shortly after returning from the graveyard to bury Eduardito, complaining of a headache. Suggesting, "It must be that you spent the day in the cemetery burying your brother," she gave him some acetaminophen tablets and sent him home. He felt worse the next day and returned. Mirna gave him more acetaminophen; he took four of them. Two days later he appeared at Myrna's clinic-kitchen and complained of a different problem—on top of headache, fever, intense itching, and acute numbness, he could barely urinate, and he was beginning to suffer from the acute pain associated with urinary retention. This had, in fact, been going on for several days. Macotera showed up later, noting that her son had acute abdominal pain. "Why don't you take him to Nabasanuka, so that the doctors can see him?" Mirna suggested. Although she injected Mamerto with the penicillin the clinic provided, she wondered about the strange symptoms. "I didn't know. They didn't give me any information about that." Afterward, "he didn't recover—he got worse. I told his parents that he must be taken to Tucupita. And that time I went with him to Nabasanuka." She told the doctors, "This boy can't stay here. You need to send him to Tucupita."

Muaina residents did not blame Mirna for failing to save Eduardito, Dalvi, or Mamerto, nor did anyone worry that treating them was endangering their children. Mirna, however, lost not only three patients but three relatives.

THE NURSES AT THE NABASANUKA CLINIC

Dear God, may this child reach Tucupita. May she be saved. May they use a special medication that will stop this disease.—Alonzo Moraleda

In Nabasanuka, working conditions for nurses couldn't have been more unlike those for nurses José and Mirna. When their shift approached, they donned white jackets and walked to a cement-walled structure with its own electrical generator. Except when the doctor was away in town or a new one had not been appointed, they worked under the direction of a physician, who generally took charge of diagnosis and treatment plans. Rather than a precarious enterprise built on the perseverance of a single individual, Nabasanuka enjoyed a dynasty of nurses starting with Florencia González de Rodríguez, who began working with Dr. Herbig in 1975 and has since retired. Her son, Alonzo Moraleda, now in his late forties, already had over a quarter century of experience in 2007 (figure 2.5). The other nurses are his cousins. Jesús Moraleda, forty-seven, Conrado and Enrique's

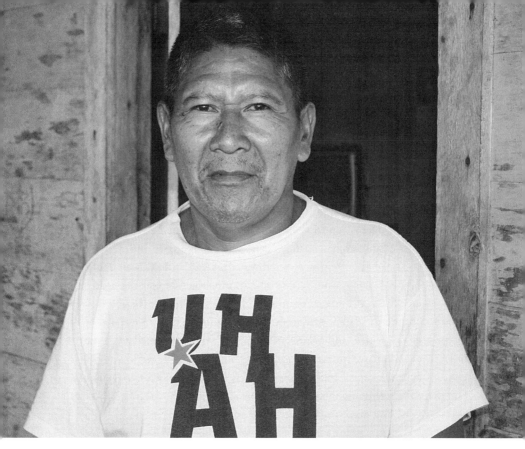

FIGURE 2.5. Alonzo Moraleda, 2010. Photograph by Charles L. Briggs.

younger brother, had worked twenty-two years as a nurse (figure 2.6). Aureliano Moraleda, Conrado's son, was in his late thirties. Alonzo and Jesús live across the river, where houses generally resemble other palm-thatched structures in the delta, but they built houses with floors and walls of milled lumber and tin roofs fitted with gutters to collect rainwater for drinking. Alonzo's is unique in that it is graced in front with a neatly painted wooden fence. Aureliano and his family live with his parents in a house next to the clinic. Nabasanuka's women nurses were all on leave in 2007–2008, and it was Alonzo, Jesús, and Aureliano who faced the strange epidemic alongside Dr. Ricardo.

Unlike the physician, the nurses were not caught entirely by surprise by the first case. Dr. Ricardo may have enjoyed more access to the two-way radio, but the nurses were deeply attuned to Warao Radio. Word of a strange death in Mukoboina, a boy with unusual symptoms that did not respond to intervention by healers, had already reached them. When the boy's little sister Yuri developed the same symptoms, word got to the clinic before she did. Describing

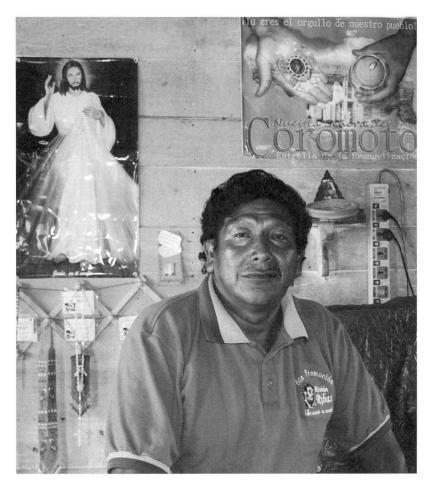

FIGURE 2.6. Jesús Moraleda, 2010. Photograph by Charles L. Briggs.

Yuri Torres's arrival in July 2007, Alonzo recalled how the staff reacted: "When the first patient was admitted, we thought it was a simple virus because there was a cold that was making its way around nearly all the communities. Well, it really surprised us! It was different—the patient presented with fever and cold [symptoms], but accompanied by tremors . . . with a very high fever. She was almost unconscious. You couldn't wake her and you couldn't touch her, because it was as if you were giving her an electric shock—thank God the doctor was around!"

The nurses ran an IV and started antipyretics to reduce the fever. Yuri wasn't breathing well, so Dr. Ricardo told them to give her an antibiotic, thinking that she might be developing pneumonia. But as one day turned into two, "the patient didn't show any improvement, and the fever didn't go down," Aureliano remembered. "At the time, we didn't know anything, we didn't think more patients would arrive." But arrive they did, and "the children cried, and how—all night long, they cried all the time. They tossed and turned; those children really suffered." The nurses labored intently, monitoring vital signs and administering medications. They tried dipyrone. When that didn't work, "We used wet towels to bring down the fever, but it was fruitless." Perhaps reflecting their own position within medical hierarchies, none of the nurses reported speculating on the nature of the pathology after their initial hunch proved incorrect. The nurses recalled sharing the doctor's sense of frustration and anxiety, feelings that did not dissipate when Yuri was sent upriver to Tucupita. Alonzo remembered his appeal to another order of healing: "Dear God, may this child reach Tucupita. May she be saved. May they use a special medication that will stop this disease." He concluded, "I felt just awful."

Treating one dying child after another took its emotional toll. Aureliano, for example, remembered one child who was rushed to Tucupita before he could administer the bottles of iv solution he had just prepared. After hearing of the child's death, he just kept looking at those unused bottles. The sense of frustration grew as the cases mounted and no advances in diagnosis or treatment were forthcoming. Parents knew the score, and the nurses listened as they lamented their children's impending deaths. Alonzo recalled, "My God, tears came to my eyes as well," when parents moaned, "My child is going to die."

The nurses had great faith in Dr. Ricardo. Jesús described him as having been "very active, very anxious to help, to make a difference" when he first arrived at the clinic. He gave talks about disease prevention, about treating water to prevent diarrhea. In these meetings, Dr. Ricardo told residents, "I'm going to help you with any kind of health problem that emerges; we'll do anything that's needed." This spirit is what prompted his initial efforts to solve the mystery, constantly pushing his superiors for results on the patients he sent upriver. One nurse recalled the rebuke that these efforts earned Dr. Ricardo from RHS's director: "'Look,' he said with an aggressive tone, 'so are you a better doctor than we are? Are you superior to us? Have you learned more than we have? You have to erase these cases,' meaning to forget them, the director told the doctor." After that, in the nurses' estimation, Dr. Ricardo didn't appear to care, was just waiting for his year of service to be up so he could leave Nabasanuka. He spoke little with the nurses and grew short tempered and sometimes irritable with the relatives who brought children with the strange symptoms to the clinic. The anger he sometimes expressed when parents withdrew hospitalized patients to seek treatment from healers began to rub nurses the wrong way. They, on the other hand, invited parents to combine different forms of treatment. According to Alonzo, "We never forbid that. When they said, 'No, the wisidatu said that he had to treat him,' I told them, 'Fine, take him or bring the wisidatu—that's not prohibited here—he can use his rattle right here.' Even I believe in that."

Aureliano said his initial impression was, "A disease has come from elsewhere, is appearing here, and will possibly finish off the Warao—we are going to die out rapidly." Having no idea what it was, they had no way to tell if they themselves might be at risk. Threading a needle into the tiny vein of a child who is crying hysterically and thrashing about is difficult, Aureliano said. "Several times I got covered in blood. I washed it off very quickly." After more and more encounters with these patients, the nurses feared that they might be endangering their families. Aureliano always left his white coat behind at the clinic, and upon arriving home, immediately undressed, asking his wife to use strong chlorine solution on his T-shirt and pants.

As anxiety increased in the lower delta, it began to encircle the nurses. When the number of dead in Mukoboina reached 10 percent, the nurses' neighbors, relatives, and other residents asked if the deaths would soon haunt Nabasanuka families, but official silence left the medical team without any means of responding. The nurses never blamed Dr. Ricardo; their rage was silently directed at officials in Tucupita. With tears of anger and sadness in his eyes, Alonzo told us he remembered thinking, "Could it be that it doesn't matter to them, it doesn't hurt them to see an indigenous child die like that?" Thinking not about Dr. Ricardo but physicians in the city, Alonzo said doubts emerged: "Could it be that the doctors aren't trying to treat them, not using the best medicines? Since I wasn't in Tucupita, I didn't know what they were doing with the patients that we sent them."

The nurses' anger turned into bitterness when word came from Tucupita that the only treatment to be used for these patients was acetaminophen, which had already proved to be useless. Jesús' reported, "In Tucupita they said we shouldn't give them anything, because they are still studying [the cases]." The nurses watched their patients burn up with fever, witnessed their excruciating pain without being allowed to provide even palliative care. This led the parents—some of whom were relatives—to think that the nurses, too, were indifferent. It was the last patient, Mamerto, who hit the staff the hardest. It was particularly hard for Jesús, with whom his nephew Mamerto had lived while studying in Nabasanuka. Mamerto's talk of his dreams of fighting discrimination had made his uncle proud. Since Elbia was from nearby Barranquita and had studied in Nabasanuka too, Jesús also knew her well. The nurses gave Mamerto more space than just the opportunity to respond to clinical questions. He talked to them about the symptoms he had observed in his little brother, Dalvi, perceptively reporting, "My legs itch, just the same."

When Caregivers Fail   93

Mamerto's final visit began at 8:00 AM. Alonzo remembered, "He had a fever, a sore throat. He couldn't swallow; he was having trouble breathing and was dizzy at times. 'I have a really bad headache, and I pass out sometimes. My whole body hurts, and it really hurts when someone touches me.'" Mamerto told Jesús that he couldn't feel his legs. The nurses spoke with Mirna, getting her account of the course of Mamerto's disease. It broke their hearts to see Mamerto suffering so terribly and be forbidden to provide him with palliative care. Jesús said, "I felt bad, really bad." By evening, Mamerto didn't recognize anyone and shifted between periods of semiconsciousness and writhing in pain. Care and power were in conflict. They knew they couldn't cure him, but they could not let Mamerto suffer. Drawing on their emotional resources and determination, breaking the rules, they eased Mamerto's pain.

From the time that the first child arrived, the nurses were frustrated that they could not contribute more to finding a diagnosis. When they first heard stories about a strange disease in Mukoboina and learned that a patient was on her way, they didn't tell the doctor: "What could we have said?" How could they translate the Warao advance warning system into biomedical knowledge that would register with a physician? In the clinic, they similarly heard the words of parents sitting beside their children or in the blue plastic seats outside, statements not elicited by doctors or incorporated into one-page summaries of the cases sent with patients to Tucupita. When epidemiologists came to investigate, Nabasanuka's bilingual nurses were overlooked. Jesús reported with obvious frustration, "They didn't even come here. They didn't ask us. We, the ones who are here, the nursing staff, we would have told them what was happening, we who have been seeing and living with the problem. They never asked us anything." Nurses from Tucupita who didn't speak Warao were sent to Mukoboina, and they didn't think to ask their colleagues for information. By the same token, however, Nabasanuka's nurses never even mentioned nurses José or Mirna, their peers who worked in lower-status facilities.

Warao Doctors: Searching for Answers beyond the Visible

We wisidatu think that this disease is too dangerous.... When there is hebu sickness, we extract it, and patients recover. But when we treat these patients, nothing happens.—Inocencio Torres

We have, thus far, presumed that readers know in general what doctors and nurses do, only adding qualifiers such as pointing out that physicians in Venezuela work as *médicos rurales* for a year between their graduation and their residencies and that nurses in Siawani, Muaina, Nabasanuka, and other parts of the lower delta are not technically nurses, if the term is assumed to refer to people who hold degrees from schools of nursing. We cannot, however, take for granted that readers are familiar with the knowledge practices of the heterogeneous class of people we refer to as healers. And lumping them under the aegis of alternative and complementary medicine would be a disservice to all.

There are about as many different types of healers in the delta as there are biomedical specialists. Much like their physician colleagues, some rank higher than others, depending on the stature of the person who trained them and the extent of their experience.[7] Most use the ritual inhalation of smoke from palm-leaf cigars filled with strong tobacco to activate their healing power and contact pathogenic spirits. The most visible specialists are wisidatu.[8] They are like general practitioners, often the first to be consulted and referring cases they cannot treat to other specialists, but wisidatu are rather like priests, holding ceremonies like the annual *nahanamu* or in response to a shared threat in order to ensure collective well-being. In addition to using therapeutic touch, breath, and singing, like other practitioners, they extensively employ large rattles. Another type of specialist is the *bahanarotu*, who can extract *bahana*, often embodied as material objects, from patients' bodies. Tirso is a highly skilled bahanarotu. A third common type is the hoarotu, who can diagnose and treat hoa. Hoarotu have extensive repertoires of songs that are based on myths. Charles became a hoarotu several decades ago while living in the Mariusa area; two friends who were among the most renowned (and feared) practitioners in the delta thought that he had potential and decided to teach him.[9]

These are the classes of practitioners that are familiar to most laypersons, so they were the ones sought out by parents during the strange epidemic. Note, however, that no one mentioned looking for a yarokotarotu, though Odilia tried herbs because her mother is a practitioner, and Florencia used them with Dalvi because she is herself skilled.[10] Generally only men can become wisidatu, bahanarotu, and hoarotu, although a few postmenopausal women are trained.[11] There are accordingly gender issues involved in devaluing the yarokotarotu's work. Among the many other types of specialists are those who have learned from people classified as criollo healers, especially those trained in *oración* (the Spanish word for prayer), or varieties associated with the "black people" from neighboring Guyana and Trinidad.[12] When pathogens cross what are perceived as ethnoracial borders, they are often deemed to be particularly difficult to cure. The most powerful practitioners often know several of these specialties. Some parents sought out as wide a variety of healers as they could get access to, while some stuck to a more limited field.

I thought, "we just can't do anything [with these patients], our techniques don't
work at all with this disease."—Inocencio Torres

The first stop in the parents' search for help in the ground zero of Mukoboina
was their neighbor, relative, local leader, and healer, all wrapped up into Inocencio Torres (figure 2.7). As wisidatu go, Inocencio is low ranking, a local go-to
for an initial diagnosis and treatment, often preceding a trip to a more distant,
skilled, and expensive healer. Zoila and Wilmer Torres brought Gabriel to their
Uncle Inocencio's house as soon as they arrived from Tucupita. They gave him
a full account of the symptoms, and Inocencio placed the boy in his hammock.
As darkness fell, the wisidatu wrapped his head in a bandana, took out his sacred rattle, and smoked a small palm-leaf cigar, activating his spirit helpers and
opening a channel to reach any hebu in Gabriel's body.

Inocencio didn't have much to go on: the only reported symptom was a fever;
no cough, congestion, or phlegm. Zoila could not recall any recent mishap. Inocencio used therapeutic touch on Gabriel's head, moving down to his chest and
abdomen, but could feel nothing. Then, singing a song that named hebu spirits,
he recruited the power of the *kareko* spirits, embodied in tiny stones that make
dimly visible sparks when moved in a circular fashion inside the rattle. Hoping
that they would reveal their names by speaking through his own larynx, Inocencio sang in the healers' sacred language, but his hands could not make out the
large soft mass of a hebu; no hebu seized his vocal cords to intone a response; the
rattle was not drawn, as if by sacred magnetism, to any afflicted spot. Nor could
he find any smaller and harder lumps associated with hoa or bahana—those he
could not extract, but finding them would help him make a referral. "*Ekida*—
nothing," he said, increasing the parents' fear and Gabriel's as well.

When this pattern was repeated over and over in the coming weeks, Inocencio began to think that a past conflict might be behind it all. He remembered
when Simón Ortega came to live in Mukoboina. Hailing from a larger, more
"modern" settlement upriver, Ortega used his political clout to secure a Fogón
Comunitario (Community Hearth) for Mukoboina—and the position of its
coordinator for himself. The Fogón Comunitario program forms part of the
Chávez government's efforts to combat malnutrition, particularly among children and pregnant women. Ortega showed up in Mukoboina with a boat full
of food that he had been given by the government. People were surprised—
someone from another area had, without their consent, obtained the only government service (and salaried employment) that was provided to Mukoboina.
But people watched and waited.

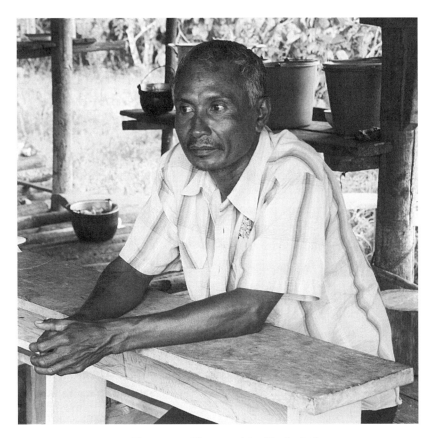

FIGURE 2.7. Inocencio Torres, 2010. Photograph by Charles L. Briggs.

The situation turned sour when, according to residents, Ortega refused to share the food. Residents complained. A complaint brought supervisors to Mukoboina and resulted in the selection of a new coordinator, Roberto Torres, Inocenio's brother. Ortega reportedly attacked his rival, verbally and physically. Mukoboinans held a meeting in which they asked Ortega to leave. Trained in various healing modalities, he can turn puffs of tobacco smoke into projectiles and send them into a victim's body. Returning one night to Mukoboina, Ortega rose near midnight, stood on the edge of the house next to Roberto's, and blew tobacco smoke in his direction. Inocencio asked, "What's going on?" Ortega replied, "Your younger brother is truly a dead man." Roberto died two days later; although the apparent cause was a heart attack, everyone knew that Ortega had killed him. Enraged, they told Ortega and his family to leave Mukoboina for good. Subsequently, word came from Volcán Port, where Ortega was living, that he promised revenge against all Mukoboinans: "Those people will all die. They will be finished off." If he had performed the bad medicine himself, healers would have been able to stop it, but Ortega reportedly paid a *curioso*, a nonindigenous practitioner, to kill Mukoboina's children.

Starting with Gabriel, Inocenio kept abreast of the experiences of other healers, both through Warao Radio and when he ran into them during trips out of Mukoboina. "I thought, 'We just can't do anything [with these patients]. Our techniques don't work at all with this disease.'" After treating Yuri unsuccessfully, he told fellow Mukoboinans, "We wisidatu think that this disease is too dangerous. When we examine them, we can't do anything. When there is hebu sickness, we extract it, and patients recover. But when we treat these patients, nothing happens. The doctors have medicines. We should take the patients to them. From now on, we have to take these patients to the hospital." When more children got sick, parents "took them to the clinic; they examined them; they gave them medicines, but things came out the same. That's when they took them far away," meaning to Tucupita, Maturín, and Puerto Ordaz. When city doctors failed as well, a collective, Mukoboinan voice emerged: "We all kept thinking, 'What's going to happen? Where did this disease come from? We want to know.' We thought, when [we took the children] to the doctors, we asked the nurses, 'What disease is killing the children? We want to know.' But they replied, 'We don't know.' We *still*," Inocencio emphasized, "want to know."

FRANCISCO PÉREZ

I never ever thought about inflicting this disease. Why would I?—Francisco Pérez

Inocencio struggled with the strange disease and lost, but people didn't blame it on him. Francisco Pérez of Heukukabanoko had a rougher time.[13] He lives on the other side of Muaina, even nearer to the coast. Widely renowned in the area as a hoarotu, he is also skilled in several other types of healing; now in his midfifties, he has been practicing for nearly three decades. As a result, Santa Rosa de Guayo parents sought his assistance in June 2008. The settlement is located not far from San Francisco de Guayo, which is nearly twice the size of Nabasanuka and has a larger clinic (see map I.1). Because they are located in a different parish (a political division), Padre Barral, residents had heard little about the strange epidemic. They took their children to the San Francisco de Guayo clinic promptly, but, according to their accounts, the medical staff did not realize that something strange was going on, and the children were soon sent home with bottles of medications. Although the parents could have called healers from San Francisco de Guayo, several of whom have considerable reputations, they traveled to Heukukabanoko to find Mr. Francisco. He saw some of the patients in his own home, but he also made repeated trips to Santa Rosa. Four children died in Santa Rosa in June and four in July. When the diagnostic techniques associated with one specialty failed, Mr. Francisco tried another. At times, the patients appeared to be getting better, their fevers and strange symptoms diminishing; Mr. Francisco thought he was on the right track. And then they died. Proud of his ability as a healer, Mr. Francisco can brag, but Santa Rosa troubled him—he felt like it was his greatest failure. He didn't even come up with a hypothesis to explain it. He just admitted that nothing he tried worked.

What happened to him in neighboring Muaina might be a case of no good deed going unpunished. During the meeting held in Muaina during Mamerto's wake, which took place less than two weeks after Mr. Francisco lost his last patient in Santa Rosa, several witnesses accused him of killing Eduardito, Dalvi, and Mamerto. It all began, they claimed, when Muaina resident Catalina Pizarro recruited Mr. Francisco's children for Muaina's school. Three months before the epidemic began, when Eduardo Pizzaro was bringing the children to school one morning, he did not hear his brother's boat approaching and they collided. All three of Mr. Francisco's children were injured, two seriously. Residents immediately took the children to Nabasanuka; the physician there sent them to Tucupita. When Mr. Francisco came looking for them in Muaina, he became irate, not just about the accident but for not respecting his right as a parent and healer to plan their treatment. Then came the angry words: "If all of my kids recover, nothing will happen. But if any die, all Muainans will die as well! Today we are crying, but soon you will cry too." Witnesses claimed that shortly afterward Mr. Francisco sent bad medicine toward Muaina "all day long, until it grew dark." A crucial detail, in the eyes of Muainans, emerged in Florencia Macotera's account of Dalvi's death: "'Dad, I'm dying. The evil healer Francisco is killing me. When I die, kill Francisco, because he's killing me.'"

A delegation of the elders assembled at the meeting decided to ask Mr. Francisco to participate in a monikata nome nakakitane dispute mediation process. Accepting this invitation was an act of courage, given the Muainans' anger. After hearing the accusations firsthand, Mr. Francisco tore apart their logic. He was, he noted, opposed to busing his kids to school in the first place. Sharing a common perception in the region that Muaina residents got all the government benefits—jobs as teachers, school boat operators, and cooks, and new houses— he complained that his children were given nothing to eat, even though Muaina receives funding for school lunches. On top of that, the government contractors hired to build new houses for Muainans—which they never finished—

tore down the school and never built a new one, leaving the children sitting on the floor in a cramped space. Turning the accusations on their heads, Mr. Francisco reported having lodged a complaint against the school boat operators with the Guayo police. The climax came when Mr. Francisco admitted that he had spoken about killing Muainans, but these were words of anger spoken after the incident. Raising hairs on the back of Muainan necks, he boldly asserted, "I have learned the words of my ancestors," referring to the source of his healing power. After enumerating the types of bad medicine he could have sent, he added, "I never thought about inflicting this disease. Why would I? My children did not die." Mr. Francisco then stepped into the shoes of an epidemiologist. If the source of the disease was bad medicine that he directed against Muainans, why, he asked, did the children he treated in Santa Rosa die? Anger and fear receded almost magically as twilight brought the meeting to a close.

AVELINO CAMPERO

My treatment is effective, and that's why patients come to me. But sometimes doctors can't cure patients either.—Avelino Campero

Elbia Torres Rivas refused to visit the Nabasanuka clinic, but she was open to other healing modalities. Her parents, Anita and Arsenio, sent for Avelino Campero, a healer who is just as renowned and versatile as Mr. Francisco. He was living in Bamutanoko, another coastal island, not far from Heukukabanoko. Mr. Avelino is a short, muscular man in his late forties (figure 2.8). His fairly nondescript appearance and generally low-key manner do not immediately give away that he has received extensive training in nearly all the indigenous and nonindigenous healing varieties found in the delta.

The trip to Bamutanoko through turbulent coastal waters in a small canoe was rough on Elbia. Upon arrival, her parents helped her trudge through some thirty meters of mud and aquatic plants, nearly carrying her to the beach. Mr. Avelino motioned them to the far side of the house. There he took out his sacred rattle as darkness fell. "Smoke was coming out of her body," he noted, referring to an effect of bad medicine invisible to untrained eyes. He worked nearly all night, smoking cigars, singing song after song, massaging her feet, legs, and head, and supercharging the rattle and then pressing it against her afflicted areas. Some six hours of treatment enabled him to remove several pathogens and decrease the pain and fever.

Elbia and her parents returned home in the blackness of night after Mr. Avelino finished in order to avoid the clouds of mosquitoes that are part of life on the island. The next morning when we visited Elbia, we were astounded

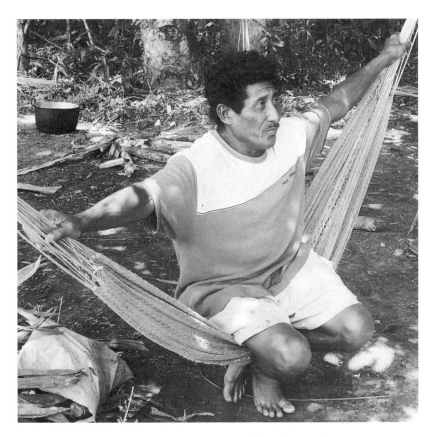

FIGURE 2.8. Avelino Campero, 2009. Photograph by Kalim Smith.

to see her contentedly chewing on sugarcane and even taking a few sips of water. Her look of fear, pain, and anguish had been replaced by a broad smile. She still reported a headache; her temperature, 38.5°C, was still elevated, but lower. Dishearteningly, when we returned that evening her symptoms had all returned. She was in great pain, discouraged, somewhere between terrified and despondent.

Mr. Avelino told us that the problem was that "on top" of the Warao pathogens he removed, she had been afflicted with a virulent type of oración, viewed by Warao practitioners as the quintessential form of criollo bad medicine. Since he had studied oración on the mainland, he would in theory be able to cure her, but this oración was *vela* or "candle." It works rather like trick candles on a birthday cake—you blow them out, but they come right back. "A candle is placed inside the body, and that's why the body burns up and the person dies. . . . The other healer keeps working so that the candles [i.e., the disease] return."

Who was responsible for this incurable pathogen? His explanation pointed to the contractors who were working in Muaina in 2008 when the three deaths occurred and Elbia's symptoms began. Elbia was collateral damage, he told us, in a conflict between the contractors and Muaina residents, who wanted fair wages, sturdy houses built according to their needs and environment, and the school, nursing station, and community center specified in the contract. In the end, Mr. Avelino likened the outcome of his practice to that of his biomedical colleagues: "My treatment is effective, and that's why patients come to me. But sometimes doctors can't cure patients either."

PAULINO ZAPATA

We did not do this. We don't do this kind of thing. Criollo people are the ones who know this stuff.—Paulino Zapata

Mr. Avelino's explanation is far less elaborate than the one offered by Paulino Zapata, who treated Inez Rivero's son Jesús. Some sixty-five years of age and one of the most renowned wisidatu in the delta, he lives on the Winikina River in Morichito, across the river from Barranquilla—the ancestral home of El Cocal residents.[14] His father, Carlos Zapata, was an acclaimed wisidatu as well (see Heinen 2009: 2). A model of medical pluralism, Mr. Paulino works in collaboration with his son-in-law, Ildebrando Zapata, who trained as a nurse (figure 2.9). They work together in a structure fitted with a table, chair, and metal cabinet containing medicines for Ildebrando and a hammock and stool for Mr. Paulino, who first diagnoses patients for hebu sickness, then turns them over to Ildebrando. Mr. Paulino sometimes assists medical personnel at the Arawabisi clinic (figure 2.10).

Mr. Paulino can be given to braggadocio, declaring himself to be the most prominent wisidatu. When speaking about the afternoon that the Rivero family placed three-year-old Jesús in his care, however, he was quite humble. The parents told him that the fever came out of the blue and hadn't responded to antipyretics. The boy's eyes looked strange. He couldn't swallow, didn't want anyone to touch him, and at times had trouble walking. "He was acting crazy," Mr. Paulino reported. No cases had appeared for a month and a half and none in his area, but Mr. Paulino suspected that Jesús had the mysterious disease. Having heard colleagues relate their experience, he knew the odds were against him, but his professional pride and curiosity prompted him to try. He grabbed his sacred rattle, but a preliminary session was inconclusive. Night is the best

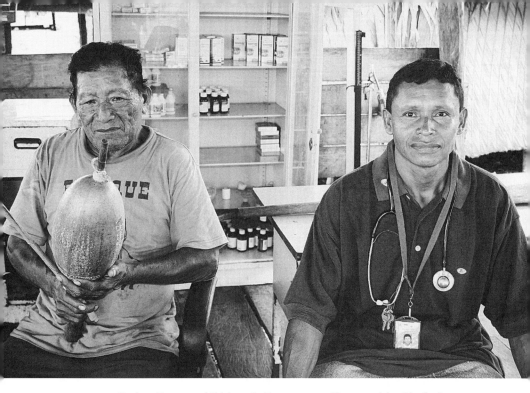

FIGURE 2.9. Paulino Zapata and Ildebrando Zapata, 2009. Photograph by Charles L. Briggs.

time to undertake extensive treatment for hebu sickness, so he asked the family to come back later. But when they returned, "He was really sick. He was in really bad shape," Mr. Paulino said softly. "He died shortly thereafter."

Questions haunted Mr. Paulino: What is this disease? Where did it come from? He did not treat Jesús's older brother Lizandro, but he spoke with several of the dozen healers who did. Mr. Paulino focused on how swallowing water induced a drowning sensation and the boys' strange, sometimes frightening, at times enticing visions. Inez's account of Lizandro's dying words was key. As death approached, he called out the names of "two criollos" (hotarao) who worked on a government project to build a new cement bridge in El Cocal. Having accused five-year-old Lizandro of stealing one of their tools, they struck him until he bled, threatening to kill him with "black magic." When he spoke their names, Inez said, their images appeared before the Riveros' house. The words of a dying patient are read in divinatory fashion as evidence of bad medicine and as revealing the culprit's identity. Lizandro's words reportedly caused the two men to fall ill; they hurriedly left the area. The government contract yielded only cement pillars and rusting steel reinforcing bars.

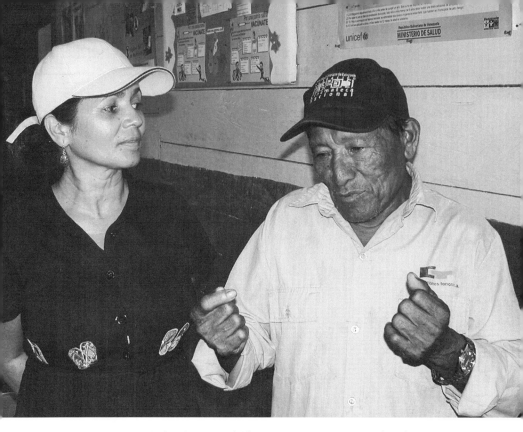

FIGURE 2.10. Paulino Zapata and Clara Mantini-Briggs in Arawabisi clinic, 2006. Photograph by Charles L. Briggs.

Like other practitioners who faced the mysterious disease, Mr. Paulino found that the evidence did not fit his diagnostic categories. Like physicians, he thought that applying broad social and political contours would never suffice to explain the epidemic unless he also took into account the specificity of the symptoms. Why, for example, did patients recoil from the sight of a glass of water? He was forced to think beyond a universe exclusively populated by human beings—patients, parents, squabbles, and government contracts—to bring in the "natural" world, to think about a time when it was still "social." Mr. Paulino asked himself, could it be *nabarao*? The term commonly refers to the delta's beautiful freshwater dolphins, but here evokes the parallel world that exists under the water and the troubled history of relations between its inhabitants and those who live above—a history in which sexuality, failed reciprocity, and menstrual blood loom large. As Candace Slater (1994) argues, exchanges between humans and creatures who live under the water—as emerging in narratives—constitutes a powerful realm of the imagination, enchantment, danger, and sexuality in greater Amazonia.

In times past, *hoarani*, people who lived beneath the water, sometimes married humans.[15] A Warao man who wished for a hoarani wife saw a woman while fishing; arising from the water, she asked him to take her home. Fishing together the next day, she invited him to visit her father's home beneath the water; as she held his hand, they arrived safely. Her parents invited him to sit on a bench (actually a pet alligator), saying, "I sent you my daughter for your wife; you must live a good life, and must now send your sister for my son." After they gave the man food and drink, the couple returned to the surface. The rift between water and surface people arose over prohibitions regarding menstrual blood, the rationale for excluding menstruating women as healers (except yarokotarotu). In Mukoboina and Siawani, women use a *nehimanoko* (menstrual house) located between home and forest when they menstruate and give birth. The water-spirit wife warned her husband that if forced to go to the menstrual house, she would die; her father would then send calamities not yet visited on surface people. When she menstruated, women forced her into the nehimanoko; by morning she was dead. Grieving, the husband returned to her father. Chastising him for not listening, he warned, "From now on sickness, accident, and death will come among your people from mine" (see Roth 1915).

Something had gone terribly wrong in 2007. An unprecedented form of sickness and death had suddenly sprung up. Mr. Paulino looked to a sort of molecular level of explanation, to the first principles of his perspective. If his account could be called mythic, it was also tied to the present: how health and housing programs of a socialist state can turn into just more disease and death. Mr. Paulino hypothesized that the problem was "not the nabarao themselves." He asserted, speaking for Warao healers, "*We* did not do this. We don't do this kind of thing. Criollo people know this stuff. They did something really terrible; they are the ones who know how. They told the nabarao. Then the nabarao came onto the land and took someone, then came back and took someone else." As we sat in his clinic/house, he suggested that patients feared glasses of water because water spirits appeared there, beckoning them to follow them into the water—to die.

The water spirit Mr. Paulino deems responsible is not a Warao woman but has blue eyes and light-colored hair; her legs form a tail when she enters the water. The image is the mermaid, *la madre del agua*. She is associated with La Llorona, who, legend has it, drowned her children and now wails as she traverses waterways, drowning other children or even adults. Mermaids appear in folktales, capturing humans, carrying them beneath the water to become their lovers or handing women over to male spirits.[16] In the small stores in Tucupita that supply the criollo practitioners, Mr. Paulino had seen images of María Lionza and her court, the spirits that "come down" to empower criollo healers.[17] The source of the wrath that led the contractors to inflict "black magic" was not sexual but material—the accusation of theft against Lizandro. Here Mr. Paulino's account questioned the idea that a five-year-old stole a tool from a contractor who had stolen government funds allocated for building a cement bridge to connect the wooden houses occupied by people close to starvation; never finished, the project left only a bizarre sculpture garden of cement and steel (figure 2.11). Braggadocio returned to Mr. Paulino's voice as he revealed his theory of the strange disease. Finally he could explain why he failed to cure his patient: nabarao do not listen to sacred rattles; wisidatu do not know the spirit names for controlling nabarao; and the etiology comes from a healing system located across an ethnic divide.

Both his and Mr. Avelino's explanations bring in the supernatural effects of discrimination and corruption. Their accounts could appear self-serving, as trying to get themselves off the hook, but they demonstrate how, much like doctors and nurses, they were sincerely trying to figure out why their healing arts had failed.

Doctors, Nurses, Healers, and Parents: The Great Divides

When children began dying from the strange disease, there was no shortage of care in the Delta Amacuro rain forest. Patients were surrounded by attentive providers, starting with their parents. Beginning with Gabriel Torres, most were treated by healers, including some of the most senior practitioners, by nurses, the local physician, medical interns, and specialists in urban hospitals. Each used the diagnostic and treatment tools available to him or her, trying to solve the mystery and save the patient's life. They all failed. Most of them were troubled by that, some deeply. Two Nabasanuka nurses were so disconcerted that they almost quit; fortunately, they overcame their despondency.

The strange cases left Dr. Ricardo, nurses in rural clinics, and healers feeling isolated, but remarkably little pooling of collective knowledge emerged. When Mirna treated Mamerto, the penultimate patient, she had nothing more to go on in the way of treatment guidelines than those available to José Pérez treating Yuri Torres in Siawani. All the nurses could do was to try to address the fever and pain symptomatically, empirically. The Nabasanuka nurses may have conferred with Dr. Ricardo, but they had nothing to share but their mutual lack of answers, having received guidelines—to use only acetaminophen—that would have resulted in less effective care if they had followed orders.

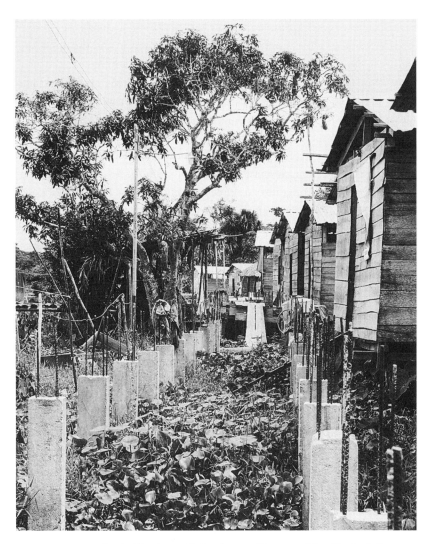

FIGURE 2.11. Unfinished bridge in El Cocal, 2008. Photograph by Charles L. Briggs.

At times, perspectives aligned. Nabasanuka's nurses identified with Dr. Ricardo's frustration regarding the official silence from above, but also identified with patients who, seeing the failure of the clinic's medicines, hedged their bets and took their children to healers. Collisions in perspectives emerged in, for example, Dr. Ricardo's frustrated inscription in the medical records that Graciano and Matilse had initially rejected his decision to send Adalia to Tucupita and instead took her to healers. More common, however, was a complete lack of intersection between perspectives and a failure to share knowledge among practitioners struggling to save the same patient. This includes the dozen healers who worked to save Lizandro as much as Dr. Ricardo and the urban specialists. These erasures structured each of the accounts of the epidemic that we heard over four years. After MPPS denied the bat-transmitted rabies hypothesis, the deaths, pain, and labor of care became only a sense of collective ignorance rather than the feeling that something had been learned: the parents say, "We *still* don't know what killed the children."

One of the most striking gulfs separated the parents from the practitioners. With the partial exception of the nurses, none of the latter devoted much effort to trying to see things from parents' perspectives. Somehow, however, parents were supposed to magically be able to see things from each practitioner's perspective—know how to comply with guidelines for bringing patients to providers, how to follow through on care instructions, allow the children to be whisked off to a city, be compliant even when hardly a word was spoken to them, when they could understand little of the language, and could not read the documents they were signing or understand intrusive procedures such as intubations or autopsies and why they were deemed necessary. They were expected to grasp these perspectives and practices, even when practitioners did their best to keep them at arm's length by working in specialized languages— healer's language as much as medical jargon—and generally articulating only outcomes, not processes: "There are no hebu," "We want to send her to Tucupita," "Your son is dead." Remarkably, the parents had to bring all of these perspectives into alignment, know how to weave together the care they provided with that of multiple varieties of healing and medical practices, know the limits and the claims to authority of each. And, finally, it was the parents, in the end, who paid the price: the practitioners may have felt inadequate, but the parents were left with the work of mourning.

3

———

EXPLAINING

THE INEXPLICABLE

IN MUKOBOINA

Epidemiologists, Documents, and the Dialogue That Failed

Dime cómo mueres y te diré quién eres.
(Tell me how you die, and I will tell you who you are.)
—Octavio Paz, *The Labyrinth of Solitude*

The parents, healers, doctors, and nurses ranged all over the map regarding theories about the epidemic. The wide scope of sites in which care was undertaken and the perspectives that guided diagnosis and treatment invited diverse ways of imagining what the disease might be and how it could be addressed. They recruited other participants in their narratives, including water spirits, candles, selfish administrators of food security programs, criollo healers willing to kill for money, government contractors turned black magic practitioners, and callous public health officials.

But what of epidemiologists, professionals charged with looking at the strange epidemic from a more distanced perspective? Free of anxieties regarding their own children or patients, they would certainly be expected to follow replicable methodologies, provide reliable data and statistics, and break free of voices telling them what they could see and whom they should tell. We need epidemiologists to sort through mountains of conflicting data in an epidemic, and—as in movies, novels, and works of popular science—we sometimes turn them into heroic "disease detectives" who can save the world as much from ignorance and politics as from microbes.[1] But the epidemiologists' participation was no less heterogeneous, no less far reaching, and no less complex than that of their clinical colleagues. Mukoboina was central to their efforts, but even when practitioners arrived there on the same boat, they were worlds apart in what they saw. Diane Nelson (2009) notes that the verb *contar* in Spanish means both to count and to narrate, and these meanings were perhaps never more closely entangled than in the ways that epidemiologists investigated the epidemic and how they represented it in reports, conversations, and statements to journalists.

The View from the Office of the Regional Epidemiologist: Quantifying the Normal

The intersection between health and political power in Delta Amacuro State lies in RHS headquarters in Tucupita. Here the director receives a steady stream of political patrons lobbying for jobs or contracts, products of the national oil income that flows through the regional government.[2] The Office of the Regional Epidemiologist, on the other hand, is located in a modest cinderblock structure in Hacienda del Medio, some five minutes away. Ensconced among stores and cinderblock and tin-roof houses, it consists of two buildings placed in perpendicular fashion. Painted bright green on the bottom and white on top, its nondescript façades are interrupted only by the strange protrusions of air conditioners. Although it is one of the most important nodes in the RHS bureaucratic structure, few people know it exists, and fewer still cross its large, unkempt courtyard.

The regional epidemiologist is among the most important RHS officials and the one who becomes the most visible in a health crisis. His office lies at the end of an uninhabited, nondescript hallway graced by dim illumination. Piles of official documents, some extending nearly from floor to ceiling, become visible; even the bathroom doubles as a space for storing mountains of official paper. The end of the hallway finally yields a human presence, a secretary who controls access to the regional epidemiologist's office, a small space with even less light but animated by the roar of a large air conditioner and graced with file cabinets, desks with computers and printers, and walls plastered with printouts of statistics and proclamations of RHS's goals and accomplishments. The assistant epidemiologist's office is adjacent. If one turns left at the main entrance, a room fairly buzzing with activity is revealed. Nurses assigned to the office joke congenially while transferring numbers between books, plot the progress of the current phase of the national vaccination campaign, and watch over the vaccines that lie in refrigerators in a back room, ready for the efforts by teams of nurses, physicians, and health workers to reach each house in Tucupita and each area of the rain forest in Delta Amacuro State several times a year with childhood vaccinations. Charles and Clara visited this space five times because Clara had been bitten by a vampire bat in Hubasuhuru. After watching Elbia die from rabies, the discomfort of seven shots in the stomach and the risks associated with the vaccine derived from animal nerve tissue, which is currently not recommended by WHO, seemed less pressing than the chance of dying from rabies.[3]

Entering the main door of the second L-shaped building yields a more extensive and spacious hallway, equally devoid of visible human presence but marked by signs indicating a proliferation of bureaucratic units that contrasts with the centralization evident next door. The building houses offices for the health directors and epidemiologists assigned to each of Delta Amacuro's municipalities: Antonio Díaz, where the epidemic occurred, as well as Tucupita, Pedernales, and Casacoima. Compiled statistics are generally distributed to each municipality by the Office of the Regional Epidemiologist, and public health politics and practices are largely determined by RHS for the entire state. The municipal epidemiologists make trips to their respective administrative areas, some scheduled and some prompted by problems, but they live and work in Tucupita, not in the areas they administer. Their offices are required reporting stops for nurses and physicians stationed in the lower delta.

The daily work undertaken in the Office of Regional Epidemiology is a monument to the pursuit of normalcy. It is the central node in a vast network that extracts numbers from local prefects, public and private clinics, and hospitals throughout the state, turning births, accidents, illnesses, and deaths into statistics. The epidemiologist can point to tables and figures that track what is "normal" for each disease, district, season, and demographic group, quickly summarizing, for example, what are often referred to informally as the "normal deaths from diarrhea" for Antonio Díaz. Deaths that occur beyond the regional epidemiologist's statistical reach become almost impossible to see, given how the office defines not only the meaning of epidemiology but also of health and disease for Delta Amacuro State.

The regional epidemiologist's tables, percentages, lines, curves, and causes of death also help to define political normalcy, given that a sudden aberration could draw the attention of local leaders, journalists, and opposition politicians. As its name indicates, RHS as a whole is regionally focused, a vital part of a political system that exchanges jobs and contracts for loyalty to political parties and their leaders. But the regional epidemiologist's work is also quite focused on Caracas, where many of the numbers he or she submits are compared with those from other states before national statistics make their way to WHO in Geneva via the Pan American Health Organization.

September 2007 was one of those moments that disrupted the pursuit of normalcy. Given that he did not receive medical attention, Gabriel Torres's death on 24 July did not cause a blip on the regional epidemiology radar screen. When his little sister Yuri died in the Nabasanuka clinic on 11 August, no alarms went off either. After that, clinicians in Nabasanuka, Tucupita, and Maturín examined Ángel Gabriel, but his death still did not throw the Office of Regional Epidemiology into crisis mode. Clinical evidence had not yet been transformed into an epidemiological pattern. On the other hand, the response to the hospitalization of his little sister Adalia, on 5 September, would shape clinical and epidemiological perspectives and actions throughout the epidemic. In Nabasanuka, her symptoms were recorded as "fever, inability to swallow, swollen tonsils with white platelets, and generalized weakness that evolved over a week."[4] After her condition did not improve with antibiotics, Dr. Ricardo proposed referring her to the Tucupita Hospital, but Graciano Florín and Matilse Carrasquero initially declined, trying another round of healers. When Adalia returned to the clinic the next morning "in a generally bad state," Dr. Ricardo sent her to Tucupita, where physicians at the Maternal-Pediatric Dr. Oswaldo Ismael Brito Wing of the Tucupita Hospital (figure 3.1) described her symptoms as sialorrhea (excessive salivation), rapid contraction movements (*movimientos tónicos-clónicos*), and difficulty breathing. After being incorporated into the epidemiologists' reports, Dr. Ricardo's observations seem to gain new precision and traction, a result that probably would have surprised him greatly.

Adalia was sent the following day to the Dr. Manuel Núñez Tovar Hospital in Maturín. There, pediatricians and toxicologists provided a "diagnostic impression" of mercury poisoning. When she died the following day, an autopsy was performed, and samples were sent to the National Institute of Hygiene in Caracas. Things were no longer normal. Given that Maturín is located in Monagas State, the regional epidemiologists for both Delta Amacuro and Monagas states followed the case closely. If the clinical evidence did not solve

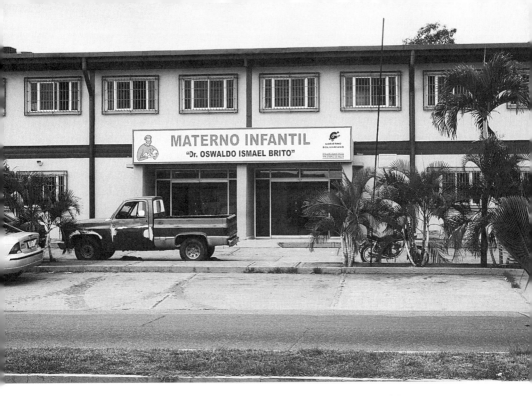

FIGURE 3.1. The Maternal-Pediatric Dr. Oswaldo Ismael Brito Wing of the Tucupita Hospital, 2010. Photograph by Charles L. Briggs.

the mystery, results from the highest-ranking laboratory would surely provide answers. This anticipation turned to frustration when Monagas's regional epidemiologist informed colleagues in Delta Amacuro that Adalia's samples "unfortunately 'got lost' in the institute" because it was undergoing repairs.[5] The results of the autopsy did arrive, and they listed the cause of death as "respiratory insufficiency due to intoxication by unknown substance."

DR. FROILÁN GODOY, RHS REGIONAL EPIDEMIOLOGIST
OF DELTA AMACURO STATE, AND SANITARY ENGINEER
WILFREDO SOSA

> It was intoxication. . . . That was what we were told by the toxicology people. . . .
> So from that point on we started looking for intoxication from mercury, looking
> for the symptoms.—Dr. Froilán Godoy

Throughout the epidemic, Dr. Froilán Godoy held the post of regional epidemiologist.[6] He has short black hair and a receding hairline, a roundish face with a prominent nose. His demeanor is serious but friendly, and he often stares straight ahead in concentration. His voice seldom departs from a low,

modulated tone, his words emerging slowly and carefully, as if he were calculating in advance the effect of each syllable, even as he mixes medical jargon
with a colloquial, man-of-the-people vocabulary. His unassuming attire does
not draw attention. Speaking with him on the street, little would indicate that
he is one of the two most important officials in Delta Amacuro's public health
system.

Despite the loss of Adalia's laboratory samples, Dr. Froilán placed his faith in
the judgment of specialists in metropolitan areas: "We referred the majority of the
patients to Monagas. I remember the first day when they said it was intoxication,
because that was what we were told by the toxicology people at that level, the
people in Maturín. So from that point on we started looking for intoxication from
mercury, looking for the symptoms." Dr. Froilán did not mention it, but Conrado
Moraleda visited him during this period to report that a number of strange deaths
had occurred and that residents were deeply worried that more children would
die. Conrado also consulted RHS director Dr. Guillermo Rendón.

Dr. Froilán acted swiftly: he formed an investigative commission and left for
Mukoboina the day after Adalia died. In the daily practices of his office, when
the epidemiologist immediately forms a commission in which he participates,
this signals that a significant threat to normalcy has occurred. The commission also included a sanitary engineer, a bioanalyst, a laboratory assistant, and a
motorboat operator. After interviewing Dr. Ricardo, the commission traveled
to Mukoboina and met with community leaders. Residents recounted the children's deaths, but the visitors concluded, "For the moment in which we visited,
there were no persons with similar symptoms."[7] Given that Henry's symptoms
only began a few days later, neither parents nor the commission noted that he
was ill. In addition to treating fourteen patients for other illnesses, the commission took nasal swabs and blood samples, which were sent to the National
Institute of Hygiene in Caracas. The document that summarizes the trip simply
reports that all samples were subsequently reported as negative, without specifying the nature of the tests, except for leptospirosis. A water sample tested for
mercury also came back negative. The commission also tried to locate other
possible sources of mercury. Although evidence for the mercury hypothesis was
hardly overwhelming, Dr. Froilán still favored it.

The commission's sanitary engineer was Wilfredo Sosa, who had long worked
for the Malarial Institute, the ministry division that focuses on vector-borne
diseases and food sanitation.[8] Some fifty-five years of age, Sosa's controlled,
slightly nervous demeanor reflected a personal caution that had enabled him to
survive political battles and keep his job for some three decades. He noted that
the commission spent nearly all of its time in Mukoboina observing domestic

spaces and everyday activities, particularly food preparation and child care. The intoxication by mercury hypothesis shaped what Sosa witnessed in Mukoboina and how he interpreted his observations:

> What I saw was a massive consumption of canned tuna fish in aluminum cans of the brand California, which is the cheapest. In several houses I saw sacks of cans and piles behind the houses. That tuna is bad, the worst; I only ate it once, when I was working in the rain forest, when there was nothing else, and I got sick. Well, that tuna has a certain level of mercury, and its massive consumption could elevate mercury levels. And we had some results, which indicated that mercury levels were high.

Sosa tied the origin of the epidemic to the same event identified by Inocencio Torres, the Fogones Comunitarios program, but the mechanism he posited was food poisoning, not "bad medicine." The brief and controversial life of the Fogon Comunitario had already been reshaped by the mercurial hypothesis into an epidemiological fact.

DR. YOLANDA OTHEGUI, DIRECTOR OF THE ANTONIO DÍAZ MUNICIPALITY HEALTH DEPARTMENT

> You see, we did all of this [investigating], but there was no mercury. It wasn't lead or anything like that.—Dr. Yolanda Othegui

Yolanda Othegui also participated in the commission.[9] A tall, graceful woman in her midforties, she conveyed a strong sense of scientific integrity and also deep emotional engagement in her work as an epidemiologist. "I would say that I was the person who was most deeply impacted, personally," she said self-confidently in a measured and dispassionate voice. Trained as physician and employed for years as an epidemiologist, she served in 2007–2008 as director of Antonio Díaz Municipality's Health Department. As the top health official in the local political jurisdiction in which the deaths occurred, she potentially faced institutional scrutiny. Her office was located in the building next to Dr. Froilán's. Unlike many of her colleagues, who call the lower delta "remote" and "difficult" and avoid spending much time there, Dr. Yolanda savored the chance to visit Antonio Díaz; she combined the air of a dedicated professional with a touch of Indiana Jones.

Like Dr. Froilán, Dr. Yolanda considered the origin of what she referred to sarcastically as the "sacred" quest to find evidence of mercury poisoning to have been the declaration by a Maturín pediatrician and toxicologist. Speaking of Adalia, she described her thought process and how she pursued her epidemiological investigation:

I myself went by boat to the girl's house, and I searched everything from top to bottom. I asked myself, "Where could the mercury have come from?" You know, when you have spent a lot of time in the area, there is always someone who can give you an idea what's going on. I looked at it from all angles. I inquired whether anyone had gone to the mines—some ten years earlier some people had gone to the mines—and had a bucket, a can of mercury hidden somewhere in the roof. So, we climbed up to the roofs to look.... And they had tons and tons of canned tuna, so we brought back some cans. We brought back food.... We took samples of canned tuna here in Tucupita from the Fogones Comunitarios. You see, we did all of this, but there was no mercury. It wasn't lead or anything like that.[10]

Dr. Yolanda viewed her participation as going beyond responding to the regional epidemiologist's initiative and the mercury hypothesis to create a new epidemiological culture, an attempt "to do something very different in the lower delta." Dr. Yolanda wanted to produce the very sort of statistics that most Delta Amacuro epidemiologists and health officials wanted to avoid. She expressed discomfort with normal epidemiological patterns: "Over a hundred children die on me each year. That is what's normal for me." This figure was at odds with epidemiological statistics presented by the Office of Regional Epidemiology, and Dr. Yolanda explained that she compiled it from notebooks she gave to the nurses working in small settlements to record births and deaths. Dr. Yolanda reports discovering evidence of the epidemic after reviewing the notebook compiled by Siawani's José Pérez. She did not, however, have a means of transforming the numbers into official statistics, nor did she publicize them. Periodically, RHS officials rotate between such posts, and when Dr. Yolanda was transferred after the epidemic ended, her initiative disappeared.

She makes a powerful claim—it wasn't specialists in Maturín who first turned clinical data on Mukoboina's children into an epidemiological event but Dr. Yolanda herself, as a result of conscientious execution of her daily work as a health professional.

ANTONIO PEÑA AND RONALDO DOMÍNGUEZ:
VACCINATORS DISCOVER AN EPIDEMIC

They [RHS] disappeared my report. When I went back to get a copy, they said
they couldn't find it.... They didn't pay much attention to me.
—Ronaldo Domínguez

Dr. Yolanda was, however, not the only RHS employee to make this claim. Antonio Peña and Ronaldo Domínguez were nurses assigned to Antonio Díaz

Municipality in 2007–2008, that is, to Dr. Yolanda's jurisdiction.[11] They live next door to one another in a working-class neighborhood of Tucupita. Their epidemiological contributions were even less visible in the RHS documents than Dr. Yolanda's. Agreeing to relate his experiences in the epidemic and on the trip to Mukoboina, Antonio immediately jumped up and said, "Let me call Ronaldo, because he was there more of the time. He will remember more of what happened." Both men appeared minutes later.

Like most delta nurses, Ronaldo and Antonio received a year and a half of training before embarking on their careers, but they had little in common in terms of physical appearance and self-presentation. Antonio, in his early thirties, retained the round curves of childhood and was self-effacing and open. His dedication to his work and willingness to explore new challenges in the lower delta led to his being selected for many assignments there. Ronaldo, forty-five, was tall, slender, and athletic; he radiated seriousness and self-confidence. Like many Delta Amacuro health professionals, the beginning of his career was forged in the cholera epidemic, serving on Clara's team. Now, after twenty-seven years of nursing, he was eager to claim a heroic role for his profession—and himself—in recounting his experience in Mukoboina. Antonio, with fourteen years' experience, demurred to Ronaldo, who was his boss as coordinator of nursing for Antonio Díaz. Jointly, they claimed credit for discovering the epidemic.

They were in Mukoboina vaccinating children, as they did twice a year. "What we found when we arrived," reported Antonio, "was the very first case: a boy who had died that morning." During a subsequent visit, they "found out about the *other* child, who had the same clinical presentation." They took the child to the Nabasanuka clinic.

Between them, the two nurses participated in nearly all of the epidemiological investigations in Mukoboina. Like Dr. Yolanda, Ronaldo portrayed his role in the first-person singular. He explored and then discarded a series of hypotheses regarding possible causes: diseases borne by mice, such as leptospirosis; mercury or lead intoxication; poisoned fruit; a bacterial infection; or something associated with what he described as a very high level of infestations of head lice and intestinal worms. He also thought in broader terms, wondering if the constant passage of oceangoing commercial vessels or the flow of contraband to Guyana and Trinidad, which includes both gasoline and illegal drugs, might have occasioned intoxication through exposures to chemicals or gasoline. He noted that parents reported that several children had been bitten by bats. Heavy salivation and seizures led him to suspect rabies, but he did not remember mentioning this hypothesis to others. He portrayed the collection of samples and their transport to Tucupita as having taken place through his initiative. Claiming to speak Warao adequately if not fluently, Ronaldo said he collected detailed data on the Mukoboina cases and gave a report to the regional epidemiologist. "Those data," he said, "were mine—but they disappeared my report. When I went back to get a copy, they said they couldn't find it." He said simply, "They didn't pay much attention to me." The early work that the two performed was clearly shaped by the rumors about Mukoboina being discussed informally in Tucupita, trying to turn them into dates, names, and other epidemiological facts.

DR. DIEGO ESCALANTE, DIRECTOR, BARRIO ADENTRO OFFICE OF EPIDEMIOLOGY FOR DELTA AMACURO STATE

Most likely a highly virulent kind of modified adenovirus, or an enterovirus of the Coxsackie type, or another type of germ that uses this route of tranmission.—Dr. Diego Escalante

Dr. Yolanda felt that the concept of normalcy and practices for preserving it had paralyzed epidemiological inquiry. She reported that that was why she suggested the idea of bringing in Cuban epidemiologists: "One of the first criticisms I leveled at the investigation we had been conducting was that we were all from here [RHS]—and we had just reverted to what we normally do." Responding to the spirit of her proposal, RHS director Dr. Guillermo said, "Let's send the people from Barrio Adentro *alone*, without us coming along." The parallel health system, Mission Barrio Adentro, brings health services to millions of Venezuelans. It includes an epidemiological component, and a Cuban epidemiologist directs activities in each state. Dr. Diego Escalante, who directed Barrio Adentro's Office of Epidemiology for Delta Amacuro State in September 2007, submitted a "Preliminary Report of a Visit to the Community of Mukoboina," dated 20 September 2007, which contains some of the most detailed and accurate data compiled on Mukoboina.[12]

Dr. Diego took along two other Barrio Adentro personnel as well as a dentist working temporarily in Nabasanuka, along with boat operators, translators, schoolteachers, and community leaders; none of the members of these last four groups, presumably all delta residents, was named. His group sought "to obtain the largest quantity of data" possible. They visited each household where a child had died, interviewed parents and other relatives, "looked for data of hygienic-epidemiological interest," "observed the surroundings," and searched for suspected cases. Houses where deaths had occurred were numbered and residents recorded in a census; verbal autopsies provided the age, gender, and dates on which the first symptoms appeared and of death. They also documented cases in nearby Hokorinoko and Sakoinoko (see map I.1). Dr. Diego's tables also documented the number of inhabitants in each house and how the deaths unfolded through time. The team ruled out spills (presumably of gasoline or oil), dead or strangely behaving birds or animals, piles of trash, and "visits by people not belonging to the community." The report lists symptoms as "elevated fever, headache, throat and neck pain, difficulty in swallowing solids and liquids in that order, salivation, trembling, deliriousness, difficulty in breathing, with forced and noisy inhalation."

Such systematic data did not, however, yield clear explanations. Dr. Diego hypothesized that an infectious disease might be to blame, "most likely a highly virulent kind of modified adenovirus, or an enterovirus of the Coxsackie type, or another type of germ that uses this route of tranmission,"[13] although they could find no direct evidence to support this hypothesis. Both types are spread from person to person. Adenoviruses cause a wide range of common illnesses. Although they occasionally result in pneumonia, meningitis, and encephalitis, they are not likely to produce a 100 percent case fatality rate. Dr. Diego accordingly argued that the adenovirus might have "modified" into "a highly virulent kind." Enteroviruses include polioviruses and the Coxsackie virus. Given that they can also lead to meningitis, which involves inflammation of the protective membranes surrounding the brain and spinal cord, it makes sense that Dr. Diego would deem both adenoviruses and enteroviruses to be possible causes. Nevertheless, his hypothesis did not account for hydrophobia (fear of water) or excessive salivation, nor did it explain why transmission would be so selective within a single household. Although the Venezuelan epidemiologists were actively pursuing the mercury hypothesis, Dr. Diego did not even mention it.

ASSISTANT REGIONAL EPIDEMIOLOGIST BENJAMÍN LÓPEZ: THE RESURGENT EPIDEMIC

. . . In a state of complete tranquility from the health point of view.
—Benjamín López

By September 2007, Mukoboina had become the center of attention for Cuban and Venezuelan epidemiologists alike. A remarkable number of professionals visited a small cluster of houses and devoted considerable attention to figuring out what killed some 10 percent of the population. What they saw was shaped by two preexisting ideas: the mercury hypothesis, sparked by observations generated by specialists in nearby centers of medical authority, and a generalized conception of indigenous people as being characterized by deficient hygienic practices, leading to diarrheal infections. No one had a clear idea what was happening. The last death in 2007 was seven-year-old Dominguito Macotera, who died in Siawani in October. Since he was not seen by doctors, his case failed to disrupt public health officials' conviction that the epidemic had disappeared. Although no one believed that they knew what had killed the children, epidemiological inquiries disappeared along with new cases.

Then on 11 January 2008, Odilia and Romer Torres took a third sick child, Yomelis, to Nabasanuka. Examination indicated an infection of the left middle ear, so she was treated with antibiotics; but Dr. Ricardo also wanted to hospitalize her "because of epidemiological precedents." An earache would not appear related to the cases of July–October 2007, but the medical staff viewed Mukoboinan children with caution. Her parents did not wish to hospitalize Yomelis, but they brought her back to the clinic two days later with a temperature of 40° C and nausea; she vomited once. Again "in view of the patient's condition and epidemiological precedents," they sent her to Tucupita, where physicians in the Maternal-Pediatric section assessed her as being "in fair overall condition, without fever, hydrated, neck painful on palpitation, and without cephalic strength," meaning that she was unable to hold her head upright. In addition, she had involuntary movements of the pupils of both eyes, excessive salivation, and her breathing produced crackling sounds.[14] Testing for Kernig and Brudzinski signs indicated neurological problems,[15] and Yomelis had trouble standing and walking. Other symptoms were reported the following day, on which she died: secretions containing mucus and pus, nosebleeds, and vomit with blood. "An autopsy was performed," with the results reported as "acute respiratory insufficiency, widespread intravascular coagulation, septicemia, pneumonia, and severe malnutrition."[16]

When Norbelys Torres of Sakoinoko was taken to the Tucupita Hospital on 19 January, physicians called the toxicologist of Maturín, who recommended sending samples to the regional toxicology center; because it was closed, the samples were sent to Caracas. The Caracas report does not mention mercury specifically, which would seem to indicate that results were negative; tests done for dengue fever, meningitis, and Rickettsia were negative. Then another child from Sakoinoko died, followed by one from across the river in Horobuhu. Eudio García died in Muhabaina, northeast of Nabasanuka. The epidemic was clearly back. Although some epidemiologists continued to pursue the mercury hypothesis, patients were not treated for mercury poisoning.

Then came a visit by Conrado and Nurse Alonzo Moraleda to the Legislative Council, which sparked a clash with RHS officials, and coverage in the local paper, *Notidiario*, that put the epidemic on record. Renewed epidemiological investigation was tied as much to that public confrontation and media coverage as to the new cases.[17] According to *Notidiario*, it was the Legislative Council—not RHS—that announced the epidemic, thereby shattering any semblance of epidemiological normalcy.

Assistant regional epidemiologist Benjamín López launched a widespread investigation on 13 February. Dr. Benjamín, a familiar figure in Delta Amacuro epidemiology, has a thin build and an angular face graced with a trim black moustache. Always well dressed and carefully spoken, he exuded an air of professionalism that he periodically—but unsuccessfully—attempted to turn into electoral success for such posts as mayor of Tucupita. He brought on board Dr. Ricardo, with Conrado Moraleda and Juan Pérez "representing the community." Dr. Froilán, accompanied by a National Office of Epidemiological Surveillance representative, arrived the next day. Teams visited thirty-seven settlements in Antonio Díaz, conducting epidemiological surveillance (looking for abnormal patterns of disease), treating patients, checking for disease vectors, fumigating, and giving talks on "proper handling of water and environmental sanitation."

Launched a week after the Legislative Council's declaration, Dr. Benjamín's intensive, seven-day investigation only mentioned two symptoms: "diarrheas and vomiting." Concluding that two toddlers had died, the inquiry otherwise produced "no data whatsoever." Two charts tabulated 211 cases of diarrhea. The notion both that water-borne diseases were to blame and that MPPS's intervention focused precisely on diarrheas was reinforced by the distribution of large blue water tanks in nearly all of the places visited; they were never hooked up to pumps that would draw water from the river (figure 3.2).

After returning to Mukoboina and Sakoinoko in mid-March, Dr. Benjamín reported both settlements "finding themselves in a state of complete tranquility from the health point of view and that it was demonstrated that the inhabitants of these communities are complying" with instructions for using the big blue tanks.[18] It is hard to imagine how this rosy assessment emerged. Mukoboinans told us that they were still waiting for answers at that point, afraid that more children would die. The report hinted that the group was looking for evidence of the strange disease, even if it was not on the official agenda. Mukoboina and Sakoinoko were each visited five times.[19] Blood samples were taken from several Mukoboinan parents and sent to Caracas to test for metals. A note indicates vaguely that lead levels were "above normal." Dr. Benjamín spent an additional five days in Nabasanuka in February. Dr. Alfredo Pineda, regional coordinator of zoonosis, instructed him in setting up traps for capturing bats. Although Dr. Alfredo had used the same trap successfully on previous occa-

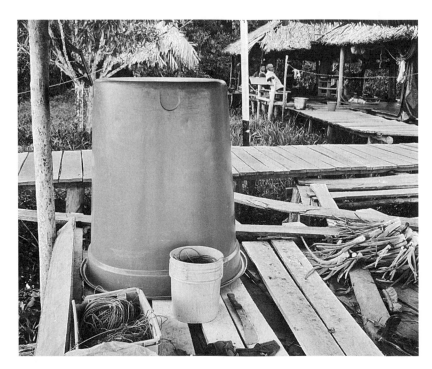

FIGURE 3.2. One of the big blue water tanks in front of Inocencio Torres's house, Mukoboina, 2010. Photograph by Charles L. Briggs.

sions, Dr. Benjamín did not capture any bats. Why? The report suggests that the regional government had denied a request for logistical support needed to more adequately carry out this research, even after allocating substantial resources for the diarrhea investigation. Another link to bats appears in an internal report dated 7 August 2008, referring to two brothers from El Guamal who died in March 2008 without receiving biomedical attention. It mentions that they "had been bitten by bats approximately a month before."[20] At least starting in February, bats were in the air and rabies was suspected, but no one was vaccinated, and no autopsy has emerged that reports having tested for rabies.

EPIDEMIOLOGY IN THE THIRD WAVE OF THE EPIDEMIC

They tried to hide the epidemic [*opacarlo*] so that it wouldn't come out in public—and this was all the way through.—Ronaldo Domínguez

From June to August 2008, fourteen children and three adults died in seven settlements; physicians examined some of the patients, and several died in hospitals. Pressed by parents, nurses, and leaders, Dr. Ricardo wrote Dr. Benjamín, the assistant epidemiologist, on 4 June reporting the death of Norma Macotera in Hominisebe. Perhaps trying to blunt the negative response he expected for reporting more cases, he used the already-familiar diagnostic category: "deaths due to intoxication by an unknown substance." The response was official silence. Of the three waves of the epidemic, the greatest number of deaths occurred in this final phase, but very little additional epidemiological investigation was undertaken.

Dr. Yolanda insisted that she never gave up the quest for a diagnosis. Public health laboratories are ranked in terms of levels of reference, indicating whose results will be considered definitive. Dr. Froilán accepted the results of the regional reference laboratory in Maturín. Dr. Yolanda, his subordinate, called a friend in Caracas to obtain current protocols for obtaining, transporting, and submitting samples, took her own samples, and pushed Drs. Froilán and Guillermo to send them to Caracas, to the national reference laboratory: "We sent samples to the Institute of Hygiene, asking them to test them for everything!" But all of the results "kept coming back negative." Dr. Yolanda then bypassed Dr. Froilán to press RHS's director. Upon reporting the advice she received from her friend in Caracas, she said that Dr. Guillermo told her approvingly, "You're right, doctor." When a diagnosis was not forthcoming, she pressed him again: " 'Might it be possible to send them abroad, to the United States, Europe, who knows!' He replied, 'Go for it, doctor!' So I looked into all ways of sending that sample. . . . I said, 'Okay, we need to know, perhaps we need to call someone who knows more than we do . . . so they can help us identify what is killing the children back in the lower delta.' " She suggested the Centers for Disease Control and Prevention in Atlanta, the reference laboratory for the Americas. Given Venezuela's tense relations with "the Empire" (the United States), the suggestion gained little ground.

Although she occupied a subordinate position through her placement at the municipal level, Dr. Yolanda declared that she never simply responded to directives from the regional epidemiologist or RHS director Dr. Guillermo. She characterized herself as the driving force behind epidemiologists' efforts to solve the mystery, as launching a creative search for causes that put her job on the line. The documents, however, give her little voice—she appears as simply one of the silent figures accompanying the reports' authors in their investigations. As a subordinate official, she was similarly invisible in public forums and in press coverage: Drs. Guillermo, Froilán, and Benjamín were the official faces of the epidemic.

This same disjunction between how subordinate health professionals envisioned their work and how it figured in official accounts is evident for Nurse

Ronaldo. He made the connection between health inequities and health/ communicative inequities, noting that the failure to address both bothered him deeply: "They tried to hide the epidemic [*opacarlo*] so that it wouldn't come out in public—and this was all the way through. I wanted to know why the children died, and when they told me that the samples had been lost, it made me furious." Ronaldo then confronted Dr. Froilán and other officials: "I told them that these were *children*, they were *human beings* who were dying." Ronaldo wanted to send samples directly to a leading researcher in the renowned Institute of Biomedicine and ask him to bring a team from Caracas to Mukoboina. He tried to send the samples himself, but said, "They scolded me. They told me that I couldn't go over the head of the authorities."

Claiming and Disclaiming Mukoboina:
Shifting Relations between Politics and Epidemiology

Mukoboina's designation as the location of the index cases and the concentration of so many deaths made it the site from which authoritative accounts must emerge. It was repeatedly turned into an epidemiological space as houses were numbered and features were mapped in terms of "whatever relationship they might have" with the epidemic. Kinship relations were redefined as connections between cases, even as epidemiological teams and different participants in the same investigation remembered Mukoboina in divergent ways. No one was looking for a Nobel Prize; we never found that anyone was motivated by the desire to contribute to scientific discovery, to publish an article in an epidemiological journal. Dr. Yolanda and Nurse Ronaldo characterized their efforts as the diligent, proactive pursuit of their daily work; while others, like Dr. Froilán, saw their efforts as simply responding to clinical findings. Even though no one claimed to know what killed Mukoboina's children, participants in the investigations often sought to position themselves as having been the first to recognize that an epidemic was unfolding, or to have found the best clues, or compiled the best data.

Epidemiologists displayed diverse affective relations to Mukoboina. All of these health professionals voiced sadness and regret. For Dr. Yolanda, these dimensions combined with the excitement, pride, and intrigue of having demonstrated both her dedication and ingenuity as an epidemiologist and her interest in solving a puzzle. Ronaldo combined all these components with both empathy and anger. He summarized his confrontation with Dr. Froilán: "And I told them that if they didn't take charge, I would, because *I am the one watch-*

ing these children die!" He implies that Dr. Froilán and other officials lacked the same empathy and commitment.

Party politics and epidemiology intersected in complex ways during the epidemic. Dr. Guillermo wielded substantial influence in electoral politics by distributing jobs and contracts so as to sustain support for Delta Amacuro's caudillo or regional power broker, Governor Micaela Montoro. He also needed to ensure that health did not become a political weapon for opposition politicians. Dr. Froilán was charged with detecting problems before they threatened the statistical construct of public health normalcy, and thus the political status quo. Disruptions of normalcy could also attract negative attention from Caracas bureaucrats and politicians, particularly if covered by the national media. Given that they played less visible roles in this matrix, politics and epidemiology came together in more muted ways for Dr. Yolanda and Ronaldo. They had more flexibility and less on the line.

By February 2008, the epidemiology-politics interface had shifted considerably. Regional elections, including for governors and mayors, would be held in August. Pedro Salazar, Delta Amacuro's first indigenous mayor, turned electoral politics on its head by declaring himself a candidate for the United Socialist Party of Venezuela nomination for governor, challenging Montoro's candidate, and thus the whole political process in Delta Amacuro, including its ethnoracial base. Dr. Ricardo, the nurses, Conrado, and others were confronted by dying bodies and by distraught, angry parents. The epidemiologists were still puzzled by the Mukoboina cases. Dr. Benjamín and zoonosis coordinator Dr. Alfredo wanted to see if bats might be part of the equation, that is, if rabies was causing the deaths. In the eyes of Tucupita politicians, however, all of these efforts were framed in terms of electoral politics. Dr. Benjamín, who had entered electoral politics in the past, was building a political base to run for Tucupita's mayor as an opposition candidate. The sitting governor and her allies thought that when Conrado and others went to the Legislative Council to publicize the deaths and demand an epidemiological investigation, they were probably acting on Pedro Salazar's orders, trying to make Montoro look bad and build support for Salazar's candidacy. Mentioning the strange epidemic became political treason. When the third wave of cases began just two months before the election, more epidemiology would simply have created more political liability. But that was moot—it just didn't happen, at least on RHS's part.

Epidemiology per se never became "just politics" during the epidemic. Except perhaps for those holding the highest RHS posts, epidemiologists grew more and more uncomfortable as more and more new cases were met with the same lack of a diagnosis and treatment protocol. But as events were interpreted by politicians and epidemiologists alike—albeit often in different ways—no epidemiological space existed apart from electoral politics. If we, too, adopted this perspective, the epidemic would be reduced to a battle between science and electoral politics, between scientific and political elites. This is the way such stories are usually told, and they emerge as tragedies of the loss of scientific integrity and suggest that the production of knowledge lies legitimately in the hands of physicians working as epidemiologists who can somehow magically remain above politics. This perspective overlooks the way that the people we have featured in this chapter brought a wide range of perspectives, preconceptions, training, and experience to the epidemic. They came to the same sites and sped away on motorboats after coming to very different conclusions. The science-versus-politics model would also ignore how their perspectives depended both on recruiting the observations of residents and reducing them to one-word answers to fill in epidemiological slots. The epidemiology of the epidemic both depended upon and was fatally undermined by health/communicative inequities, much like the work of the journalists we examine in the next chapter.

4

H E R O E S ,

B U R E A U C R A T S ,

A N D

A N C I E N T

W I S D O M

Journalists Cover an Epidemic Conflict

This topic is completely taboo for us.
This issue was handled at the highest level.
—Ministry of Popular Power for Health press official,
quoted by Carmen Buenaventura

In February 2008, *Notidiario*, Tucupita's newspaper of record, put the epidemic in the public eye when it published three full-page stories on Antonio Díaz Municipality, two focused on the strange epidemic and one on diarrheal diseases. In August, the mysterious epidemic became one of the most prominent health stories in the history of the Venezuelan press, perhaps dwarfed only by coverage of the cholera epidemic of 1991–1993 and discussion of HINI (swine flu) in 2009. It was nearly everywhere in the national press, not to mention in newspapers, on television programs, and on websites worldwide. The leading opposition newspaper, *El Nacional*, put a reporter on it virtually full-time for a month, and *El Nacional*, *Ultimas Noticias*, and BBC Television sent reporters to the lower delta.

The role of journalists in creating and circulating stories of the strange disease was complex. Their coverage was organized by professional ideologies, by concerns with independence, newsworthiness, balance, and objectivity. In speaking about their work, they emphasized professional differences, that is, their sense of providing a unique journalistic perspective that distinguished their work from that of physicians, state officials, and others. Their takes on the epidemic and their engagement with it were no less heterogeneous than those of physicians, parents, or healers. If we were to talk about these journalists' perspectives apart from what they wrote, we would miss one of the central points they made in speaking with us: they insisted that the most important things they had to say about the epidemic were contained in the articles themselves. This chapter weaves together the reporting that emerged in February and August 2008 with comments by journalists, particularly the reporters for *Notidiario* and *El Nacional* who produced the most influential coverage. We draw both on interviews and on our own observations as protagonists in the events, including media ones, that unfolded in August 2008.[1]

One of the reasons that the news coverage of the epidemic is so important for our story is that the work of journalism requires being finely attuned to differences of training and practice: seeking out people with quite different perspectives and attempting to grasp what they did and why. The reporters' jobs revolved around both connecting people and words and drawing attention to the gulfs that separated them. In reporting the words and actions of nonconventional news sources—particularly Conrado, Enrique, Norbelys, Tirso, and other delta residents—journalists opened up possibilities for exposing health/communicative inequities as well as provided key resources for the official effort to keep them in place. The reporters' general reliance on medical authority and government officials, however, ultimately secured official attempts to reestablish the communication status quo.

Notidiario*: "Servicing" Government Agencies, "Equilibrating"
Opposing Perspectives, and Educating Delta Readers*

You have to have laboratory results. You can't make that claim.
—*Notidiario* journalist Leo Romero

Notidiario is a quintessential small-town paper. Although the corporation that owns it is based in Puerto Ordaz, reporters and readers are firmly located within Delta Amacuro State.[2] It is published six days a week from a small office in a multistory building a few blocks from Tucupita's central plaza. *Notidiario*'s circulation averages 7,000 daily copies, sold mostly in newspaper kiosks, small stores, and by vendors walking up and down Tucupita's streets. Insofar as there is a public sphere in Delta Amacuro, an arena of communication and debate about issues of common concern, *Notidiario* defines it. Caracas newspapers, such as *El Nacional*, also arrive every day at kiosks in the central plaza, which get swarmed in the late morning. Several radio stations have large local audiences, but primarily it is a story in *Notidiario* that turns a subject into a topic of discussion and debate for Delta Amacuro residents.

The paper's founding reporter, Oscar Marcano, had been writing for *Notidiario* for a quarter century in 2008. In his sixties, Oscar has black, curly hair with traces of gray above an angular face with a prominent nose. His tall, strong build and bronzed skin reflect years pursuing stories on the streets of a town on the edge of the rain forest. He speaks with a confidence that springs from enjoying uncontested status as the state's senior journalist. Leo Romero writes many of *Notidiario*'s health articles. He is of medium height with an athletic build and a youthful face that belie his forty years. Oscar's rapid speech is marked by pauses and intonations that evoke a serious and reflective bent, as if he were writing a regional history of journalism for us on the spot. Leo's words, in contrast, have an off-the-cuff quality. According to Oscar, the initial impetus for including health reporting in *Notidiario* came from "specialists," surgeons, cardiologists, and pediatricians who wanted to find a way to transmit information "to people, to families." Asserting that the health reporting has been "very successful, tremendously," Oscar cited as evidence seeing health articles cut from *Notidiario* pasted on walls in clinical facilities throughout Delta Amacuro.

Three types of health-related articles appear in *Notidiario*. One details diseases, treatments, preventions, and the like. Some content is provided by "specialists," including a weekly column by a leading local pediatrician. Oscar noted that when these sources do not yield sufficient health stories, "We go to the Internet." This first type of coverage embodies most directly what Leo described as *Notidiario*'s primary role with respect to health: "to circulate, to inform, to educate: . . . the people must be educated." It is framed in general, apolitical terms; articles generally make little or no reference to Delta Amacuro or health inequities; no articles on the epidemic took this form.

Oscar referred to the second type as "performing a service for the [RHS]." Although *Notidiario,* like most small papers, does not have any health reporters per se, much of Leo's reporting focuses on RHS's programs and activities. Either the RHS director, his secretary, or another official, such as the regional epidemiologist, will call Leo, brief him about an upcoming event, such as a visit to a particular health center, a vaccination campaign, or the inauguration of a new facility, and invite him to RHS headquarters. In Oscar's words, the director "calls him, [Leo] goes, he gives him the information, and [Leo] edits the information and gives it directly to the newspaper." No press releases are involved, and, by *Notidiario* policy, material is not taken over the telephone but through a recorded interview. Two of the articles published in February 2008 were of this type.

The last type is the *denuncia*, a public performance of a complaint or accusation. *Notidiario*'s policy, in Oscar's words, is that "our door isn't closed to anyone": any individual or group can show up at *Notidiario*'s office to make a denuncia. A reporter will tape record a statement and take a photograph. Officials have the right to respond; the governor herself often did just that during the epidemic. Oscar noted, "There are denuncias that we have just sat on in order to avoid a confrontation with [the governor].... There are things that you can see she takes personally, which is silly." Leo added this cautionary note: "When you make a denuncia, you need to know how to do it; you need to do it well."

The mysterious epidemic first became the focus of media attention when Conrado, Nabasanuka nurse Alonzo, and several parents appeared suddenly in Tucupita. When the second outbreak, which started in January 2008, rekindled anger over the lack of a diagnosis, Conrado, as health committee president, and Alonzo approached Dr. Ricardo, Nabasanuka's Consolata nuns and priests, teachers, and other residents. Meeting in the chapel, they decided that Alonzo and Conrado should raise the stakes by going to Tucupita. Even after having been rebuked by his superiors for taking the disease so seriously, Dr. Ricardo risked writing yet another official letter to RHS.

The trip's goal was to involve a new set of official agencies in order to provoke broad recognition of the epidemic, including media coverage. Alonzo and Conrado delivered a copy of Dr. Ricardo's letter to Tomás Rivas, a member of Delta Amacuro State's Legislative Council and a Caracas-trained radio journalist. While he visited Nabasanuka researching stories for his radio program, Conrado told Rivas about the epidemic; he was seen as a good potential ally. Rivas took the letter to fellow legislator José Fernández, an educator who teaches the Warao language in Tucupita. In his late thirties, short, with small eyes and a disarmingly serene demeanor, Fernández was, like Rivas, something of a political anomaly—having been elected due to his support of social causes rather than his obedience to Governor Montoro. (Each served only one term of office before the political machine booted them out.) Rivas convinced his council colleagues to pencil a new item "regarding a disease that is finishing off the children in Antonio Díaz Municipality" into the agenda for the meeting scheduled for that day. The council unanimously decided to hold a public hearing; RHS's director and the regional epidemiologist were scheduled to appear on 7 February.

An article appeared in *Notidario* the following day, titled "Emergency Due to Infectious Outbreak in the Lower Delta." The front-page photograph of Conrado addressing the Legislative Council was highly remarkable: a person classified as indigenous pictured in a powerful pose, speaking, documents in hand (figure 4.1). The story, on page 3, contains a similar image as well as one of Conrado and Alonzo posing with the council's president. However, the text, not authored by Leo, places Conrado (misidentified as Manuel Moraleja) in the background in what is depicted as a confrontation between the Legislative Council and RHS. Conrado and Alonzo enter as "indigenous representatives of the affected communities who presented in detail the grave situation." Their intervention is thus assimilated into the usual story of confrontations between rival politicians. Two mechanical failures—cases in which children died en route to Tucupita when the fluvial ambulance broke down—are cited as having led parents to lose faith in RHS. The article then shifts to presenting RHS's position: it had conducted epidemiological investigations and "had at no time neglected the situation," which it attributed to "possible toxic or infectious agents." The confrontation became a war of numbers, with officials—statistics in hand—claiming twelve deaths and Conrado and Alonzo eighteen. Legislator Fernández supported Alonzo, arguing, in a statement not quoted in the article, that the witnesses are the parents themselves, nurses, and leaders "who live there and keep tabs on who is dying. They aren't going to lie!" The final word in the article is given to legislator/journalist Rivas and other legislators, who called for action by national and regional health officials.

To some extent, the article fits into the denuncia frame, a public statement that exposes inadequacies with government agencies, albeit one delivered in the Legislative Council rather than *Notidiario*'s office and that included an official rebuttal in the same story. Even if they are cast as players in a drama dominated by government institutions, the recognition that an indigenous nurse and a layperson produced knowledge about an epidemic was remarkable, as was the idea that the council—rather than RHS—would declare an epidemiological emergency.

The author of the *Notidiario* article did not follow up on the story, nor did legislators. Officials of RHS soon generated rumors in the form of epidemiological explanations that attributed the deaths to actions taken by "the Warao."

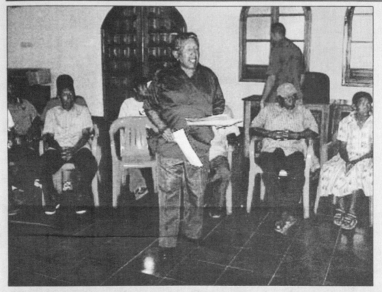

NOTIDIARIO
EL DIARIO DEL DELTA Y DEL SUR DE MONAGAS

Tucupita viernes 8 de febrero de 2008 — Año XXIV Nº 7.630 — *Depósito Legal pp 83-0249* — Bs 1000 Bs.F. 1,00

Emergencia por brote infeccioso en el Bajo Delta

Tucupita.- Miembros del Parlamento regional se reunieron de emergencia con representantes de los organismos rectores de salud del estado Delta Amacuro a objeto de enfrentar una situación epidemiológica que ha causado la muerte a una docena de niños en cinco comunidades indígenas ubicada en el Bajo Delta , Municipio Antonio Díaz, declaró la presidenta del órgano legislativo, Ledys Carrasqueño Cañas, quien estuvo acompañada de los legisladores: José Barreto, Luís Alfredo Marín, Tomás Barreto, Yoel Ramos y José Gregorio Toro. N/3

FIGURE 4.1. Conrado Moraleda appears on the front page of *Notidiario*, 8 February 2008.

In doing so, they normalized strange deaths from unknown pathogens via well-established stereotypes. One rumor claimed that Warao parents had caused the epidemic by giving their children rotten food taken from the dump. A second claimed that the deaths resulted from eating a poisonous fish known as the *tamborín*. A third rumor focused on the consumption of poisonous fruit. Julio Mondragón, a former RHS director, offered both the fruit explanation and a fourth assertion—that indigenous healers were killing their own patients—on a radio broadcast. This latter went beyond the common stereotype that Warao people refuse to visit doctors because they believe in "witches" to assert that Warao healers are not only ineffective but engage in practices that are criminally injurious.

Public health professionals working in Tucupita circulated these explanations in conversations with colleagues, politicians, and friends and through occasional radio broadcasts, where health professionals spoke as individuals rather than for ministry offices. The explanations gained broad circulation in town and the lower delta. By purporting to explain the mysterious deaths, they helped to overcome RHS officials' acknowledgment that they could not diagnose them. Moreover, they shifted blame away from problems with the public health system and onto the shoulders of indigenous residents. The lack of official status limited, however, their potential for countering Conrado's and Alonzo's disruption of RHS's control over the production and circulation of health knowledge. The dominant narrative that an accusation of health problems constitutes a political move was soon exploited by opposition politician Rafael Pérez to attack officials. In a short article that is a classic denuncia, here taken by reporter Leo, Pérez cites Mondragón's radio broadcast, challenging the poisoned fruit and healer malpractice "hypotheses." Pérez asserts that it is common knowledge that "indigenous people in this area are dying from hunger and from abandonment on the part of this government, which does not attend in any way to their more urgent needs, which are: health, food, potable water, and broad-based attention to their problems."[3] Pérez then demands an end to "talk of hypotheses and suppositions" and calls for "studies by experts, epidemiologists, universities, and scientists on the true origin of these deaths."

Next came a full-page article by Leo, published with three vivid color photographs on 20 February. A classic example of the "service to RHS" genre, Leo recalled how it began: "RHS sent an invitation to the local media here in Tucupita, and I went as Notidiario's representative. They invited us and we went to cover this activity." The "activity" was a visit to Nabasanuka by Ministry of Popular Power for Health (MPPS) vice minister Mariela Martinelli and RHS director Guillermo Rendón. A high national official's visit to the lower delta is a newsworthy event in the public health and political worlds of Delta Amacuro. According to Leo, the visit "was very educational. As a journalist, I am not accustomed to that kind of area, the sort found in the lower delta, which are a little neglected [descuidadas]. I really liked the motive for the trip: we're going to investigate, we're going to the place to listen to what the people have to say, [to see] what is happening. So we arrived where there were families whose children had died from the presumed disease, so then [RHS officials] asked them what happened." Leo outlined what he learned and how it shaped his perceptions:

> Look, they had vomiting, diarrhea. They lay down in their hammocks and didn't want to eat. They didn't want anything. The clinical picture, the physicians say, was five days in the hammock: you don't eat, you don't drink liquids, all you do is just defecate and vomit. This leaves the body debilitated, in a critical state that can even lead to death. And it is even worse at an early age, five, six years of age or less. The body has no resistance. . . . Certainly there exist life circumstances that are very difficult for anyone.

The trip, the epidemiological investigation that it reported, and the story Leo filed on returning to Tucupita turned "the emergency situation in which the delta community is living at this moment" into a problem of diarrheal disease, one that could be addressed by analyzing water samples and "controlling the ingestion of water" through household-by-household hygiene talks and the delivery of large blue plastic tanks.

Leo reported speaking with some of the same parents whose narratives are presented in chapter 1. In the parents' testimonies that our team recorded, vomiting was mentioned in eight (21 percent) accounts and diarrhea in six (16 percent); in Leo's story, however, the fever, paralysis, hydrophobia, excessive salivation, seizures, and strange visions all disappear. In the 8 February article on the council meeting, Dr. Guillermo states that RHS had been investigating "the origin of the strange pathology" since July 2007 and that work was "continuing through the present." By the visit to Nabasanuka one week later, the disease had evolved into diarrhea. How could the pathogen have mutated so quickly? Leo's 20 February article describes the investigation as part of a Strategic Plan for Epidemiological Intervention, which he lauds as "very ambitious." The article reports that Vice Minister Martinelli "personally inspected the activities undertaken by this multidisciplinary working group."[4] Vice Minister Martinelli, whose red cap and T-shirt made the visit's political significance clear, demonstrated her concern in a photograph taken inside the clinic as she leaned over an infant placed on an examining table. The "epidemiological intervention" constituted a response to both the public debate and media coverage, imposing both a new epidemiological frame and creating an elaborate backdrop for a visit by a vice minister and journalists.

The day after the article appeared, RHS director Dr. Guillermo invited Leo to his office, where he, regional epidemiologist Froilán Godoy, and assistant epidemiologist Benjamín López gave statements that appeared in a 22 February article, "Wisidatus Don't Cause Deaths of Indigenous Children." Here, diarrheal disease has disappeared and deaths in Mukoboina "from some species of intoxication, produced by an unknown substance" are back. The article's focus is on the three officials' efforts to register their concern with "some commentaries" that blame the epidemic on wisidatus.[5] To the contrary, asserts Dr. Benjamín, "We believe in the behavior of the Warao doctors, who possess an ancient culture that has always existed." The article pictures the three RHS officials and includes archival shots of "a traditional Warao doctor" and "indigenous communities." Denying that the wisidatus had caused the deaths implied, however, that wisidatus could have killed their patients. The article kept alive Mondragón's other hypothesis, the notion that the deaths might have been caused by eating poisonous fruit. Far from the 8 February front-page image of Conrado, this story projects a voiceless, homogenous indigenous population infused with "an ancient culture that has always existed" and whose health problems can only be sorted out by nonindigenous health officials.

The articles on diarrhea and wisidatus provide classic examples of *Notidiario*'s RHS service genre: responding to the director's call, visiting RHS offices, and participating in an RHS-sponsored tour to get "the information," edit it, and give it "directly to the newspaper." Statements by Oscar and Leo indicate, however, that they saw the situation more complexly. Oscar said that *Notidiario*'s policy calls for "always listening to various parties," asserting that no one is shut out of the newspaper's pages. Leo similarly argued that "the role of the press is to give recognition to both sides," to report "in an objective manner, as objectively as possible." He told Charles, "We always go to RHS, to hear the official side. There are two sides. You need to hear both sides." Interestingly, most of Leo's articles do not follow this principle: the "service to RHS" genre does not appear to open up space for controversy and does not require looking for another "side." Speaking about his *Notidiario* articles on the epidemic, Leo framed them as having reported

> as much the side of the indigenous people who asked for an explanation, a clarification of the deaths, as whether or not there would be actions so they wouldn't happen again, whether there was an epidemic or a disease decimating that population, and the other side, for RHS to find the solution, what it was doing and what was happening.... All of this coverage included the positive and the negative, because remember that I as a journalist must create an informative equilibrium, getting both sides.

In short, Leo characterized the council article, like Pérez's denuncia, as attacks on the government; achieving "an equilibrium" required not only devoting space in the council article to Dr. Guillermo's reply but also publishing two full-page articles in which only RHS speaks.

It would be easy to explain this unbalanced balance in economic terms. Oscar noted that *Notidiario*'s sales just pay for the paper on which it is printed; local businesses do not provide much advertising revenue. Accordingly, he said that what keeps *Notidiario* afloat is income from publishing official announcements paid for by Delta Amacuro's government. A strictly economic argument would, however, oversimplify a complex relationship between journalistic and medical ideologies. The reporters were able to do relational work, to explore different perspectives, but only insofar as those perspectives could be assimilated to one of two preexisting subject positions or sides—that of the regional government or of its political opponents. Individual voices could only enter as synecdoches, parts that represent a larger political whole by serving as spokespersons for one side or the other. The idea that the deaths could not be neatly subsumed by partisan politics was simply unthinkable; they were, in essence, demedicalized, treated like other types of controversies, at the same time that RHS's medical authority was privileged.

Leo laid out for Charles the legitimate and the unacceptable types of health-related *denuncias*: to declare that there are cases of fever "in my community" is okay, "but we can't say that it's yellow fever—I am not a physician who can say that it's yellow fever.... You have to have laboratory results. You can't make that claim." By definition, "indigenous communities" lack the authority of "Western medicine." By performing a service for RHS and creating an "equilibrium" simultaneously, *Notidiario* could both incorporate competing voices and assist RHS officials in reestablishing their monopoly over the production and circulation of epidemiological knowledge.

The Second Outbreak—of Media Coverage: The National and International Press

Why speak of politics if what the Warao are asking for is an investigation?
—*El Nacional* reporter Carmen Buenaventura

It would be hard to imagine two more distinct journalist contexts in Venezuela than *Notidiario* and *El Nacional*. *Notidiario* is the local paper in what is seen as one of Venezuela's most politically and economically marginal regions; *El Nacional*, centered in Caracas but read throughout the country, was until recently considered the national newspaper of reference. Life for *Notidiario* reporters revolves around political dramas associated with the *caudillo*, the personal power and patronage network vested in the person of Governor Montoro; the words "Chávez," "socialist revolution," or "PSUV" never emerged in epidemic-related stories or interviews with journalists. In contrast, *El Nacional* is positioned at the heart of national politics.

El Nacional was founded in 1943. After the 1958 fall of dictator Marcos Pérez-Jiménez, it was deemed center-left. After Chávez became president in 1999, it became closely identified with the anti- Chávez opposition, thrusting it into the center of what has been termed the "media war" between Chávez supporters and the opposition. *El Nacional* served for decades as a key site for training health and science journalists who were obtaining degrees at the Central University of Venezuela. During the cholera epidemic of 1991–1993, *El Nacional* health reporters enjoyed a particularly close relationship with the minister of health, and the newspaper published a prodigious number of articles on the epidemic.[6] In 2008, Carmen Buenaventura, a graduate of the Central University of Venezuela's School of Journalism, was one of *El Nacional's*—and the country's—most prominent health journalists. In her thirties, with shoulder-length blonde hair, light skin, and brown eyes, she had been on *El Nacional's* health beat for nearly a decade. Her reporting appeared in *Ciudadanos*, a daily section that includes business and crime as well as health.

After drawing up its detailed report on the epidemic and creating a document containing epidemiological details, on Sunday, 3 August 2008, our team spent two days traveling from the delta to Caracas. The six of us entered the lobby of the MPPS headquarters on Wednesday, 6 August, and requested an interview with MPPS minister Col. Rafael Serrano, in which we planned to give him our report and ask MPPS to send a multidisciplinary commission to investigate the epidemic. We were all government supporters. Enrique was an official in Chávez's PSUV. Norbelys was newly appointed as a nurse/EMT in MPPS's Office of Indigenous Health. Clara had served as director of MPPS's National Fight against Dengue Fever. Conrado was the president of Nabasanuka's health committee. Charles had taught in the government's public health school in Maracay and had appeared on Chávez's television program, *Aló, Presidente*. Our efforts deeply reflected the spirit of the Bolivarian Revolution and its commitment to the health of low-income and indigenous populations.

Rosenda Mandagno, coordinator of the Office of Indigenous Health's Plan Delta, descended the stairs and greeted us. A social worker, Rosenda identifies herself as Wayuú, that is, as a member of Venezuela's largest indigenous group. She has long, straight black hair and attractive features, and on that day wore a long, bright orange dress. "The vice minister will see you. What resources are you requesting?" Conrado replied, "We're not here to beg. There is an epidemic in the lower delta; the six of us investigated, and we are here to give the minister a report and ask him to send a commission and stop the deaths." She looked confused and phoned upstairs. She turned to us again, but now her face was less friendly. "We thought the visit was by some Warao with a problem, coming to ask for something. We didn't know that you were making a complaint [denuncia]." "It's not a complaint," replied Enrique. "We're here to deliver a report." Rosenda replied, "They will not receive you or your report." "Why?" asked Enrique. "You should have taken your complaint to the RHS in Tucupita and not come to Caracas. They have not informed us about any such epidemic in Delta Amacuro." "We did inform them, twice," Conrado responded, "but the director didn't do anything about it. So we decided that we had to come here directly."

Security staff members emerged from an adjacent office, frowning, their body language hostile. "We're not going anywhere," Enrique stated angrily, "until they receive us and review our findings." He took out eleven photographs showing delta families affected by the epidemic. "These are parents whose children died," he stated defiantly. "Here is a young woman dying from this disease. We're not going anywhere!" The standoff lasted two and a half hours. Two high-profile witnesses appeared: Carmen Buenaventura of *El Nacional* and Hector García, the *New York Times* correspondent for the Andean region, who happened to be in Caracas that day. Conrado, Enrique, Norbelys, and Tirso were suddenly in the middle of a media maelstrom that would continue for several weeks. Though they had never met a reporter before, decades of reflecting on racism, health, and injustice and dreaming of a better world welled up inside of them to produce powerful and articulate words in their second language, Spanish.

Each projected a distinct, personal voice to the press. Enrique's anger flamed white hot, often directed straight at RHS director Dr. Guillermo. The language of socialism, the indigenous social movement, and his brother Librado's passionate engagement with social justice issues saturated his often-poetic declarations. Conrado's sober, calm, modulated voice produced close descriptions of watching patients die and accounts of appeals to RHS officials. Tirso spoke in a collective "we Warao" voice, providing moving accounts of Delta conditions. Norbelys, the youngest member of the group, used a poised and confident voice; unlike Conrado, Enrique, and Tirso, hers had not been seasoned in political meetings.

Two and a half hours later, the stalemate broke. Officials agreed to meet with Conrado, Enrique, Norbelys, and Tirso alone. At first they refused, arguing that the team had always operated collectively and that we would not split up. When it became apparent that these were the only circumstances under which a meeting could take place and the report delivered, they took the elevator upstairs and entered a conference room where the director general of epidemiology, Rómulo Pérez, was waiting with two of his assistants. In his mid-fifties, he wore thick glasses, his black balding hair pulled back and gelled. The four outlined the results of the investigation and stated their demands. Enrique passed around the photographs of Elbia, her family, and other parents, one by one. He noted gravely, "We are experiencing a threat to the Warao people." Pérez's reply, in their estimation, was insulting. They were again placed in the frame, "What have you come to beg for?" Dr. Rómulo told them that he had never been informed about any such cases, that they lacked the knowledge and authority required to make such statements, and that they should never have come to Caracas. "It was very hard, but we defended ourselves," Norbelys recalled. Then María Márquez, director of the Office of Indigenous Health, appeared. She confirmed that Dr. Ricardo had informed her of the strange deaths. "Then the tone of the meeting changed completely," recalled Norbelys. Dr. Rómulo, Dr. María, and their staffs examined the report carefully and discussed what should be done. "The ministry has accepted your report," stated Dr. María, "and it has named a commission, headed by Vice Minister Martinelli and Dr. Rómulo. It will investigate the situation thoroughly. Indigenous representatives will be included on the commission and in future planning. We see these results as a quite positive outcome."

As the team was preparing to leave MPPS headquarters at nearly 9 PM that night, the head of the Ministry of Popular Power for Indigenous Peoples (MPPPI), Margarita Taller, sent an assistant to escort us to her office. Tirso, Norbelys, Enrique, and Conrado all rankled at what they perceived to be a dismissive attitude on the part of Minister Taller. The meeting proved largely confrontational, although it ended with a promise to provide hammocks with mosquito nets that would protect against bat bites. From this point on, government officials did not express interest in further meetings, leaving open a space that was taken up by an avalanche of interview requests from national and international journalists.

The next morning, the team rose before 6:00 AM and turned on television news programs that featured the story of the epidemic, drawn from the morning papers. Charles saw the headlines as he picked up breakfast for the team. It was clear that their voices had grabbed the journalists' eye, ear, and nose for news. Health journalists for elite newspapers had treated four indigenous, working-class Venezuelans and their physician/anthropologist collaborators as producers of health knowledge and credible actors. In *El Nacional*, Carmen Buenaventura notes in her first article on the epidemic that "the community decided to create a commission" after RHS failed to act. Her lead quotes Conrado: "For us, this is a monstrous disease. We don't know where it came from. It is painful." Citing the team's statistics, Carmen characterizes Conrado's goal as "dejar registro," to "put [the epidemic] on record." Stereotypes of politically passive, easily duped indigenous actors who cannot make sense of biomedical knowledge appeared, at the time, to be swept aside. The article recounts the symptoms and epidemiological hypotheses that led to the rabies diagnosis, then adds Tirso's observation that "the eyes die before the body." Enrique, emerging as the team's most explicitly political voice, is given the last word. Positioning himself as strongly pro-government, he is quoted as saying, "I have come to bring the clamor of the Warao people. The patience of our Warao brothers and sisters has reached its limit. We form part of the revolutionary project, but it appears that the health revolution has not reached the Warao. We have not committed any crimes, nor are we trying to offend anyone. And we know that the president doesn't get this kind of information." The article concludes with both an invitation and a challenge: " 'We invite the president to attend our funerals,' he stated sadly. He added that they would not leave the capital before receiving an answer to take to their brothers and sisters."

El Universal published a map, a prominent headline, and a one-paragraph summary on page one. Health reporter Ramona Herrera had not been at MPPS, but she requested a copy of the report, which forms the focus of her story, which stresses the element of mystery, the strangeness of the epidemic, the lethality of the disease, and the possibility that it could extend into new areas: "In many communities, they are afraid everyone is going to die." Hector García's *New York Times* article notes the U.S. connection, highlighting Clara and Charles's employment at the University of California, Berkeley, and previous work on the cholera epidemic. Mentioning that "the Warao leaders and the Berkeley researchers emphasized that they all supported Mr. Chávez's policies and that their intent was not to smear his government," García quotes Norbelys's angry statement: "We traveled by bus 16 hours to Caracas to make the authorities aware of the situation with the hope of getting some response.... And we are met with disrespect on every level, as if the deaths of indigenous people are not even worth noting." A statement by Enrique brings health inequities to the fore: "All we request is for authorities to respond to this disease as they would if it occurred in a rich district of Caracas." The *Times* article turned the epidemic into a global story.

The photographs that appeared were arresting. *El Universal* sent a photographer to MPPS headquarters, but he arrived after the chosen team members had gone upstairs to meet with the MPPPI minister and the iron gate to the ministry had swung closed. He encountered Charles and Clara outside the gate, waiting out the meeting. Thinking of the parents' and Enrique's charge to disseminate photographs of the children, Charles gave him several photographs from his flash drive. The next morning, *El Universal* featured his picture of the dying Elbia comforted by her mother (figure 1.19).

Carmen Buenaventura invited the team to appear the next morning on a program she hosted on a national channel, *Fe y Alegría Radio*; here Conrado, Enrique, Norbelys, and Tirso became even more articulate. They were intimately familiar with this medium—radio was the primary medium reaching the lower delta before DirecTV. Clara joined them for part of the live national broadcast. Energized by the print coverage, they kept copies of *El Nacional* and *El Universal* in front of them. Enrique saluted MPPS for agreeing to fully investigate the epidemic and praised Taller for her commitment to send mosquito nets: "For the first time in history we have an indigenous person at the head of a ministry." Tirso and Conrado were more critical, outlining the shortcomings of Delta Amacuro officials. Clara put a human face on the epidemiological statistics and recommended providing mosquito nets and vaccinating anyone bitten by bats. Carmen stressed RHS's political vulnerability: officials acted, he said, "very badly. This is a negative verdict for regional health authorities for not having responded in time—this could have been avoided."

The conversation continued after the live interview ended. Carmen researched the story that she was writing for the following day's paper, but it soon became clear that her agenda was much more ambitious: she had already negotiated with *El Nacional* to visit the lower delta. Although the newspaper has always been very conservative about providing travel expenses, they had approved her proposal to spend a week there. The trip would involve no small personal commitment, for Carmen had recently given birth. Meeting in the studio after the broadcast, she put her proposal to Conrado, Enrique, Norbelys, and Tirso, who promised to take her to Mukoboina, Santa Rosa, and elsewhere.

Upon leaving the station, the team received several more invitations from journalists, including one from the vehemently antigovernment television channel Globovisión, which we rejected. Another was from an Associated Press reporter in Caracas, who had read Hector García's *Times* article. A Californian in his mid-thirties with a youthful face and longish brown hair, Paul Oliver was waiting for us across from the pristine white National Assembly building in a back booth at a steakhouse that cultivates romantic images of Venezuelan cowboy culture. After eliciting some good quotes from Conrado, Enrique, and Tirso, Oliver asked for access to Charles's photographs, having seen the ones published in *El Nacional* and *El Universal*. After the interview, Oliver rushed off to cover a press conference by Minister Taller; he was surprised we had not been invited. Taller acknowledged the team's visit, expressed her concern, and declared that 6,500 hammocks and mosquito nets would soon be delivered to the delta. The team then met an *El Universal* photographer who pictured us in front of the impressive National Assembly building.

The story Paul Oliver distributed over the AP wire appeared the next day in *Ultimas Noticias*, a Caracas tabloid that juxtaposes government and opposition perspectives, and in many newspapers throughout the world, often accompanied by photographs of Elbia Torres Rivas and her family. Oliver's story contains an important new angle provided by a major figure in rabies research, Charles Rupprecht, then chief of the rabies program at the U.S. Centers for Disease Control and Prevention. Oliver quotes Dr. Rupprecht as noting that the diagnosis was reasonable and that the outbreak was similar to those in Brazil and Peru. Rupprecht also adds an environmental dimension: "environmental degradation" through mining, logging, or dam construction projects might have led vampire bats to seek an easy source of blood—humans. Oliver also cites Daniel Bausch of Tulane University as agreeing that the symptoms suggested bat-transmitted rabies; both urged a vaccination program.

The impact of this national news coverage on Delta Amacuro State's political landscape was cataclysmic. The moment the team arrived at MPPS headquarters, calls went out to RHS director Dr. Guillermo: national officials felt blindsided by the news that an epidemic had remained undiagnosed for a year. "What's going on in Delta Amacuro?" they asked. Copies of *El Nacional* and *El Universal* quickly arrived in the small kiosks in Tucupita's town square, delivered by assistants to Dr. Guillermo and Governor Montoro. That very afternoon, 7 August, RHS held a press conference that featured not just Drs. Guillermo, Froilán, and Benjamín but three others as well: Diego Escalante (the Cuban epidemiologist who submitted the report on Mukoboina), Wilfredo Sosa (the sanitary engineer), and Julio Mondragón, the RHS official who broadcast hypotheses about fruit and wisidatu. The takeaway appeared in the title of the article *Notidiario* published the next day: "There Is No Epidemic in Antonio Díaz."

The story's lead pinpoints information on "a disease that has still not been identified" as having originated in "a website and national print publication." The article quotes Dr. Guillermo as both denying that the deaths had occurred and then attributing them to the "probable causes" of diarrhea and pneumonia. Asserting that extensive investigations had been launched that very week, he states that he was "not certain which data or statistics the supposed investigators and groups of physicians used to endorse or confirm their statements."

The article ends with an apparent threat in the director's voice: "These self-proclaimed scientists should be reminded that to undertake any investigation or medical examinations in indigenous areas they must inform health authorities of the objectives and plans to be undertaken in the investigation, because they will otherwise have to account for their actions to the Office of the Public Prosecutor." Dr. Guillermo forgot to mention that Charles and Clara had visited him in July before leaving for the lower delta and that we had been in frequent contact with Dr. Ricardo and the interns. Back in Caracas, several team members' cell phones rang as relatives and friends in Tucupita reported proliferating rumors: "They're waiting for you, and they are going to lock you up!"

The following day's *Notidiario* reprinted Herrera's *El Universal* articles of 7 and 8 August. The latter focuses on MPPS's commitment to send a commission to the delta, also mentioning that autopsies had been performed but had not produced a diagnosis, "nor had the obligatory notification [to the parents] been provided." *Notidiario*'s front page, however, bore the headline "Prosecutor Investigates Complaint Regarding Indigenous Deaths," accompanied by a photograph of prosecutors Principia Centella and Roberto Antonio Guzmán holding a copy of the *Notidiario* article containing RHS's denial. Guzmán and Centella stated that their "superiors" had commissioned them to "initiate an investigation into the matter" and announced plans to order Clara, Conrado, and Enrique to testify regarding "where they obtained the data disclosed in the newspaper article, given that this is very delicate."

The enraged RHS response pointed to a wave of emerging attacks by government officials. We were therefore surprised by an invitation to appear on 8 August on the program *En Confianza*, a widely viewed noontime interview program aired on the Chávez government's most prominent channel, Venezolana de Televisión (VTV). Half a dozen stylists and makeup artists greeted the team, dusted us with powder, and combed our hair. Once we were ushered into a waiting room, an *En Confianza* assistant warned that space limitations would permit only three participants on set. Norbelys and Tirso wanted a break from media attention; Enrique and Conrado would participate throughout; Charles and Clara would each appear for half of the fifteen-minute interview.

Host Ramón Martí—serious and distinguished-looking in a white shirt, brown sports jacket, and glasses—opened with the announcement that "terrible things" were happening to lower delta residents, adding, "We'll see if we can offer them solidarity after listening to them." A sensitive interviewer who obviously felt moved by the story, Ramón portrayed it positively. After Conrado described the epidemic and the failure of officials in Tucupita, Enrique emphasized that the team had come to Caracas only after "having exhausted all of the regular channels, because regional authorities in Delta Amacuro State appear immune to the pain and the feelings of the Warao people." He stressed that the team's goals were not to complain [denunciar] but to provide the central government with information and to "claim our rights as they appear in the Constitution of the Bolivarian Republic of Venezuela" and the Organic Law of Indigenous Peoples. Charles noted that working with the team had been "one of the most profound experiences of [his] life," recounted the community-based epidemiological investigation, and described Mukoboina. Clara asserted that the team's work constituted "a great success for the revolution" due to its origin in a popular struggle, and she outlined possible measures MPPS could take. Asked to wrap up by "giving a message to Venezuela," Enrique stated his solidarity with the revolution, giving the thumbs-up gesture. He added that "the revolutionary project in health has not reached Delta Amacuro State, specifically the indigenous area," but also praised MPPS and the Ministry of Popular Power for Indigenous Peoples for responding positively. He credited the team with "having fulfilled its commitment to fulfill the task it was given by the indigenous community."

Despite the attention it customarily gives to health, the pro-government daily, *Diario VEA*, remained notably silent on the epidemic. Many print-oriented Chavistas avoid *El Nacional* and *El Universal*; the Oliver article reprinted in *Ultimas Noticias* reached many members of this audience, given the paper's nonaligned stance. Chavistas who are more oriented to television than print news generally avoid news programs on the oppositional commercial channels. Thus, VTV is a key venue for connecting government supporters. The team's fifteen-minute interview on a popular VTV show complemented what had emerged in other media, and few Venezuelans remained unaware of the epidemic. At the same time, the interview further infuriated Delta Amacuro officials.

After three tumultuous days in Caracas, in the wake of the anxious telephone calls from relatives, Conrado, Enrique, Norbelys, and Tirso left for the bus terminal on Friday afternoon. No seats were available, so they returned to the hotel just as we received a call from Leo Casagrande of ViVe TV, a government television channel created to give women, ethnic minorities, and low-income populations greater media presence. Hailing from the Andean region, Leo fell in love with journalism in high school. His appearance is rather nondescript, but his idealism and creative reporting had won him awards for finding innovative ways to use popular voices and perspectives to rethink health and other foci. Having arrived at ViVe only months earlier, he quickly embraced the idea that journalism could leave both corporatist and statist agendas aside and put "the people" on camera. He had seen the press coverage on the epidemic, and he wanted to cover the story.

Years of suppressed anger about health inequities were erupting inside Enrique. On ViVe, he lodged a direct attack on a powerful public official—Guillermo Rendón. Possibly jeopardizing their own jobs, Leo and the director of ViVe's news division ran this statement on a six-minute news segment that first aired on 11 August. The on-camera reporter emphasized "the extensive work that the Bolivarian government has performed in health" and Clara's assertion of the team's "commitment and close association with the revolution," thereby attempting to deflect angry official reactions. Editors wove the interviews with team members together with footage Charles provided of Elbia Torres Rivas, her relatives' efforts to save her, and her wake. It was broadcast repeatedly.

Over the weekend of 9–10 August, articles in the national press announced the government's emerging line of attack: a war of diagnoses and numbers that also helped reporters turn the story into a political controversy, thus sustaining its newsworthiness. For Carmen's 9 August story, a quotation from National Assembly Deputy Representative María Luz Figueroa, herself trained in Warao herbal healing, provides the headline: "It's True That Our Warao Brothers and Sisters Are Dying." In the story, Dr. Guillermo is quoted as countering, "It's true that they die, but from diarrhea and from hunger, because they don't have a treatment plant for potable water and they don't have anything to eat, because there are no jobs in that area."[7] Dr. Guillermo recycles the diarrhea discourse he used in February, adding that he had never received any information on the thirty-eight deaths, and "at no point had he authorized any commission whatsoever to investigate." Aware of at least seven deaths in Mukoboina, officials investigated, he says, "but we found absolutely nothing." Dr. Guillermo diagnoses "the real disease" in Antonio Díaz as caused by pervasive fecal contamination, a situation in which "that municipality is socially sick." He thereby indicts the Antonio Díaz Municipality administration of Pedro Salazar, indirectly blaming him for the lack of sanitary infrastructure. His statement also constitutes a political shot across the bow, given that Salazar was running against Governor Montoro's hand-picked candidate for governor. The article introduces the principal nonhuman actor in the story, quoting leading Venezuelan bat expert Omar Linares Prato as saying that a species of vampire bat, *Desmodus rotundus* (featured in a fang-bared portrait), was the likely vector for rabies transmission.

A story filed by another *El Nacional* reporter on 11 August focused exclusively on MPPPI Minister Taller, who opened up the statistical attack that would become one of the government's leading strategies for discrediting the team's work. She is quoted as asserting, "I don't think there could have been so many deaths," arguing simultaneously that such high numbers would have alerted health authorities and that the deaths could have been from other causes. Her closing quote surreptitiously introduces one of the most charged terms in the Chavista lexicon: "Warao people have suffered greatly due to the imperial onslaught." Carmen's 12 August story reports that Delta Amacuro epidemiologists had documented ten deaths as early as September 2007. She includes the names and ages of the children who died, noting that "all of the symptoms presented by the 10 children coincide with the findings made by the specialists Charles and Clara Briggs."

On 13 August, MPPS minister Col. Rafael Serrano gave a rare press conference where he advanced Taller's statistical attack. Reporting on the press conference, Carmen writes that after recognizing that thirteen had died, Serrano declared that "the victims reported [*denunciadas*] by those people" were really deaths that had occurred in previous years. When Carmen asked him the cause of the deaths, he responded, "some from diarrheas, others from different causes," painting the team as epidemiological incompetents who got the numbers wrong and confused normal causes of death with rabies. Covering his bets, however, Serrano "confirmed that a new shipment of rabies vaccine will be sent to the area." Serrano advanced two interpretations of the deaths. He asserted, first, that "indigenous people have different customs," thereby taking readers back to the 1992–1993 cholera epidemic in Delta Amacuro and the discourse of cultural difference that became its lasting epistemological residue. Second, Serrano turned Taller's cryptic allusion to "the imperial onslaught" into a full frontal attack: "Apparently there are people who are not Venezuelans who are making this complaint." International news reports, he continued, "invite reflection that those who exploited indigenous people for more than 500 years and made them into slaves have come to make a big fuss about something that happened months ago and about which the President and the Ministry had already taken action.'"[8] Serrano had repositioned Charles as an agent of the empire, the United States, thereby explaining the entire affair as an attack lodged by the U.S. government against Venezuela.

Charles and Clara had returned to Tucupita several days earlier. Charles received a call on his cell: "Hóla, Carlos, it's Carmen. Can you talk? Did you see what Serrano said about you? Can you give me a reaction?" At the time, Conrado, Enrique, and Norbelys were in the lower delta and Tirso was at his daughter's home. "We are pleased that the minister himself has commented on the epidemic," Charles began, noting again that the team had not made a denuncia but had delivered a report.

But I consider such remarks, spoken by a high public health official, to be irresponsible. It is irresponsible to imply that indigenous leaders, such as Conrado, Enrique, Norbelys, and Tirso, would need a gringo, a foreigner, to tell them what to say and what to do, denying their role of leadership in organizing this response. It is irresponsible to reduce real deaths of real human beings to the status of a political scandal. It is irresponsible to blame unconscionable health conditions and the limitations of existing public health facilities on the "different customs" of indigenous peoples, thereby blaming parents and "their culture" for their children's deaths. And, finally, it is irresponsible not to have done one's homework before making a public statement. It is widely known that this supposed "agent of the Empire" has enjoyed legal residency in Venezuela for nearly twenty years, has worked alongside Warao leaders for two decades, has appeared on President Chávez's program *Aló, Presidente*, and is a Chávez supporter.

In the following day's *El Nacional*, Carmen quoted Charles's statement nearly verbatim. The only omission was telling: given the paper's oppositional stance, she omitted Charles's reference to his support of the socialist government.

Ramona Herrera's 16 August *El Universal* article opened up a new perspective on the epidemic. She cites Guyanese health minister Leslie Ramasammy as saying that in Guyana "'a not unusual number' of deaths have been detected," which, as in Venezuela, "some scientists and experts have attributed to rabies, for which reason they will collaborate with Venezuela to determine the cause" of the epidemic. If it is rabies, Guyana "will rapidly carry out an immunization plan in the most exposed communities, which are indigenous peoples, miners, and loggers of African origin." Herrera contrasts this position with that of MPPS, "which rather than responding to a possible epidemic, had chosen to discredit the researchers who conducted the study and minimize the situation in the Lower Delta." A sidebar reports that Warao people lack access to the rabies vaccine. Calling Charles that evening to ask for a comment on the story, Carmen phrased an accusation as a joke: "You cheated on me!," implying that he and Clara had tipped Ramona on the Guyanese story.[9] A reporter for the Spanish news service Efe, however, had made that contact. Health reporting is, unsurprisingly, no less competitive than other beats; Carmen felt that the relationship she had built with the team implicitly entailed an obligation to pass along new story leads exclusively to her.

State officials worked feverishly to sustain their counterattack. Perhaps the least effective maneuver in the statistical campaign emerged when Governor Montoro asked Carmen to interview her. The resulting article's lead quote has

Montoro lowering the number of dead to seven. Carmen reminds Montoro that her own office had already stated that the number was nine. Caught off guard, Montoro then attributes the number to MPPS. Carmen counters that the ministry had placed the number at twelve. Montoro then defers to MPPS. After denying that anyone had died after February, Montoro states that a successful vaccination program had been undertaken, thereby confusing routine infant-child vaccination with rabies prophylaxis. When Carmen uses the term "epidemic," Montoro declares, "It is not an epidemic. . . . For that to be the case, there must be a significant number of deaths, even if we accept that there are dead children." When Carmen questions the governor's understanding of the technical sense of "epidemic," Montoro again defers to "specialists" and goes on to assert, "Some say that it is due to fruit from a particular tree; others the little tamborín fish, which if you don't take out something-or-other is poisonous."

Carmen asks, "If the Warao had not made a complaint, would this have been kept under the table?" Montoro: "We have not hidden it, and now those people went over there and made political statements." Carmen: "Why speak of politics if what the Warao are asking for is an investigation?" Montoro then implies that team members were backing a different gubernatorial candidate, alluding to Pedro Salazar, adding, "There are so many things that are behind all of this, but I am not going to say what they are," hinting at broader conspiracies. Even card-carrying, dyed-in-the-wool Chavistas were surprised. "It's not only embarrassing," a loyal Chavista and friend of Clara and Charles in Tucupita remarked, "it scares me to think that she is running our state—what ignorance! We have become the laughingstock of Venezuela."

A call on Clara's cell phone confirmed *Notidiario*'s 9 August article: Principia Centella of the Third Prosecutor's Office of the Justice Ministry with Jurisdiction over Environmental Crimes in Delta Amacuro State informed her that she must appear for questioning in connection with a criminal investigation for "environmental crimes against the state." Centella grilled her for three days on every tiny detail of the team's work, releasing her periodically when Tucupita's power outages interrupted the proceedings. They tried to intimidate her, looking for discrepancies that might warrant prosecution in connection with "an extremely serious affair," the criminal character of which was never specified. Agents appeared from the Dirección de los Servicios de Inteligencia y Prevención (DISIP), a widely feared intelligence branch of the Ministry of Justice, which had inaugurated its own investigation. Charles and Tirso kept vigil each day outside the office, both attempting to ensure that Clara was not spirited away and awaiting their turn.

A 19 August *Notidiario* article by Manuel Martínez headlined "Excessive Contradictions in Case of Indigenous Deaths" juxtaposes the interrogation—without quoting the prosecutors or the results—with the *El Nacional* interview with Governor Montoro, which it characterizes as "having sparked many expectations and generated great confusion due to the different versions, confrontations, and controversies created by individuals and characters, governmental, community, indigenous, and political sectors and others, who have demonstrated more interest in benefiting personally, as nearly always happens, from the plight of the Waraos, than in finding a solution or at least a palliative, to the disease that affects what are, now and always, the least protected members of our population." The article reports the DISIP's visit to the prosecutors' office to demand a copy of the criminal charges, which, Martínez notes, had never been drawn up. Noting that autopsies on the children would be required by law, he attributes their absence to the shortage of pathologists and the remoteness and "difficult access" of the "indigenous communities in which they were buried," overlooking the fact that many of the deaths occurred in the hospital and that several autopsies had been performed whose results were not released. Making fun of the presumptive diagnosis of rabies, Martínez contrasts the delta's geography to that of Transylvania, concluding that Count Dracula has no delta relatives and that "the Bat Family swears on a pile of crosses that it had nothing to do with the deaths." Weaving together legal and medical vocabularies with highly colloquial language, the story first normalizes the situation as political maneuvering and then turns it into a joke.

After their return from Caracas, Charles and Clara became increasingly uncomfortable with their media visibility, including active efforts by opposition politicians (including ex-health ministers) to recruit them and by right-wing television stations who sought interviews and statements that would provide them with political ammunition. Crucially, Conrado, Enrique, Norbelys, and Tirso were in the lower delta and could not be reached by reporters. After feeling so positive in Caracas about opening up a space in the press in which indigenous health knowledge and leadership was positively portrayed, the withering attacks in *Notidiario* and on Tucupita radio stations had left the four feeling vulnerable and angry. The story was turning into an old, familiar narrative: two nonindigenous professionals fighting on behalf of a poor, silent, suffering indigenous population. Fostering this story would have undermined the very struggle for health/communicative rights that Conrado and Enrique had launched, and accordingly Charles and Clara stopped returning calls from reporters.

Charles and Clara returned to the lower delta from 18 to 21 August to regroup as a team and report to the parents on the trip to Caracas. Recounting the reprisals directed against them by government officials, Conrado and Enrique wanted out of the limelight.

A Journalistic Expedition to the Heart of the Epidemic

This image is engraved in my memory, an image of resilience, human fortitude, of ancient wisdom.—*El Nacional* reporter Carmen Buenaventura

Carmen told the team in Caracas that her first article on the epidemic had prompted her editors to devote prominent attention to the story "as long as it lasts." They allowed her to devote her exclusive attention the story, and *El Nacional* published an article almost daily for a month. Speaking for *El Nacional*, she commented, "This is our focus [*tema*]—for us, this is very important." When she visited the lower delta, accompanied by a photographer, Conrado, Enrique, Norbelys, and Tirso took her to many of the places where the deaths had occurred, including Santa Rosa de Guayo, where many of the parents retold their stories (figure 4.2). The result was five full-page stories in *El Nacional* over six days, each on the front page of the Ciudadanos section. In negotiating with her editors, Carmen had argued, "This needs to be a complete series of at least a week." The section's front page ordinarily rotates daily between crime, business, and other desks, but the other editors ceded their priority.

Carmen's 26 August story features Mukoboinan parents Matilse Carrasquero and Odilia Torres, both pictured, retelling the story of their children's illnesses and deaths, including their accounts of symptoms. The article conveys their demand to hear from government officials what had killed their children, as well as their request for a nursing station. Repeating Taller's statement that she had sent 6,500 hammocks with mosquito netting, Carmen notes that those provisions had only arrived in some of the places in which children had died and that, in Mukoboina, each family received only one. She quotes an unnamed resident who complained, "This is a mockery, as if I might know which child will be bitten by a bat tonight." A photograph on the paper's front page pictures the row of new tomb-houses in Mukoboina's cemetery. The 27 August article widened the series' scope to include Muaina, Santa Rosa de Guayo, and Horobuhu, again providing articulate voices of parents and including their photographs; a sidebar recounted the story of Elbia and Mamerto.

A shift occurred on 28 August with another story, "When We Want to Hurt Someone, We Use Our Ancestral Knowledge." Here Lourdes Rodríguez, MPPPI's Delta Amacuro representative, acts as the storyteller, recounting the Muko-

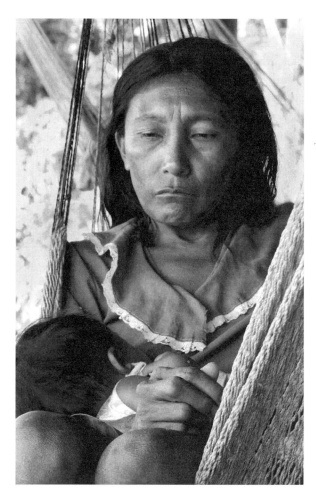

FIGURE 4.2.
Sinergia Torres
of Santa Rosa de
Guayo, shortly after
the death of her two-
year-old daughter,
2008. Photograph by
Charles L. Briggs.

boina narrative of bad medicine that resulted from the Community Hearth conflict (chapter 2). She asserts that this narrative encapsulates how "indigenous people" think about health and attempt "to explain the inexplicable." When the team was drawing up its report, Enrique proposed that "witchcraft" be left out, knowing that including it would reproduce stereotypes. Rodríguez resurrected the narrative for Carmen precisely as the government sought to discredit the team's report and counter the notion that indigenous laypersons could legitimately produce knowledge about health.

This attribution of health problems to a cultural barrier that left indigenous residents incapable of learning hygiene and accessing health services dominates most of Carmen's remaining articles. The 29 August story focuses on a mother who lost seven of ten children, six to "diarrhea, fever, and vomiting." Although structural factors, such as the lack of sanitary infrastructure, are mentioned, the problem is represented as being due to cultural preferences: "They say they don't like the taste of potable water." Efforts in specific settlements to teach residents hygiene purportedly did not meet with success. Again MPPPI's Rodríguez, who has no medical training, provides the epidemiology. The article features a color photograph of a three-year-old whose head is so covered in what appears to be scabies that it is worthy of an illustration in a medical textbook; the caption suggests that his relatives didn't know the name of the disease and had abandoned treatment before he was cured. The 30 August article repositions the familiar cultural impasse story in the Tucupita Hospital. Carmen quotes her sources, an MPPPI-provided translator and a Capuchin priest, as saying, "Indigenous people don't trust Western medicine, and when they finally decide to come to a health center, then they are mistreated." Ending on an upbeat note, the final article lauds the solar panels that light up houses in the Santa Rosa de Guayo area.

After reading the series, Enrique and Conrado felt betrayed by the reporter they most trusted and with whom they had spent considerable time. In Caracas, Carmen had appeared to grasp what they were saying about what had brought them there and what they hoped to accomplish. It was a remarkable convergence of perspectives. After the trip to the delta, their trajectories diverged— or perhaps it was revealed that the intersection was only a mirage. What had happened?

Reporting on the epidemic—most significantly visiting Mukoboina, Santa Rosa, and other settlements—had become, in Carmen's view, one of her most satisfying and important experiences as a journalist.

> I admired a journalist who traveled to all of the revolutions of Africa, to the most lost, unknown countries in Africa. But [after viewing the delta], I said, "you don't have to go so far away to see this divorce between what we recognize as Western civilization and things that happen in your own country, about which you have no idea. . . ." We have everything here in Caracas, we have all the advantages, in comparison. On the one hand it engendered in me a lot of admiration and, on the other, the awareness as a Venezuelan of how little we know about the situation of the indigenous people: all of this was a discovery.

Discovering multilingualism proved to be "a culture shock" for her: "It had never occurred to me that I would need a translator. It surprised me." Another striking feature was "to see the resignation" of a mother whose child dies from a diarrheal disease, "who sees it as almost natural." In her criticism of conditions in Tucupita Hospital and how indigenous patients are treated, Carmen saw evidence of this same sense of passive resignation. She contrasted this scene with patients in major city hospitals who complain about the lack of medicines or other problems, who demonstrate "a more combative attitude." At the same time, Carmen vividly recalled watching Enrique stand in the front of his boat at night in the rain, like a statue: "This image is engraved in my memory, an image of resilience, human fortitude, of ancient wisdom." The figure of cultural difference, resignation, the naturalness of infant death, and the Noble Savage are precisely the stereotypes that Conrado and Enrique were actively countering in their investigation of the epidemic and their trip to Caracas.

Ironically, what made the epidemic so newsworthy for Carmen was how it formed, in her view, a striking departure from this baseline of otherness, timelessness, hopelessness, and resignation. Women protested these deaths, unlike those from diarrheal diseases, because, Carmen told Charles and Clara, "If a child dies from that disease, they can't get over it because we don't know what it is." The baseline for determining the newsworthiness of deaths from the strange disease was the stereotypic assumptions that naturalize unconscionable rates of infant mortality, rendering them not newsworthy. Similarly, Carmen was struck by the "valor" apparent in the team's "having made this almost biblical trip to Caracas and going to the ministry. . . . It certainly produced a very powerful sense of empowerment." Coming from a world characterized by resignation, "the absolute firmness with which they acted" formed such a striking departure from the ordinary that it could become a major story.

In Caracas, Carmen saw Conrado, Enrique, Norbelys, and Tirso as articulate, thoughtful individuals, not simply as exemplars of a homogeneous and alien population. They took her to the delta so that she could see how what they had done had sprung from critical perspectives on everyday inequalities, from ongoing efforts to rethink health and citizenship and to imagine new futures. In introducing her to Odilia, Matilse, and other residents, they wanted to give her the opportunity to listen to other thoughtful individuals who possess agency and complex worldviews. In short, they were recruiting her to the long-standing project launched by Librado Moraleda to confront anti-indigenous discrimination. What Carmen saw there, however, were the stereotypes that sustain the very inequities so visible in the epidemic.

After Carmen returned from the lower delta to Tucupita, it was MPPPI representative Rodríguez who recycled the standard narrative turning the Mukoboina story into proof of an impenetrable cultural divide between savage bellicosity reflected in the "ancestral wisdom" of witchcraft on the one hand

and the cold biomedical rationality of doctors on the other. The parents' complex narratives of collaborating with doctors and nurses presented in the first two articles gave way to reinscription of stereotypes and a pessimistic view that rendered Conrado's, Enrique's, Norbelys's, and Tirso's intervention inexplicable and their utopian vision unthinkable. Herein lies the source of Conrado's and Enrique's bitter reaction.

For Carmen, the experience as a whole was positive and transformative, and she believed that her reporting was remarkably successful. She received "an unthinkable" number of e-mails from readers, almost uniformly positive. The articles became the focus of daily talk shows; breaking with her usual practice, she appeared on a number of them. Although *El Nacional* "is not given to congratulate" its reporters, "to recognize or appreciate anything," she received a letter from the administration thanking her and congratulating her for her excellent work. She was so proud of her reporting on the epidemic that she submitted her articles to a major international journalistic competition.

The Epidemic Becomes Yesterday's News

There Is No Rabies (*Rabia Selvática*) in the Indigenous Warao Population.
—MPPS press release

And then it all ended—officially, that is. On 21 August, Vice Minister Martinelli placed a one-page statement on the MPPS website and distributed a press release titled, "There Is No Rabies (*Rabia Selvática*) in the Indigenous Warao Population." Reporting results from the MPPS commission that visited the delta, she stated, "There is no record of patients having died as a result of bites from bats or any other animals." Nevertheless, "health authorities will continue to conduct research in order to determine the causes of death of members of the Warao ethnic group."

No empirical evidence was offered, including results of tests on the captured bats. No press conference was called. Inquiries from reporters went unanswered. Hector García of the *New York Times* complained about the lack of empirical evidence; by only filing a brief note, however, he suggested that the story had run its course. Charles and Clara's response to the AP's Paul Oliver reflected the fact that they did not want to keep the story alive by attacking Vice Minister Martinelli: "The UC Berkeley researchers . . . welcomed the government's findings and said their only interest is determining the cause of the unidentified illness. 'We made a presumptive diagnosis,' Mantini-Briggs said Friday. A Venezuelan who has long worked among the Warao, she said, 'The important thing is for them to clear up the causes of the deaths.'" His 280-word story was reprinted in newspapers around the world and on such Internet sites as Yahoo! News.

Carmen tried to bring the story back to life. Every time Minister Serrano gave a press conference, her first question pressed him on Vice Minister Martinelli's promise to release the results of the commissions' investigations and explain the cause of the deaths. Carmen took her queries to MPPS's press corps. They told her, "This topic is completely taboo for us. This issue was handled at the highest level." After Serrano resigned, Carmen did not pursue it further. Remarkably, the opposition press played a leading role in enabling the very government they despised to dispose of what officials took to be a major threat to their authority: a strong assertion of health/communicative rights. We return to this issue in chapter 8.

part II
———

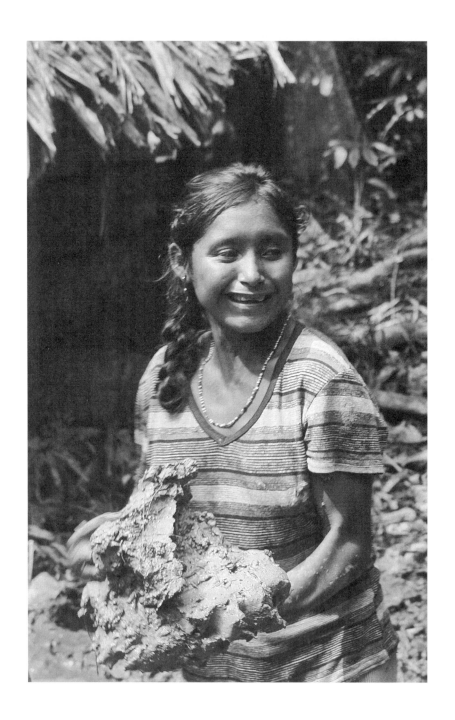

NARRATIVES, COMMUNICATIVE MONOPOLIES, AND ACUTE HEALTH INEQUITIES

Although the mysterious epidemic involved a unique configuration of viruses, bats, cats, chickens, cattle, and human bodies, it nonetheless has important commonalities with epidemics that kill millions each year with HIV/AIDS, tuberculosis, malaria, and other diseases. Part I offered a kaleidoscope of the viewpoints taken up by sets of actors discussed in turn—parents, doctors, and so on—each bringing in different perspectives on what transpired. Part II shifts to a more reflective, analytic mode, using tools provided by thinkers in the fields of medicine, anthropology, public health, psychiatry, and sociology, even as it continues to build on the insights provided by the people who faced the strange epidemic. Their narratives, their efforts to make their knowledge mobile and circulate it, the work of their mourning, and their challenges to health/communicative inequities all yield striking new insights into the mechanisms that produce such health problems as well as the sorts of collaborations that can help circumvent future "mysterious epidemics." Part I was tightly focused on the events and how participants perceived, talked about, and acted on them; the following chapters shift focus frequently between the epidemic and broader issues it raised. In these chapters we attempt to sharpen—but not to explain away—these mysteries and discern the breakthroughs they can yield. In sync with Michel de Certeau (1984), the shift from part I to part II is less a movement from facts to theory than an attempt to expand on the insights forged by people in the delta in building a new analytics of health.

Learning to Appreciate the Social Lives of Stories

The parents' demand, "Tell me why my children died" has outlived these deaths and even the epidemic itself; it still resounds through the lower delta. The stories they insisted on telling detailed how they cared for their children and how they labored to enlist others to help save their lives. As Garro and Mattingly (2000a, 27) suggest, rather than being about illness per se, such stories "are better characterized as being about a life disrupted by illness"; the stories we heard in Mukoboina, Muaina, and elsewhere recounted how lives, individual and collective, had been shattered by multiple illnesses and deaths. They quintessentially embodied a quality that Byron Good ascribes to illness stories in general, a "subjunctivizing" character that has "the potential to recast reality in relation to the unexpected, the non-ordinary, a predicament, the mysterious" (1994, 164–165). Rather than ending when the children died, their accounts grew longer and longer, because they also revolved around the occasions on which the parents sought to tell people what had happened and hear what others had learned. Over and over, the parents stressed that the failure to listen to their narratives and respond had greatly exacerbated their pain, seeming to compound the biological death of their children with a social death. This deafness did not affect only them but thwarted efforts by doctors, nurses, epidemiologists, and healers to diagnose and stop the epidemic. These narrative inequalities did not simply reflect but helped produce acute health inequities and their profound consequences. In attempting to sort out these issues, following the parents' guidance can help us greatly extend scholarly insights.

When health problems are deep, pervasive, and intractable, imposing the sorts of narrow limits and hierarchically structured rights to tell, listen, and request stories that emerged in the epidemic is tantamount to putting blinders on any search for its cause. Our analysis points to how narratives are crucial means of X-raying the way that forms of care, bodies, and human dignity circulate and how they get incarcerated by ethnoracial and other inequalities. Narratives constitute crucial sites for shaping relational identities and revealing and crossing ontological perspectives. They do not simply represent links between care and communication but reshape them continually. If, as Garro and Mattingly (2000b, 261) suggest, "one of the things that . . . narrative constructions do is demarcate the parameters of appropriate responses to deal with illness," who gets to tell stories, when, and how are crucial. Conrado and Alonzo demanded to tell their story in a politically visible setting in Tucupita; when policies and practices did not change—and official efforts to diagnose and stop the epidemic virtually disappeared—Conrado, Enrique, Norbelys, and Tirso claimed the right to narrate in MPPS headquarters in Caracas and in meetings with reporters. Officials emphatically told them—and the two of us—that such a narrative act was a criminal act, not a part of the fundamental right to health. You may have rights to health, they implicitly declared, but we hold a monopoly on health/communicative rights.

Linguistic anthropologists and conversation analysts have argued that narrative is a collaborative enterprise. Even when a single person is designated as the primary narrator, others, including people who are cast as audience members, often shape the unfolding story by expressing interest in particular details, challenging events or assessments, and even adding content. This was certainly true of the narratives of the epidemic, not just the ones performed in Mukoboina and Muaina but many told by doctors, nurses, healers, and others. Our analysis of collaborative narrative goes much further. Parents, patients, healers, other residents, nurses, physicians, epidemiologists, journalists, politicians, and others coproduced a vast network of circulating narratives about the epidemic.

Scholars generally envision narration as an aspect of communication, of the representation of medical facts, rather than as part of care; narratives are accommodated insofar as they achieve limited instrumental effects, especially providing and summarizing diagnostic detail and building trust in the physician or in enabling scholars to extract accounts of health-related phenomena. Here we present a different point of departure. We attend to the coproduction of narratives and medical subjects and objects in a range of contexts, including clinical medicine and epidemiology. Second, like Mattingly (1998), we see narratives not as representing care but as co-produced with it. Third, differential rights to tell and circulate health-related narratives, to structure their content and their effects, is a powerful dimension of health/communicative inequities and a powerful shaping influence on health inequities. Scholars are no less caught up in this matrix than anyone else. Finally, because narratives and health inequities are coproduced, the former provide particularly revealing insights into what creates health inequities and obstacles to care. In the case at hand, the narratives we presented in previous chapters not only describe what happened but also can help us think about why the deaths occurred and why it took so long to diagnose the disease.

Focusing on narratives as a source of epidemiological information may seem to go against ways of talking about science and medicine that have exercised considerable influence over several centuries. The role of Newton, Boyle, and others in shaping modern science in northern Europe in the seventeenth century was preceded much earlier by the emergence of the "social fact"—observations that appeared isolated, objective, and easily extracted from the contexts in which they were produced and the interests, opinions, and social positions of the people who inscribed them (Poovey 1998). Starting in the nineteenth century, numbers and diagnostic categories came to quintessentially embody what science studies scholar Bruno Latour (1988) has referred to as "immutable mobiles," objects of knowledge ideally capable of traveling anywhere without shifting reference or losing significance, with the category of rabies providing a prime example. Both numbers and categories purportedly escaped from the constraints of language; they thus maximally contrast with narratives, which appear thoroughly enmeshed in the specifics of tellers and audiences.

In the late twentieth century, narratives made a significant presence in the field of medicine. Criticizing medical education for erasing patient perspectives, Arthur Kleinman (1988) argues that clinicians can gain important insights into their patients' experiences of illness and explanatory models by listening to their "illness narratives." He reasons that "the sensitive solicitation of the patient's and the family's stories of the illness, the assembling of a mini-ethnography" is "a core task in the work of doctoring" (Kleinman 1988, 10, xiii). By soliciting patients' narratives, physicians can gain access to "the lived experience of monitoring bodily processes" (4). Making space for narratives told by patients and family members came to play a significant part in constituting today's "patient-centered medicine." Good and DelVecchio Good (2000) note that becoming "competent" as a physician is intimately caught up with learning to tell particular types of stories about patients, oneself, and other doctors and learning not to include details deemed medically irrelevant. It involves learning to disattend to ways that patients try to narrate their diseases, even while pretending to be listening attentively.

The power dynamics in situations where doctors control both care and narrativity have the potential to increase health/communicative inequities if, as Elliott Mishler (1984) urges, communicative processes themselves are not held up for critical scrutiny. Michael Taussig ([1980] 1992) writes critically that Kleinman's approach can "reify the consciousness of the patient"; interestingly, Taussig does not place the interview setting he used in constructing his argument—and his own self-presentation as both physician and anthropologist—under the same critical scrutiny.

Critical medical anthropologist Nancy Scheper-Hughes's research on organ transplantation has revealed how illegal practices of organ procurement threaten the lives of poor donors. Her work envisions narratives as springing from biomedical events, and she defines the discursive epicenter quite precisely: "Organ donors represent a social and semiotic zero" (Scheper-Hughes 2002, 55). From experiences with organ transplantation, representations of events should radiate outward through open discussion, accurate media accounts, and professional discourses to global publics. She decries how the transplant industry's suppression of donor voices, as well as "urban legends" and sensationalist press stories, have disrupted this necessary communicative circuit. Her research revealed a powerful nexus of health inequities and health/communicative inequities centered on the limited rights of poor "donors" to expose misrepresentation, malpractice, and illegality. In previous work, Scheper-Hughes (1992) closely links obstacles to the circulation of stories that poor mothers tell about losing babies to the structural factors that lead to high levels of child mortality. The stories of "organ theft" she collected, on the other hand, were produced to fit the needs of brief encounters and for subsequent mobilization by an anthropologist, not to situate the social lives of the narratives and efforts by patients and their relatives themselves to confront health/communicative inequities.

Social scientific attention to narratives has also drawn on sociologically based perspectives of ethnomethodology and conversation analysis. By listening to recordings of "doctor-patient interactions," researchers have abstracted a sequence that moves forward from an opening to identification of the presenting complaint, examination, diagnosis, and treatment and eventually to a phase that closes the interaction (Heritage and Maynard 2006). This research is often used in training physicians to learn how to interact with patients and family members, to be more attentive to patients' attempts to contribute diagnostically relevant information and the way power differences shape obstacles to care (Waitzkin 1991).

No matter how much time a physician devotes to hearing a patient's narrative, however, he or she exercises substantial control over who narrates, the form it takes, and how long the story proceeds. Good and DelVecchio Good quote a U.S. medical student's insightful observation: "Clearly I'm being told my job is to control that interaction. There's a message, very strong, that if you let the patient take over . . . you don't get anywhere, you ask an open-ended question, but you guide. You give the illusion of the patient controlling the situation when in fact you're controlling the situation" (2000, 56).

Recordings of conversations between the parents and Dr. Ricardo or physicians in urban hospitals are absent, but written records provide a measure of what clinicians deemed significant. References to details elicited by physicians, those fitted into the slots provided by medical narrative accounts, such as the prior deaths of siblings and descriptions of symptoms, are common. Parents' actions appeared noteworthy when they were perceived to be resisting physicians' recommendations: "The treating physician decided to refer her [to Tucupita], but the parents refused and proceeded to discharge the patient against medical advice." Dr. Ricardo and the medical students commented on visits "to the wasiratu [*sic*]." That clinicians had such a narrow ability to listen to their patients seems all the more remarkable to us after having ourselves faced the task of diagnosing the epidemic. Our concern was to gain as deep and broad a set of details as possible about the disease, and the ability of parents and other residents to provide this material and present it in compelling narrative form impressed us. Deciding in advance which details were relevant and how they fit together seems counterproductive in such situations. Neurologist and writer Oliver Sacks (1985) suggests that in medical narratives it is the pathology rather than the "human subject" that is the central character. Herein lies not only a source of conflict with the parents' narratives but also a major problem for biomedical narrators: it is hard to bring the pathology on stage when you have little idea as to its identity.

What patients say to practitioners helps shape the quality of the care they receive; learning to narrate their own bodies, to play the "sick role" (Parsons 1951), is central to displaying "competence" as a patient (Harvey 2008). A landmark study of U.S. health inequities stated that African American and Latino/a patients receive inferior treatment compared to Caucasians; it pointed to clinicians' perceptions of their patients' ability to understand what they are told and to turn physicians' recommendations into behavioral changes as one factor that contributes to this gap (Smedley, Stith, and Nelson 2002). The quantity and perceived quality of patients' questions also enter into such judgments. A study of Spanish-English medical translation analyzed how translators often fail to translate many of the patients' questions, leading English-speaking physicians to think that Spanish-speaking patients are less "active," less interested and involved in the therapeutic process than English speakers (Davidson 2001).

A major limitation of research on the role of narrative in medicine is that scholars generally tie narratives too closely to clinical contexts. This constraint has largely thwarted awareness of how professional domination is also evident in narratives that emerge in public health contexts. During the 1992–1993 cholera epidemic, RHS officials encapsulated what were projected as indigenous perspectives on medicine, healing, life, and death in stories about how cholera was spreading. Although these narratives presumably came from delta residents, our research demonstrated that they were often created by health professionals and that they helped structure public health policies, clinical practices, and responses by politicians and citizens.[1]

Insofar as public health policies are evidence based, that evidence is primarily epidemiological and statistical. Policies are generally proposed, debated, and enacted within the walls of public health's institutional spaces, limiting participation largely to professionals and politicians; patients and their narratives seldom enter, except as repeated by public health insiders. Popular narratives do sometimes become visible in health education and promotion; emerging in what are generally deemed to be the least prestigious sectors of public health departments, such narratives are often taken as erroneous conceptions to be displaced by hypodermic injections of biomedical knowledge (Dutta 2008). Both the cholera and rabies epidemics provide classic examples of how what are presented as popular narratives are used in proving why patients, rather than authorities, are to blame when health problems are exposed, not as suggesting clues for developing more creative and effective policies and practices.

Conrado's and Enrique's interventions in Tucupita and Caracas suggest that when laypersons do bring narratives regarding health problems to officials, responses often center on quelling what is perceived as a challenge and producing more authoritative official accounts. Chapter 3 documents Mukoboinan parents' struggles to interest epidemiological investigators in listening to their narratives and to induce the visitors to share their own interpretations. Epidemiologists misconstrued residents' frustration after being rebuffed as evidence of "the community's closed nature" (*lo cerrado de la comunidad*), as a refusal to share information. This impasse thwarted diagnosis and added greatly to the parents' anguish and anger. The epidemic provides a dramatic example, but the common deafness of public health professionals to the value of popular narratives as sources of valuable knowledge—rather than popular misconceptions—is hardly limited to the delta.

Social scientists also create their own narrative monopolies. Eliciting a narrative in an interview is like scheduling a C-section: researchers don't have to wait until stories appear, possibly at inconvenient times or in ways that might not fit their needs; rather, they can stage them in events that are largely under their control. The questions they ask shape the content and structure; follow-ups, along with expressions of interest or glances at the list of questions, signal how long responses should be ("could you tell me more about that?" versus "thanks, let's move on.").[2] Good social science interviewers attend to the emerging interaction, but their participation is largely oriented toward providing content for the texts they want to publish. The technologies chosen—audio recording, videotaping, or note taking—reflect the desired types of analysis and texts. Researchers obtain almost complete rights to decide subsequently which parts of the interviews to use, how to interpret and recirculate them, and what ends they will serve. Consent forms may limit these rights, but, once signed, the intellectual property generally belongs to the researcher. Ethnographers are sometimes open to stories that do not fit their expectations, but such detours are shaped by their interests, such as leading to a more creative, prestigious publication.

Whether a week or a year had passed since their child died, telling the story once again in the presence of neighbors and leaders like Conrado, Enrique, and Tirso was incredibly important to the parents. This act of public witnessing suggests the applicability of the Spanish term *testimonio*, which describes narratives that spring from pressing, often life-or-death concerns of people who have experienced poverty, exploitation, or violence. John Beverly (2004) notes that the term suggests an act of testifying, which accords well with the way that Conrado and Enrique created meetings that were meant to transform the parents' words into matters of public record. A testimonio, Beverly (2005, 548) argues, "takes the form of an I that demands to be heard and recognized," a protest against class and ethnic hierarchies that silence or exclude "subaltern" voices.

Remarkably, narratives focusing on epidemics or acute health inequities are seldom given the same sort of attention as those associated with political violence; what happened in the delta points to the importance of such narratives as well as how they can challenge political-economic, health, and communicative inequities. In such classic testimonios as *I, Rigoberta Menchu*, the context of narration is created largely by the researcher, and the stories fit the researcher's visions of what a story should include to make it appear authentic and enable it to have an impact. Such testimonios are generally presented as extraordinary narratives, not as part of the tellers' everyday narrative practices. By contrast, the parents' narratives were set in the rhythms both of everyday life and care and of coping with an extraordinary, mysterious situation. Telling the story of the deaths had formed part of the daily work of mourning and forging healthier futures long before our meetings took place. The two of us did not occasion these acts of narration, nor was our role in structuring them central; rather, both the context of their performance and the imperative that the information circulate were occasioned by the parents' demand, "Tell me why my children died." If testimonios are to be of value as tools for addressing gross social inequities, then it is important to make sure that their telling, inscription, and circulation is not part of a scholarly or other extractive, decontextualizing agenda but enters into the everyday economy of narration and the ends that different tellers and audiences seek to achieve with them. We must appreciate, as Das (2007) suggests, their silences and interruptions rather than immediately turning them into the sorts of narrative structures told from beginning to end where all parts seem to fit together and satisfies the expectations of audiences who view such situations from afar.

Mishler (1984, 1986) emphasizes fostering more egalitarian interview situations in both medicine and social science, creating narrative exchanges that can challenge power inequalities. Waitzkin's (1991) work points to the possibility of using power inequalities in clinical settings as a means of examining the effects of broader political-economic inequities on health rather than simply reproducing them. Dutta (2008) utilizes subaltern narratives and perspectives as fundamental tools for recasting health communication. Popular epidemiology uses "lay ways of knowing" in analyzing environmental and other health problems (Brown 1997). Community-based participatory research generates partnerships between laypersons and public health professionals in conducting inquiries and disseminating results (Minkler and Wallerstein 2008). Paul Farmer (2003) has used narratives in refocusing the attention of global health audiences on health inequities and to press for broader access to appropriate care. He retells stories—from those of the first people to die from HIV/AIDS in a small Haitian village to those told by U.S. epidemiologists—in making sense of how viruses, racial inequalities, and explanations intersected during the epidemic's early days (Farmer 1992).

Even as scholars have come to appreciate the important role of narratives in clinical medicine and public health, some fundamental questions remain. What characteristics infuse narratives with value? How might narratives be viewed as a fundamental part of care rather than simply representing it? What kinds of lives do narratives live as natural/cultural objects? And what can tracing the links between narratives and care contribute to studying acute health inequities and designing policies aimed at ameliorating them? In order to answer these questions, scholars and practitioners alike need a new point of departure.

Let us begin with the insights from Menéndez (2005, 2009) that we discussed in the introduction, particularly those regarding *autoatención*, the labor we perform on a daily basis in attending to our own bodies and those of our family members and coworkers. He argues that physicians depend on the work that family members do but seldom acknowledge; the previous chapters pointed to how even the parents' extensive labor performed for their children got erased or pathologized. Dutch philosopher Annemarie Mol (2008) outlines the "logic of care," the flexible, collaborative, quasi-experimental efforts, knowledge, and practice in which people interact with the world, each other, and bodies in preventing and coping with health problems. Our eyes, ears, and hands—not to mention our brains, nerves, hearts, and joints—are all tied to monitoring our own corporeal states and those of persons within our circles of care. We touch ailing partners, children, and elderly parents, move bodies that cannot move themselves, clean their noses, wipe off feces, bathe them, introduce food or pills, touch foreheads, and use technologies.

Let us extend these insights by drawing on Walter Benjamin's classic essay, "The Storyteller." Master craftsmen of the Middle Ages, he argues, learned their trade and repertoires of stories simultaneously. Accordingly, hand, mouth, and ear came together for them and their clients as the production of material goods fused with the circulation of narratives "in the milieu of work" (Benjamin 1969, 85, 91). Benjamin argues that the sensorial aspect of storytelling, "by no means a job for the voice alone," also involves the hand that unites narrative and labor "with its gestures trained by work" (102).

The work that interests us is the work of care that unfolded in the homes of families and healers, just as in clinics and hospitals. No less than for craftsmen, the work of care, labor, and narration are deeply imbricated. We look, listen, and talk, extracting material for narratives: "How are you feeling this morning?" "How many times have you gone to the bathroom?" "Does your head still hurt?" Our hands and eyes are tied to our mouths and ears in composing narratives designed to travel in particular ways. Touching a forehead, taking a temperature, listening to a cough, and delivering a spoonful of cough suppressant are all simultaneously forms of care and elements in the narratives that may be subsequently performed: after dialing 911, saying, "No school today!," or collaboratively producing a narrative with a clinician. Accordingly, care stories are entwined with forms of care, constructed by those in contact with bodies, revolving around their temporalities ("She was getting worse . . ."), appearances, and subjectivities. As acts of care continue, stories grow and move, multiplying the intersections between descriptions of acts of narration and of care: "My daughter told me she didn't feel well. Then I saw the rash. I called my mother, and she said, 'That doesn't sound good: take her to the doctor right away.' So here we are."

Basic features of narratives interweave them finely with forms of care. Richard Bauman (1977) and Dell Hymes (1981) stress the emergent quality of narrative performances. Each time a parent told a narrative, it was tied to the particular setting in which it unfolded—whether in the Nabasanuka clinic, a presentation to a healer, or an appeal to a mother. Rather than reflecting a fixed context, performances help structure interactions and how participants perceive them. Events of narration and narrated events, in Roman Jakobson's (1957) terms, are related iconically, meaning that the feeling, sounds, and space of the scenes recounted come to reshape the present even as this iconic effect works backward, folding features of performances into senses of the past.

In the powerful passage in which Florencia Macotera described Dalvi's death, she used her arms, eyes, and body to map the spaces in which he sickened and died onto the space around the white plastic chair in which she was narrating; her body became his as, gesturally, she inscribed each symptom on it (figure 1.13). Acoustically, the account was a dialogue that alternated between her own and Dalvi's higher-pitch voices. Her face reflected his shifts between fear (of the Power Ranger monsters), desire (recounting his dead cousin's promise, "There are movies up there. There are cartoons"), and compassion ("for you I won't die"), with the term of address "Mama" marking each shift into Dalvi's voice. At the same time, narratives model processes of circulation: parents and epidemiologists alike included the story of how they obtained the knowledge they were repeating and when, where, and to whom they had recounted it previously. Stories thus revolve around both situatedness, retaining their ties to contexts of care and performance, and circulation, how knowledge and bodies traveled. Parents pointed to futures of various sorts, particularly their frequent demand, "Take our words to Chávez!" and an end to health inequities and health/communicative inequities.

The way Florencia wove Dalvi's voice into her own points to another feature of narratives: how they project the interpenetration of multiple subjectivities, voices, and perspectives. M. M. Bakhtin (1981) reveals this heteroglossic character of narratives, analyzing how a single story purporting to represent a single perspective is shot through with other stories, times, places, and perspectives. V. N. Vološinov (1973) points to the centrality of reported speech to narrative, the complex and multiple ways that utterances attributed to characters are quoted or reinterpreted. He argues that reported speech does not juxta-pose preexisting identities and voices but analyzes, characterizes, and often essentializes them relationally. As Florencia quotes Dalvi, she imbues his voice with remarkable compassion and maturity, projecting a dying nine-year-old comforting his mother and attempting to dull the sharp edge of the grief she will feel. When Dr. Roselia quotes Elbia or Indalesio as saying that Mamerto "couldn't go pee," adding that "those were the colloquial words of his relative," she accentuates both the professional, medicalized perspective she attributes to herself and the lay, seemingly childlike voice she is quoting. When Conrado describes the meeting that took place in RHS headquarters in February 2008, he reverses this type of relationality: He quotes both his own initial presenta-tion, "We came here to say that the children continue to die, and we can't see that you are taking steps," and how an official responded, "Everything these Indians say is a lie. We give them medicines, but these Indians always steal them and the gasoline. They don't know anything and they are just gossips." Conrado then interpreted the officials' words: "They were scolding us as if we were chil-dren." Conrado projects himself as making a factual, sober assessment of health problems and the official as insulting, uncaring, and irrational, reversing the standard relational definitions. Conrado uses this reported exchange to project how officials responded to the epidemic and to map a shift in his own voice and affective posture: "I didn't come here to fight—or to be insulted. But if you want war, you'll have war!" (*¡Pero si eso es lo que ustedes quieren, entonces aquí va a ver candela!*) Looking closely at narratives enables us to locate the moments at which relational definitions—such as doctor versus patient and indigenous versus nonindigenous—continually are produced, examined, and contested.

One of the central preoccupations of scholars of narrative is time. Labov and Waletzy (1967) define narratives as correspondences between linear sequences of clauses and actions, giving a story the feeling that the events happened in the order that the words are unfolding. Bauman (1986) suggests that events do not preexist narratives; rather, senses of boundedness, discreteness, and continuity of events are themselves largely created in narratives. Briggs (1988) shows how such grammatical features as tense and aspect create complex temporal con-tours of narrative actions, particularly placing audiences in the middle of actions as they unfold and making them seem to extend indefinitely into the future or suddenly cutting them off, converting them into an inaccessible past. Paul Ricoeur (1980, 167) invokes Heidegger in arguing that in narrative "temporality springs forth in the plural unity of future, past, and present." Das (2007) urges us, however, to think of time in narrative not as representation but as work, a suggestion that accords well with our Benjaminian framework.

Rather than a "plural unity of future, past, and present," the parents, particularly those who lost multiple children, seemed to be lost in the inaccessibility and disarticulation of pasts, presents, *and* futures. The pasts they constructed were populated by sequences of acts of care and efforts to find help, the narrative logics, linearities, and teleologies unraveled by the utter failure of all efforts to save their children, pasts that remained ghostly through the failure to ever get a straight answer in response to their demand, "Tell me why my children died." The presents that the parents constructed were dominated by what seemed to be the inevitability of a future in which these pasts would be repeated. Over and over, parents returned from the urban hospital or the graveyard to find that "the same fever, the same disease" was claiming another child. One can certainly hear a unity of future, past, and present as Florencia reports observing that Dalvi's symptoms were appearing one by one in Mamerto: "I can see that you will not recover. Your brother Dalvi has been dead a week, and you have the same disease." This is, however, a grim, lethal fusion of temporal horizons. The only way that this "unity" could be escaped, it seemed, was by resisting the temporal and spatial logic, as in Yordi's resistance to Dr. Ricardo's request to send him to Tucupita: "Mommy, I don't want to go. If I go, I'll die." It is in this context that we hear Elbia's statement to her parents, after returning from Puerto Ordaz with Mamerto's body and his symptoms: "I'm not going to any clinic. I'm going to die in my home."

If narratives help to shape the temporalities of care, who gets to construct their temporal features is crucial. When does the story begin? For health professionals, the story generally started with the onset of symptoms and ended with the child's death. Parents and other residents started earlier, looking back to conflicts surrounding government contracts and environmental destruction from cattle ranchers, as well as disputes with neighbors. The temporal parameters of the narrative slots that parents could fill in when speaking with clinicians and epidemiologists were so narrow that there was no room for their observations regarding a chicken die-off a year previously, or the wave of nocturnal bat attacks, or the bat bites received by the patient a month or two earlier. Enrique constantly pushed the epidemic's temporal boundary further back, pointing to the negative effects of colonialism on delta settlements, starting with Columbus's arrival in 1498. In doing so, he opened up the sorts of historical, political-economic, and cultural issues that critical epidemiologists like Breilh (2003) and medical historians like Anderson (2006) argue are crucial for finding the roots of health inequities. When clinicians and epidemiologists imposed narrow, a priori temporalities, they ensured that the epidemic would not lead to broader scrutiny of the deplorable health conditions in general or of the policies that sustain them. Residents and leaders like Conrado and Enrique pushed for narratives that also included futures, efforts to recognize the value of delta residents' lives and to prevent future deaths.

Complex iconic webs of the labor of care and the labor of narration travel with patients, relatives, healers, and health professionals. Like bodies, stories are examined and evaluated. Some narratives or parts thereof are excluded from clinical spaces ("I hate to interrupt you, but let's get on with the examination"); some elicit praise ("Good thing that you decided to come in to see me immediately!") or condemnation ("Can't you recognize a simple cold? Why are you in the ER asking for antibiotics!"). Benjamin writes, "traces of the storyteller cling to the story the way the handprints of the potter cling to the clay vessel" (1969, 92). Rejecting a narrative or reducing it to details given in response to physicians' questions can be construed as rejecting embedded forms of care and the people who provided them. In the case of the epidemic, each increase in the medicalization of care correlated with an increase in the degree of rejection of these narrative/care assemblages, culminating in the imposed muteness of parents in urban hospitals. Epidemiologists seemed to be on the same page here with clinicians: they invited details designed to fit into their narratives, but otherwise rejected the parents' labors of care and narrative. Again, it seemed clear in countless interviews that rejecting narratives and denigrating the parents' labor of care increased their pain and sustained the resulting anger and devastation right through to the present. The deleterious effects of these rejections of care/narrative conjunctions is hardly limited to the parents: when the case summaries, letters, and entreaties that Dr. Ricardo sent to his superiors were met with silence, both his and the nurses' efforts to provide more effective care were thwarted.

Relationships between care and narration are not static. Indeed, how care unfolds is structured narratively, as Mattingly (1998) argues. The way parents and patients such as Yordi Torres responded to symptoms was affected by accounts of what had happened to previous patients. Epidemics can also be imbued with narrative structures, as Rosenberg (1992) and Lindenbaum (2001) argue. The diarrheal disease investigation of February 2008 indicates that the work of epidemiology can both respond to and anticipate not just broad and general narrative structures but specific narratives, including news stories. The articles on fruit and wisidatu responded to rumors that circulated in Tucupita, just as Carmen Buenaventura's coverage was informed by MPPS representative Rodríguez's stories of sorcery and culture. The cholera stories suggest how long a narrative can outlive the context of care in which it emerged, even losing its connection to a particular disease. For many parents, seeing the shocking evidence of autopsies on their children's bodies led them to retell stories of care in urban hospitals as tales of torture. Even as they wove narratives and care together intimately, the parents often questioned relationships between knowledge and care—as did healers, doctors and nurses, epidemiologists, and journalists—in confronting the failure to save their children's lives. The interventions we are making in these pages do not reveal intrinsic, objective connections but rather enter into this shifting, uncertain, and powerful field of connections and disconnections.

Even as they are tied to care, these narratives also have their own social lives. A useful analogy comes from the literature on objects and materiality. Arjun Appadurai (1986) notes that scholars learn little about objects when they see them as inert things that are simply inserted into human lives; he argues for the need to investigate the social lives of things, or, as Kopytoff (1986) adds, their biographies. Narratives similarly have social lives that extend beyond individual contexts and narrators. After the epidemic ended, stories about it continued to circulate, expand, and contract, some features taking on new forms of significance and guiding relations of care even as other dimensions seem to float out—like the current of the Orinoco tributaries—into a vast sea of forgotten narratives.

Health Inequities, Narratives, and the Temporalities and Teleologies of Care

The preceding discussion could be interpreted as yet another plea for clinicians, public health practitioners, and scholars to pay more attention to narratives, but this is not our point. Like forms of care, stories were everywhere, engulfing everyone. Just as diagnosis and treatment failed, narratives failed as well: their proliferation and rapid circulation only seemed to create more barriers between the people who needed to link knowledges and perspectives. Some narratives, like those about poisoned fruit and fish, created more pain for the people who lost children, piling social deaths on top of biological deaths. Our goal in tracing how care and narrative were linked is to think through the role of narrative in this mystery and see if the process can yield any insights into how care and narrative can come together more productively.

What could be termed a methodological point is in order. Most scholarly studies of narrative and health focus on one type of site, such as clinical ones, or elicit narratives in multiple places (such as clinics and homes) without documenting the narrative economies that exist in each and how narratives move (or fail to travel) between them. We drew on our observations during the epidemic and subsequently on time spent with the families and their neighbors, extensive interviewing, MPPS documents, media stories, and other sources, not to mention decades of work in the delta as physician and ethnographer, in tracing these narrative/care alignments and gaps. This is not to say that we have been able to construct a totalizing, definitive account that maps all forms of care and all narratives and their routes of circulation and effects. To the contrary, each new perspective increased our appreciation of the complexity and consequentiality of these connections and the way that our own positionalities sometimes facilitated, sometimes impeded, but always shaped our ability to document them.

As we tracked stories, we discerned two major ways that their circulation thwarted collaboration. First, most participants expressed fairly clear ideas about care, structuring what form or forms of care they thought most appropriate to diagnosing and treating the disease. They clearly differed with respect to their breadth and degree of flexibility, with the parents exhibiting the broadest, most plastic, but most uncertain ideas about what types of health modalities might be of value in saving their children's lives. Even as this issue formed a major topic of debate, few of our interlocutors seemed to have thought much about how care should be narrated, even though—as part I suggests—the differences between narrative modes and the algorithms used to link narrative and care were no less diverse. As we have argued throughout, positing a chasm between communication and healing and reserving causal status and ontological priority to the latter seems to have shaped this lack of explicit attention to how fashioning care/narration connections provided a crucial mechanism by which different perspectives on care were transformed into opposing ontological positions, creating barriers to linking efforts to diagnose and control the epidemic. It is here, once again, that Conrado's and Enrique's insights—which prompted them to organize the investigation—point to what can be achieved by critically engaging both health and health/communicative issues simultaneously.

We will use psychoanalysis, specifically the concepts of displacement, condensation, and projection, in elucidating a second dimension of these obstacles to more fruitful exchanges of narrative/care relations.[3] *Displacement* refers to a transfer of meaning from one domain to another, thereby shielding the displaced object from consciousness and explicit discursive representation. Perhaps the central example of displacement was the effect of the Maturín toxicologist's mercury hypothesis as it displaced attention to symptoms, environmental conditions (such as the proliferation of vampire bats), and events (such as the bat bites). Similarly, the legacy of the cholera narrative, with its construction of "the Warao" as unhygienic and parents classified as indigenous as being unconcerned with their children's health, displaced many of the specific features of this epidemic in the images of poisoned fruit and fish, adenoviruses or enteroviruses, and a massive epidemiological investigation of "normal" diarrheas.

Condensation refers to cases in which one symbol becomes so prevalent and charged that it comes to reorganize a host of others. Condensation emerged when autopsies came to form a crucial condensed symbol that reorganized how the parents and local representatives thought about all dimensions of care and communication associated with physicians. The wide circulation of narratives that described parents' experiences of opening coffins to discover that their children's heads had been "split . . . open from front to back" turned autopsies into a condensed symbol that prompted other parents to refuse to take children with other symptoms to the Nabasanuka clinic.

Finally, disarticulations sometimes emerged through what psychoanalysts would call *projection*, such as when epidemiologists attributed their diagnostic failure in Mukoboina and their unwillingness to listen to the parents' narratives to "the community's closed nature." Crucially, the stereotype that was distilled from the cholera epidemic—depicting "the Warao" as incapable of understanding what doctors say or acting in keeping with biomedical rationality—continues to provide a pervasive form of projection, one that makes it harder to see RHS's role in sustaining health inequities and health/communicative inequities.

Even as they were deeply embedded in health inequities and broader social and political-economic injustices, these narrative/care conjunctions and disjunctions were closely entwined with communicative inequities. In Caracas, Venezuelan doctors, public health officials, and barrio residents all speak Spanish, but only some of them have the symbolic and financial capital to access professional vocabularies. Mission Barrio Adentro emerged when these differences of language and perspective came together in horizontal exchanges of ideas between planners, physicians, and residents that continued, at least in the mission's early years, on a daily basis. In the delta, the lay/professional divide is greatly augmented by how the nonindigenous/indigenous binary is entwined with the opposition between Warao and Spanish languages. The power attached to "the national language" structured the vastly greater mobility of narratives told in Spanish.

Officials' attitudes toward "translation"—that is, toward multilingualism and linguistic/social inequities—were telling. Their failure to appreciate the importance of translation and to credit the nurses' crucial role as translators, along with the use of motorboat operators as translators, not only impeded knowledge exchange but also signaled the imposition of linguistic as well as other forms of health/communicative domination. A bilingual nurse not only would know Spanish and Warao but also would have access to dimensions of the onto-logical perspectives and semiotic practices associated with biomedical and heal-ing specialties. Considering translation to be a minor, mechanical issue pointed to a pervasive disinterest in residents' ontologies and the narratives and other forms they used to explore them. A large literature documents how closely lan-guages and social identities are related; when relations between languages (or language varieties) and racialized populations are substantial, dismissing a language and associated discursive practices constitutes rejecting stigmatized social identities.[4] Health professionals were hardly alone here. *Notidiario* em-ploys no Warao-speaking reporters. When she arrived in the delta, Carmen Buenaventura was "surprised" by multilingualism—"It had never occurred to me that I would need a translator." The idea that fellow citizens might not speak Spanish produced a sense of an Otherness not easily reconcilable with a shared identity as Venezuelans. When the connection between a national iden-tity and a national language just seems to be natural, less-than-full citizenship is often conferred on those deemed unable to engage with what Benedict An-derson ([1983] 1991) characterizes as the forms of "print capitalism" (particu-larly newspapers and novels) that embody conversations between citizens in the national language. Here cultural constructions of language—often called language ideologies—go hand in hand with those of medicine, amplifying the potential of each for extending and naturalizing inequities.

Exploring more deeply and broadly the labor of care and the labor of narra-tion has much to offer. Such narratives embody the complex relations between "models of" and "models for" that Geertz (1973) outlined. In their capacity as models of, narratives purport to iconically mirror acts of care and communica-tion that have occurred, reporting what happened. Some claim to be direct and transparent, as, for example, the detailed reports of symptoms, tests, and communications or tabular representations of cases emerging in the epidemi-ologists' reports; others, particularly parents' narratives, constantly announced their opacity and uncertainty, a wealth of details constantly inflected by "We just didn't know" and "We still don't know." All narratives are selective and in-terpretive, choosing details that seem relevant, deciding on starting and ending points that exclude actions that lie outside them, including particular places and actions and excluding others, and using particular modes of indexical cali-bration. At the same time, narratives of care are models for constructing disease, health, care, communication, and relations between people, viruses, animals, and environments in particular ways. Their linearities and teleologies seem to require particular actions of care and communication. Narratives attempt to shape futures, such as the immediate unfolding of a clinical interaction or media story or more distant, utopian futures where health is not experienced as a site of violence and gross inequity.

Like so many other aspects of what happened in the epidemic, a detailed look at care/narrative relations can engender pessimism, optimism, or both. The narratives were rich sources of insight into the epidemic, yielding a host of clues about what was killing the children. They also provided extremely powerful X-rays of health and health/communicative inequities. Tracing how they circulated and when they became immobile enabled us to pinpoint how relational ontologies were reproduced, frequently in ways that impeded intersubjective links and knowledge exchanges. It became clear that acts of listening to narratives with presence of mind is just as important as acts of performing them. Nevertheless, structural barriers impeded the circulation and appreciation of narratives, from sharing clues about the nature of the disease and how it was spreading to what the narratives could tell us about why such catastrophic health problems and health inequities arise and why they are so difficult to disrupt.

The parents' demand, "Tell me why my children died," and Conrado's and Enrique's insights and interventions point to the potential of exploring care/ narration relations for rethinking and reorganizing health systems. Acts of telling stories were not just descriptions of health/communicative inequities but interventions into this economy of death and discourse. Acts of narration constituted assertions of health/communicative rights. Inequities of care and communication do not just fade away, of course, once narratives expose them. When these narratives, particularly the ones told by the team in Caracas, were deemed criminal acts of political subversion, their political effects were limited at every turn. Nevertheless, they did circulate, and, still alive, their potential for disrupting health inequities and health/communicative inequities perseveres.

A number of broader lessons also emerge. Health/communicative rights must include rights to tell one's health-related story in the settings where policies and practices are debated. Social and political change rarely emerges when issues remain invisible. A more fair distribution of rights to shape the languages in which debates emerge is also required; if stories only count when they are clothed in the language and narrative structures privileged by clinical medicine or epidemiology, stories and storytellers will be ranked hierarchically, and most will lose their potential for shaping new ways to confront health problems. Health/communicative rights also include access to insert one's narratives in arenas seen as quintessentially public, to gain access to media coverage and political meetings. More broadly, when a situation of acute health inequity is denied a public, when efforts to generate a sphere of visibility, concern, and debate are suppressed, both health inequities and health/communicative inequities will continue to haunt clinical practice, epidemiology, and policy making, suppress relationships between modalities of care, and exacerbate the impact of disease.

6

———

KNOWLEDGE
PRODUCTION AND
CIRCULATION

Much that happened during the course of the epidemic points to what a tricky, uncertain process knowledge production and circulation can be. By July 2008, people had been dying from a strange disease for a year. During periods in which new patients were appearing, parents, local leaders, doctors, nurses, healers, and epidemiologists were all looking for clues, and news of the epidemic continued to be the lead story on Warao Radio. Parents in other areas of the delta knew the symptoms that riddled the bodies of children in Muko-boina, which healers had tried to treat them, about the Nabasanuka nurses' and Dr. Ricardo's frustrations, and how autopsies had "split" their bodies. Everyone was angry, confused, and frustrated—and scared. Questions that were never asked and barriers of silence thwarted pulling information together. The symptoms pointed toward one diagnosis. The government denied it. Although MPPS never produced an alternative, it largely succeeded in taking "bat-transmitted rabies" away from delta residents as a way of thinking about the deaths.

Why weren't conclusive connections made? We could advance ignorance, cultural difference, corruption, political interest, or ethnoracial discrimination as candidate explanations, but simplistic analyses cannot account for a situation in which there were no villains, no monsters (except perhaps the disease), and no saints. Determining how so much knowledge about the epidemic could have been produced and circulated, only to leave nearly everyone angry and confused, requires a fresh analytic approach.

Care and knowledge are both important. Sometimes physicians and patients collaborate in treating a case "empirically," meaning they try to find something that works even in the absence of a diagnosis. Sometimes, of course, there is knowledge without care, diseases for which no treatment is available, or when patients and physicians decide to use only palliative treatment in the final stages of life. But usually, the relationship between care and knowledge is more intimate, partial, and tense; the mysterious epidemic can provide insight into complex care/knowledge connections. Parents, other relatives, healers, nurses, and doctors provided lots of care that assumed a variety of forms, but it all failed, at least in terms of keeping people alive. The parents, patients, local leaders, nurses, doctors, healers, and epidemiologists presented in part I all tried to produce knowledge, and they all claimed to have produced evidence that might help sort out the epidemic. Just as the efficacy of forms of care was contested, so too were all knowledge claims. The use of herbal medicines, a rattle, and a song could as easily be construed as either potentially killing or curing the patient; the high technologies used in intensive care units could be considered torture or therapy. Equally, trying to bring in ideas about social conflicts over government jobs and vengeful water creatures could reflect privileged knowledge or fatal ignorance. The six team members were—and continue to be—right in the middle of all this.

This chapter looks more broadly and analytically at how care and knowledge were related, in part by thinking about how people standing next to one another in relationship to the same dying or dead body made overlapping and sometimes competing claims. If gaps between diverse perspectives thwarted diagnosis and exacerbated the epidemic's devastating impact, then exploring how these gaps were produced is crucial. Some accounts traveled broadly, while others—including most of Dr. Ricardo's observations—never got off the ground. What made some accounts mobile and others immobile? What were the costs of mobility and the circuits that shaped or channeled circulation? Here we must account for the making of nonknowledge—the active production of gaps in knowledge, forms of concealment, and labels that frame particular content as superstition or ignorance—as much as that of what gained the status of knowledge.

Analyzing Relations between Bodies, Knowledge, and Participation

Existing work in science-technology-society (STS) studies, medical anthropology, linguistic anthropology, and studies of globalization has opened up aspects of the problem of mobility and circulation. What is still needed, however, is an analytic that helps sort out how people make claims to knowledge, which we define loosely as the ways in which they attempt to add to the stock of observations and analyses, how they frame their contributions as credible and worth repeating, and how one set of knowledge claims impacts others. Philosopher and semiotician Charles S. Peirce's work proposes three types of signification—symbolic, indexical, and iconic—that offer a starting point for analyzing relations between diseased bodies and statements about them. In developing a framework for making sense of how knowledge claims are produced and circulated, this chapter draws on Peirce and on sociologist Erving Goffman's notion of participation frameworks and work on circulation. Thinking through the epidemic, focusing particularly on Mukoboina, can suggest how to build on Peirce and other scholars in coming to appreciate more fully how bodies, environments, contexts, and knowledges are coproduced.

SYMBOLIC AUTHORITY: LANGUAGES OF KNOWLEDGE

In one sense, "Tell me why my children died" demands a response in the language of biomedicine: it calls for a diagnosis. Most delta residents are at least passively multilingual in the languages of healing, meaning that they can engage with and repeat key terms from the powerful languages of healers and doctors without themselves being able to claim fluency in either. In the throes of the epidemic, they wanted interlocutors to acknowledge both the care they provided and the value of their children's lives; but, perhaps primordially, they still wanted a diagnosis. This is the single most important link between the perspectives of all of the people discussed—including ourselves: everyone wanted a diagnosis.

Here we enter the Peircean world of the symbol, "a sign which refers to the Object that it denotes by virtue of a law" (Peirce [1940] 1955, 102). A law, in this sense, is not enacted by a political body but is a relationship between a "sign vehicle" (or signifier) and a referent that is established by convention and exists apart from the context and social identity of the person invoking the symbol. From the start, the strange disease produced disorder, both corporeal and conceptual; a diagnosis promised to restore order. Accepting one diagnosis would rule out competitors: if it was diarrheal disease, then it was not mercury poisoning, intoxication from poisonous fruit or fish, or a strange, undiagnosed disease. A diagnosis would also provide valuable etiological resources, offering vast possibilities for making sense of such things as bodies, environments, foods, animals, and the failure of all the treatments used. A diagnosis would recruit infrastructures and institutions in particular ways, confirming the authority of some actors and ontological positions and casting others as failures. These statements apply no less to healers than to physicians: both groups have their own diagnostic categories. A diagnosis that gained wide acceptance could be transformed into prestige: "It was a hoa; I named it and extracted it!" "From the time the first patient arrived at the clinic, I suspected that it was X; and now I have confirmed it!"

The quest for a diagnosis theoretically put everyone on the same page. Systems of diagnosis should involve criteria that are not tied to particular individuals or contexts but operate consistently over space and time. A classic work by Bowker and Star (1999) cuts to the heart of these issues of knowledge, categories, contexts, and mobility. They note that such things as diagnostic categories are "boundary objects" that are held in common by actors occupying distinct social spheres but are defined and used in different ways by distinct groups of actors. A diagnosis can travel across social borders and maintain a sense of stability and yet be flexible enough to accommodate itself to each space it comes to inhabit. They additionally argue that employing modes of classification involves building what we will refer to as complex indexical histories, that is, particular assemblages of practices, epistemologies, technologies, materialities, and political interests. For example, physicians and epidemiologists should ideally have chosen the category that best matched the disease's signs and symptoms. But one reason that rabies is often not diagnosed is that physicians are more likely to invoke categories that they use on a regular basis, not those which they have never seen outside a medical school textbook. Similarly, invoking certain categories would unleash unwanted public health and political consequences. For example, a diagnosis of cholera, if confirmed, would require notifying the World Health Organization, getting bad press, terrifying residents, and probably the loss of jobs for top officials if an epidemic emerged. RHS officials wanted a diagnosis, but they didn't want just any diagnosis and certainly not one—like rabies—that seems to be tied to a long, culturally charged history of slobbering, unvaccinated dogs, thereby drawing negative attention from national and international health officials and journalists. Diarrheal diseases, on the other hand, are "normal" in this "indigenous area"; such a diagnosis would not be news and would not attract unwanted attention or highlight political vulnerabilities—particularly during an election year.

However, thinking about these diagnostic categories as boundary objects raises the possibility of creating a falsely egalitarian impression: not all boundaries are equal. Diagnosis involves what sociologist Pierre Bourdieu (1991) refers to as symbolic capital. For Bourdieu, the term points to the way that professional epistemologies, vocabularies, and practices require training in specialized educational institutions, such as schools of medicine and public health. The importance of symbolic capital and the status it affords becomes painfully clear when, for example, physicians scold patients for organizing their narratives around what they themselves deem to be relevant symptoms and what they propose as diagnoses and treatments. Patients are supposed to narrate only what they are experiencing, leaving it to the doctor to decide which details are diagnostically relevant and which diagnostic hypotheses should guide narration, physical examination, testing, and treatment. Delta healers can be equally dismissive of noninitiates who claim to know that a hebu, hoa, bahana, or other illness is present.[1] In the meeting in Muaina, healers did not share any of their technical vocabulary or detailed explanations with noninitiates. The limited symbolic capital associated with their training in simplified medicine generally limits delta nurses to invoking only a limited range of diagnostic categories—and to do so only when a physician is not present. A crucial premise for RHS, which often became explicit, is that "the Warao" are so lacking in biomedical symbolic capital that "they" are incapable of thinking and acting about health and hygiene. Healers devalued the parents' explanations because they lacked the symbolic capital associated with initiation and lengthy training. At the same time, both health professionals and healers appropriated knowledge elicited from parents and used it in their diagnostic and treatment efforts. Before Conrado and Enrique launched the team's investigation, no one appeared to think that the parents might have something valuable to offer when they demanded to tell detailed stories of their children's illnesses and deaths.

Linguistic anthropologist Asif Agha (2007) shows that this issue involves more than one-to-one pairings of particular statuses and specialized vocabularies (or registers); rather, everyday language use involves an active process of "enregisterment" in which words, statements, and practices become reflexive models of what are projected as particular types of persons. The regional epidemiologist's juxtaposition of medical terminology, colloquial expressions, and terms used by RHS insiders didn't just confirm his status as a physician and epidemiologist but also constructed him as a powerful medical and political figure at the center of a regional network. Some statements about the epidemic were "enregistered" as imbued with authority, whether clinical, statistical, or that associated with healers, even as others drew their force from invocations of entitlement, a sense of ownership emerging from telling one's own story, or empathy, as projecting particular types of liberal affects, such as pity (see Shuman 2005). Venezolana de Televisión host Ramón Martí added solidarity, a key feature emerging from Chávez's discourse and the socialist revolution. In other words, appeals to authority were not the only way to structure an account of the epidemic. Parents often pointed to their lack of symbolic authority: "I don't know" what killed Ángel Gabriel. "They didn't tell us. I have no idea." The symbolic authority associated with the search for a diagnosis provided all participants with a common vocabulary and goal at the same time that it stratified modes of knowledge production, creating impediments to producing and sharing knowledge.

INDEXICAL CALIBRATION: MEASURING
RELATIONS BETWEEN BODIES AND PERCEPTIONS

At the same time that they invoked the symbolic mode, knowledge claims also drew extensively on what Peirce (1932, 142) refers to as indexicality, the projection of an "existential relation" between a sign vehicle and its object. Peirce notes that "an *index* is a sign which refers to the object that it denotes by virtue of being really affected by that Object"; an index becomes "a sign of fact" (142). If a sign bears an indexical relationship to an object taken to be real, its presence offers proof of the existence of that object. Indexical relations are often shaped contextually, tying signs to aspects of the situation in which they emerged, including now absent contexts ("My daughter said to me before leaving for Tucupita [Hospital], 'Mama, I'm dying. I'm leaving you. I'm dying. I'm dying'"). In the epidemic, accounts revolved around quite different sets of objects—primordial spirits, social conflicts, pots of mercury, toxins, vectors, or microbes—at the same time that all accounts projected the same indexical point of origin: the same dying and dead bodies. All of the accounts, even denials that there was a mysterious epidemic, made claim to the same bodies. Nevertheless, as observers from Robert Hertz (1960) to Allen Feldman (1991) to Talal Asad (2007) to Charles Hirschkind (2008)—among many others—have argued, positing dead bodies as an zero point for calculating indexicality can be as precarious as it is productive.

Nevertheless, participants presented different types of indexical relations, that is, contrastive assertions regarding existential relationships between knowledge and bodies. Chapter 5 mentions the importance of temporality in organizing narratives, in shaping what got included and how notions of agency and causation were structured; temporal relations also figured strongly in shaping knowledge claims. One important feature of many parents' accounts was that the narrator was present from beginning to end. In her narrative, Florencia followed Dalvi through every moment and in every space in which his illness unfolded, even as she missed Mamerto's final days. Santa Torres's narrative marked her sadness at having to stay in Mukoboina to take care of her youngest, thereby missing the last chapter in the account of Yanilka's illness and death. This was, essentially, an indexical rupture, and she made a point of noting it.

Of interest here is the brilliant Russian literary theorist Mikhail Bakhtin's work on chronotopes, the ways that narratives project particular configurations of space and time. Generally, the parents shared a chronotope, one that revolved around a trajectory starting at home, moving to nearby healers and/or nurses, the Nabasanuka clinic, Tucupita Hospital, larger urban hospitals, and the cemetery, with each place linked in chronological order. If a child did not pass through one of these time/space slots, it was there in the story nonetheless, as an absence, such as in the accounts of parents whose children didn't make it to the clinic, in Alfonso Torres's decision to take Yanilka directly to Tucupita, and in Elbia's resolute refusal to leave home. The epidemiologists, even those who jointly participated in investigations, had vastly different chronotopes. Of the individuals who narrated their participation in the first epidemiological investigation in Mukoboina, the nurse, Antonio Peña, located his contact with sick children in the temporal parameters of the vaccination campaign that brought him to the settlement; for the sanitary engineer, Wilfredo Sosa, locating piles of tuna fish cans prompted him to broaden the time frame to that of a government food security program; and the mercury hypothesis lead Dr. Yolanda to start with gold mining that had taken place ten years earlier in another part of the delta. Nevertheless, everyone agreed on one chronotopic feature: Mukoboina was the epidemic's ground zero.

An important related point is that different participants privileged different moments as the focus of their attention. Mothers stressed the moment they perceived the first symptoms. Fathers, less responsible for the care of small children, knowing more Spanish, and less vulnerable to sexual abuse in cities, accompanied the children to Tucupita and Maturín or Puerto Ordaz; they stressed the patients' final days and hours. Dr. Ricardo's and the interns' accounts were intensively centered on the clinical encounter. The toxicologists and regional epidemiologist Froilán Godoy placed their bets on the times when samples were extracted and laboratory results obtained. The epidemiologists never worried about getting close to bodies: juxtaposing observations and results from blood tests, autopsies, and environmental samples provided them with what they saw as the most important means of linking bodies and statements. All along the way, different modes of perceiving bodies and symptoms, different senses and technologies were involved.

These competing cartographies of time, space, perception, technologies, and bodies provided the terms in which narrators infused some accounts with authority and cast others as rumor, superstition, ignorance, or criminal behavior. Projecting ministry spaces and activities as providing the only possible loci for counting bodies and creating knowledge about them gave MPPS minister Serrano, RHS director Dr. Guillermo, prosecutors Centella and Guzmán, and other officials ways to undergird their assertions to journalists that the team's numbers were false, its diagnosis mistaken, and team members' actions criminal. What we refer to here as *indexical calibration* encompasses both this process of projecting privileged points—temporal, spatial, technological, and so on—at which bodies can produce knowledge and how actors calculate their degree of proximity to those bodies and their modes of rendering them legible. Some narrators of the epidemic proclaimed—in clinical encounters, documents, statements to reporters, and interviews—their privileged access to what they characterized as particularly important sites: finding the first cases, having data on the most cases, or having laboratory and autopsy results in hand. Others' stories focused on the teller's failure to gain access to these critical points, the most striking example being Dr. Ricardo's recurrent observation that his ability to produce knowledge about the disease—and to treat his patients—was thwarted by the absence of summaries of clinical, laboratory, and autopsy reports and advice from specialists. Rather than a stable and fixed point, these indexical calibrations constitute overlapping forms of "knowledge and practice that construct death differently as an object of reflection, appropriation, and experience" (Hirschkind 2008, 54), fashioning particular pasts, presents, and futures for each death and positioning interlocutors and audiences in relation to them.

Individuals differed widely with respect to how much they incorporated multiple ontological perspectives in their calibrations of the relationship between bodies and diagnosis. Dr. Ricardo included both his clinical observations and whatever he could glean about the findings of epidemiologists and the examinations and tests performed in urban hospitals; the parents' observations occasionally entered into his account, but those of the nurses with whom he worked—let alone the Warao healers with whom he unwillingly shared patients—never entered his cartography. The parents, on the other hand, regarded the forms of care they provided along with those of healers, nurses, Dr. Ricardo, epidemiologists, and urban specialists as all generating points at which their children's bodies could yield knowledge, although bitter experiences in urban hospitals and discovering autopsies often led them subsequently to reclassify what took place there as abuse, not knowledge production. Some indexical calibrations turned others' knowledge claims into simple, unthinking, and mechanical acts of accompanying sick bodies, expressions of ignorance, or political strategizing. Journalist Carmen Buenaventura credited parents, doctors, and epidemiologists as all potentially producing knowledge about the disease, but only when it emerged from perspectives that were directly associated with their social roles; given her classification as indigenous, MPPPI representative Lourdes Rodríguez could legitimately speak about Warao "ancestral knowledge" in Carmen's five-part series on the epidemic, but she cut Governor Montoro to shreds when that politician tried to play epidemiologist, repeatedly pointing out imprecise statements on numbers and causes of death and contradicting RHS's own statements. Carmen characterized Montoro's interview to us as "horrible."

PARTICIPATION FRAMEWORKS: SHAPING ROLES IN THE PRODUCTION OF KNOWLEDGE

Simply having been there—being present at a particular spatiotemporal juncture in the course of a patient's illness and treatment—was not the sole consideration in shaping the nature of claims to knowledge production. Central points of convergence and disarticulation are revealed by what sociologist Erving Goffman (1981) refers to as "participation frameworks."[2] In the Nabasanuka clinic, parents, nurses, and physicians all shared the same space and the same goal: figuring out what was killing the children and saving their lives. Given the vastly different roles in which they were cast, however, coparticipation produced deep inequalities in the status each was assigned in knowledge production and how they were positioned in particular parts of the facility. Dr. Ricardo assigned parents a role that authorized them to answer the diagnostic questions that he directed at them, but he then claimed the remaining process of making knowledge and determining its treatment implications. When parents departed from this role by incorporating the possible contributions of healers, Dr. Ricardo characterized the parents as having failed to act in accordance with the only role they could appropriately fill. When they left home in search of help, the parents encountered situations in which they were granted little say in how participation frameworks were structured. They were saddened and sometimes angered by how these frameworks greatly reduced what they could contribute and their interlocutors' capacity to listen to them.

"Tell me why my children died" challenged these participation frameworks and demanded a collaborative search for alternatives. Mukoboinans asked to participate actively in epidemiological investigations, to play distinct but horizontally structured roles in knowledge production. When reduced to being objects of observation and respondents to brief biomedical questions, they rejected this proffered role angrily. More broadly, the parents' cry challenged the unilinear directionality of knowledge production that emerged in the epidemic: evidence produced by nurses, doctors, and epidemiologists in the delta traveled to Tucupita and, sometimes, to Maturín and Puerto Ordaz, but nothing seemed to come back. Their challenge thus coincided with Dr. Ricardo's request that health officials and urban specialists send the results of their investigations back to Nabasanuka, thereby potentially enabling him to treat patients more adequately and respond to the parents' demand to know what caused the deaths. The parents insisted that journalists include them in the participation frameworks they constructed, both as valuable sources and as intended readers, not cast them as being out of the loop.

Many scholars have expanded on Goffman's account of participation frameworks, but they have generally limited the scope of their analysis to social interaction, primarily face to face. Patients and caregivers were, however, embedded in much broader participation frameworks. Think of the refusal by seven-year-old Yordi: "Mommy, I don't want to go [to the clinic]. If I go, I'll die." Yordi had overheard numerous narratives told by Mukoboina parents who talked of Ángel Gabriel's death in Maturín and how children and parents had interacted with doctors and machines; all of these in situ participation frameworks had been packed into the narratives told in Mukoboina homes. Rumors and news articles produced in urban spaces shaped the roles that emerged in the delta; autopsies threatened to turn Dr. Ricardo and Conrado into RHS lackeys, to extract them from the roles of clinician and advocate.

Participation frameworks are similarly shaped by institutional hierarchies: Dr. Ricardo's ability to produce and receive knowledge about the disease was limited by his position as a *médico rural*, meaning that he was a low-status, newly graduated doctor working far from the urban centers that are the privileged sites for the production of medical knowledge. Dr. Yolanda far outranked him, but in the reports on the epidemiological investigations she enters into knowledge production only as a name included in lists of participants.

As MPPS minister Col. Rafael Serrano and regional health director Guillermo Rendón angrily reminded the team, participation in the production of knowledge about epidemics and health conditions in "indigenous areas" is limited to MPPS personnel and persons they authorize, thus asserting a particularly muscular and explicit participation framework.

Dr. Guillermo asserted that public health officials, none of whom identified as indigenous,[3] have a legal right, backed by criminal sanctions, to determine the participation framework for who produces knowledge about health conditions "in indigenous areas." There is a telling contradiction here. Delta Amacuro is a Venezuelan state. Antonio Díaz is one of its four municipalities. These are political designations that lack any special ethnoracial status. In the early 1990s, the Union of Indigenous Warao Communities pressed the government, unsuccessfully, for land demarcation that would give title to the entire lower delta collectively to Warao people, in other words, to truly turn it into an indigenous area. Pedro Salazar, who served in 2008 as mayor of Antonio Díaz, is classified as indigenous. Salazar was trying to make Dr. Guillermo's words come true, trying to create a municipality in which the rights of the majority of residents, who are classified as indigenous, lie at the center of political and administrative agendas. At the same time that Salazar accepted the ethnoracial binary as a central social fact, he sought to turn it on its political head. When he declared his candidacy for governor in 2008, Salazar threatened not just the caudillo leadership but a political-economic system that uses the ethnoracial binary as its fundamental logic, as a means of turning national allocations designated for the rain forest into a source of enrichment for political elites in Tucupita and preserving caudillo electoral dominance.

Governor Montoro and other officials accused us of cooking up the epidemic in order to back Salazar's candidacy, using the logic that turns all aspects of life in the state into manifestations of partisan politics. Her claim was empirically incorrect, but the political analysis was not entirely off base: by documenting an epidemic and taking this knowledge to Caracas, Tirso, Norbelys, Enrique, and Conrado threatened the political status quo—more fundamentally than Salazar did—by contradicting the stereotype that lies at its core and drawing attention to the perseverance of policies that reproduced just the sorts of political and ethnoracial inequities that President Chávez was actively challenging. Dr. Guillermo's statement was an attempt to reassert the ideological status quo by asserting that the ethnoracial divide is pervasive, real, and legally grounded, and it provided nonindigenous officials with exclusive rights to make public statements about and design policies for people designated as indigenous. In the end, Montoro's gubernatorial candidate won, and the mayor

Montoro chose for Antonio Díaz was not only a faithful caudillo politician but also an heir to the legacy of criollos who were widely deemed to "own the Indians" in the area. Thus, at the same time that participation frameworks were performatively shaped in each interactive setting, they simultaneously incorporated knowledge about the epidemic produced in different times and sites as well as how this knowledge had become the central vehicle for constructing and contesting the perceived chasm between indigenous and nonindigenous populations and structuring its political-economic fruits.

Grasping the place of participation frameworks in creating knowledge about the epidemic also entails taking on a challenge associated with STS and posthumanist work questioning the restriction of analysis to human actors. Parents, local leaders, healers, doctors, nurses, and epidemiologists all made claims to participation in knowledge production, even if their contributions were assessed in quite different ways. But technologies can also be considered to have played a role: hearing "a crackling sound" in a patient's lungs required access to a stethoscope and training in how to listen. Testing for bacteria, viruses, or toxins required other instrumental participants. Wisidatu used rattles in their diagnostic efforts. More broadly, a complex question relating to the role of viruses, bats, cattle, and other nonhumans is whether they were knowledge producers or just objects of human words and actions. Our first sign that something strange was going on came when Clara and Charles returned to the delta in July 2008 and saw a cat in Tirso's house. Asking why he had adopted a cat led us to another nonhuman actor: "Lots of bats were coming in the house and biting people." Clara remembered how a woman in Hanakanaima, near Santa Rosa de Guayo, responded to our question about unusual occurrences. "I remember a woman there telling me that she had seen a dead tiger in the forest; it didn't have any marks on it that would explain the death." "A tiger doesn't just drop dead for no reason," Conrado replied. "One time I found a dead howler monkey, which seemed really strange to me. Never in my life had I seen a howler monkey that seemed to have died for no reason. And I found a dead sloth and a tiger, too. People were really surprised. They asked, 'what is going on with these animals? Why are they dying like this?'" People tried to read these animal deaths as ways that nonhumans were contributing to knowledge, providing clues that were related to the human deaths.

This issue produced an epistemological rupture and a point of disalignment as the team was drawing up the report to take to Caracas. Tirso registered discomfort with the emerging epidemiological formulation—"more than thirty-eight Warao have died in Delta Amacuro State in 2007–2008 from a disease believed to be bat-transmitted rabies"—precisely because it cast all nonhuman actors into the status of agentless threats to human health. He lodged his objection by telling the Myth of Bat (*saha are*).

> I'm going to tell a tale told by our ancestors about the transformation of the bat. People back then lived in the forest. Back then there lived a young man who seemed just like everyone else. Nevertheless, when everyone else went out during the day to fish, hunt, and do other kinds of work, he stayed behind. He slept all day long. But when the others returned in the evening, that's when he went out to fish, to hunt, to harvest moriche palm starch. When daylight came, he would return, slip into his hammock, and go to sleep.
>
> They asked him, "Why don't you go out with us during the day?" "I can't," he responded, "because I can't see during the day"; for him it was like the darkness. The others found this behavior strange, but they didn't do anything about it.
>
> In time, they gave him a woman to marry. At dawn, her parents would go out to harvest moriche palm starch. She told him, "Come on, let's go with my parents." "No," he responded, "I won't go, it's dark, I won't go." She went out alone with her parents. When they came back, he would go out, alone.
>
> In time they realized that at night he was going out and looking for women from the same community. He would lie down with them and suck their blood and suck their blood, and they were dying. Every time he lay down with a woman and sucked her blood, she would get sick and die. And so a number of people were dying like this.
>
> The leaders of the community saw what was going on, and they said to one another, "We have to kill this fellow, because he's finishing off the women." So they grabbed him and they killed him, and then they cut up his flesh and burned it. And after it had all burned, they threw some over here, some over there, some over there, and some over there.
>
> And when they threw his burned flesh all over, that was the transformation of the bat, the burned pieces transformed into bats, they were the same color as bats. And that is the story of the transformation of the bat, that's how our ancestors used to tell it. And that's why bats like people's blood.

In the middle of drafting a report, Tirso had produced a classic Dracula story. Like Paulino Zapata's account of water spirits, Tirso's bat myth provides an example of Amerindian cosmologies, as analyzed by anthropologists Philippe Descola and Eduardo Viveiros de Castro. Building on fieldwork among "the Achuar," Descola (1996 [1986]) draws attention to contrastive ways of representing relations between humans and other beings. Descola separates perceptions of similarity and difference between humans and nonhumans along the dimensions of interiority, "intentionality, subjectivity, reflexivity, the aptitude to dream," and physicality, subsuming "form, substance, physiological, perceptual, sensory-motor," and other characteristics (2009, 150). Breathing new life into the old anthropological notion of animism, he characterizes it as an "ontological route" in which different species are perceived as sharing similar interiorities and fundamentally different physicalities.

Viveiros de Castro argues that Amerindians picture the relationship between humans and other creatures through what he calls "perspectivism," according to which persons, animals, and objects are defined relationally by how they "apprehend reality from distinct points of view" (2004, 466). He contrasts this perspective with Western "naturalism," springing from Francis Bacon's work in the seventeenth century, which, he suggests, posits an active human sphere that exists apart from a separate, passive domain of nature. As opposed to the evolutionary perspective of Western "naturalism" and its construction of people as animals who became human, Viveiros de Castro argues that Amerindians see animals as humans who "lost qualities inherited or retained by humans" (Viveiros de Castro 2004, 465). Viveiros de Castro argues that myths provide guidelines for thinking about particular animal species and their specific relationships to human beings, a point made beautifully by Tirso's performance; indeed, bat would seem to be just the sort of mythological/animal being that Viveiros de Castro has in mind.

Tirso's myth performance challenged the "tenacious assumptions" (Gordon 1988) of the biomedical perspective implicit in the bat-transmitted rabies formulation, disrupting the way that "naturalism" constructed both bats and humans. The diagnosis placed vampire bats on one side of a natureculture polarity, characterizing them as only gaining relevance to humans by becoming a disease vector. On the human side of the equation, the diagnosis presented the epidemic as affecting individual human bodies, viewed in biological, apolitical, asocial, and ahistorical terms as affected through a causal, mechanistic, and linear relationship between a single pathogen and a single disease. The subjectivities and forms of agency of the patients dropped out of the epidemiological picture. Webb Keane (2013) suggests that if ontologies are taken to be sets of beliefs about the world, they are enmeshed within efforts to establish ethical parameters for living within these worlds. Tirso's objection to centering the remainder of our work on biomedical ontological presuppositions exposed the ethical issues that we were bracketing and demanded that they be debated.

Tirso's intervention could be read as a bat-centered critique, as *Desmodus rotundus*'s own challenge to his simultaneous reduction to a rabies vector and his scapegoating as the cause of a year's legacy of social and physical death. Perhaps more precisely, Tirso located the epidemic in a complex history of bat-human relations of desire and affect. The mythic intervention suggested that human and bat subjectivities were formerly not similar, as Viveiros de Castro's broad generalization might suggest, but rather have long been engaged in a collective and intimate history of difference, of sharing spaces, resources, and bodies through exchanges of blood and violence. Unlike the epidemiological formulation, the mythic performance drew attention to the subjectivities of contemporary bats: why had they suddenly turned on humans more frequently? Why had their bites turned fatal? Bat's agency becomes a product of both its nature, nocturnal and hematophagic, and the jealousy and violent acts of men, of patriarchal relations in which men worried about bat "'finishing off the women.'" Rather than coming out of nowhere in 2007, the epidemic thus comes to form a new chapter in this long record of violent interactions, one that cried out for analysis of its own historical specificities at the same time that it could be informed by keeping this broader trajectory in mind.

Tirso's intervention would push us to look more closely at recent bat–human interactions, where it would seem that bats are learning more about humans in the delta than vice versa. *D. rotundus* tends to feed on the same person or persons over consecutive nights, often at nearly the identical site on the body. How do bats locate the same individual and even the same place to bite each night? Research suggests that, in addition to echolocation (or "bio radar," as it is often called), *D. rotundus* can read human breathing sounds like we read human voices, performing "a rather sophisticated analysis of the sounds based on multiple parameters," despite their quite low volume (Gröger and Wiegrebe 2006). The bats land; climb the ropes holding the hammock; slide down; approach the person's face, head, finger, or toe; make the puncture; and lap up the blood, often without waking the person. If the person does not awaken and the bite is hidden in the scalp and does not break a large blood vessel, the human participant in the encounter might never know that it has occurred. Accordingly, bat-transmitted rabies could kill only one or two family members and leave the others unaffected.

Similarly, healer Zapata's explanation of hydrophobia in terms of mythic relations between humans and water spirits (chapter 2) might lead us to place it solidly within Amazonian animism or perspectivism. Several major problems emerge, however, in jumping to this conclusion. First, as G. E. R. Lloyd (2012) suggests in a discussion of Descola and Viveiros de Castro, ontologies are never evenly shared across societies, but are always multiple and taken up to varying degrees. Second, recall that Zapata collaborated with his nurse/son-in-law in treating the same patients and that he worked with doctors and nurses in the Arawabisi clinic. Similarly, Tirso's extensive work as a healer did not preclude the possibility of entering into biomedical spaces: he spent months trying, unsuccessfully, to obtain adequate biomedical treatment for his wife, Surdelina, when she was diagnosed with cancer. Accordingly, the idea that ethnoracial identities and ontological perspectives correlate one-to-one, that there is a one-ontological-perspective-per-person rule simply falls apart. Perspectivism and animism rest on "late structuralist" assumptions and broad generalizations (Turner 2009) and resurrect old binaries that posit a cultural chasm between what are projected as indigenous versus Western social worlds (Ramos 2012). Our work on the cholera epidemic demonstrated that delta residents could partake deeply of knowledge systems and practices associated with both biomedicine and healing, sometimes weaving them complexly (Briggs and Mantini-Briggs 2003). Moreover, Zapata's explanation integrated mythical water spirits not only with "non-indigenous" forms of spirit possession healing but also with a critique of the colonial exploitation of delta communities by corrupt government contractors. As Menéndez (1981) has long argued, biomedicine and indigenous healing are not non-overlapping autonomous universes, but are continually defined in relational terms, a sort of intimacy and opposition not altogether unlike human–bat relations. The myth and the epidemic both point to how boundary-objects—here sleep, blood, hydrophobia, and such neurological abnormalities as seizures and hallucinations—constitute critical points in which relationality is constructed anew.

In his performance of the bat myth, Tirso asked a pointed question: if bats attack people on a regular basis, why would their bites suddenly begin producing cases of a fatal disease in July 2007? Paying attention to the history of bat–human intimacies again yielded ways of thinking through this question more productively. The Gilbert et al. (2012) study conducted in the Peruvian Amazon found that some unvaccinated individuals had been bitten by bats and exposed to the virus, but developed rabies virus–neutralizing antibodies rather than symptoms; in other words, the bite bites seemed to have vaccinated rather than killed them. The researchers attributed the ability to survive exposure to the virus by some individuals to a number of factors, including genetics and the quantity of rabies viruses introduced. We do not have the same kind of serological data for the delta; a member of the group that did the study in Peru was interested in investigating the epidemic in the delta, but the Venezuelan government was more concerned with stopping knowledge production about the epidemic than in expanding the range of people participating in it.

Bringing Gilbert et al.'s research into dialogue with Tirso's critique can open up some interesting possibilities. Why did the bats begin to attack humans so frequently in 2007? Our epidemiological questions revealed that all of the chickens died in many of the affected communities during the same period, developing what people described as "flu-like" symptoms and falling to the ground, dead. There was no avian influenza in Venezuela, but the Newcastle virus—which can wipe out chickens but causes no human illness—was evident in eastern Venezuela at the time and could have killed the chickens. Herein lies another intimacy: humans and their chickens both provide food for the same vampire bats. Gilbert et al. (2012, 212) suggest that the elimination of livestock, such as pigs or cattle, can lead to increased bat attacks on humans. When the portion of the bat's blood bank represented by the chickens suddenly disappeared, they probably relied much more heavily on humans. The chickens die out and the strange deaths of tigers, howler monkeys, and sloths in the forest not only formed part of these cross-species intimacies, but were making their own inadvertent contributions to producing knowledge about the mysterious epidemic. The cats that suddenly started to appear as pets in 2007, expressly invited into delta homes to keep the bats out, similarly formed part of the same ecology of blood, flesh, and knowledge by catching bats cruising through homes.

Thus, Tirso's indigenous cosmopolitics (de la Cadena 2010) constituted a spirited critique of biomedical authority and challenged the health/communicative inequities it upholds. Even as it raised fascinating questions about how bats are enmeshed with human sexuality and sleep, Tirso's intervention pushed the boundaries of knowledge production beyond people who could claim biomedical authority to include not only other humans, but also bats, chickens, cats, tigers, and other species as well. It opens up a larger question: was this multispecies exchange of knowledge, blood, and death pointing us to some sort of larger environmental shift, one that goes beyond the possible introduction of Newcastle virus and the viral content of *D. rotundus* saliva? This is another mystery that has outlived the deaths.

ICONIC TRANSPARENCY:
MAKING ACCOUNTS THAT MATTER AND MOVE

We examined above two types of Peirce's signs, symbols and indexes; Tirso's strategic interruption points toward a third. For knowledge to count, it must be codified. Hayden White pinpoints the issue in his analysis of historical writing. Historians, he argues, imagine the past in particular ways, then create narratives that purportedly mirror past events. This results in what Peirce (1932, 142) calls icons, where signifiers and their objects are related not through law-like systemic relations (symbols) or contextual features (indexes) but through the "iconic relation," in which signs share at least one quality or perceptible property with the objects they represent. Iconicity can infuse narratives with a powerful sense of versimilitude, a capacity that Taussig (1993) explores as mimesis.

We were not present when parents felt their children's foreheads, Dr. Ricardo heard "crackling sounds," medical personnel in Puerto Ordaz drew blood and conducted autopsies, or healers touched rattles and hands to patients' bodies and sang. The one exception was Elbia. Clara and Norbelys participated actively in her care until the hour she died. For the other children, what was available to us came through personal narratives, epidemiological reports, tables, photographs, laments, one-page clinical reference sheets, laboratory results, newspaper articles, and lots of commentary. These accounts focused simultaneously on a particular body and on how people produced knowledge about it; they projected indexical calibrations, forms of symbolic authority, and participation frameworks in particular sorts of ways—placing tellers, writers, and photographers within them, often at the center.

Bruno Latour (1987) argues that scientific narratives insert the very object they represent into texts through figures, tables, and photographs; iconicity lies at the center of such techniques. A framework developed by Richard Bauman and Charles Briggs (1990) builds on Bakhtin (1981) in suggesting how textual iconicity works. People build iconicity into narratives by, first, extracting fragments—words, observations, numbers, affects, medical registers, and the like—from forms of care, epidemiological investigations, newspaper articles, rumors, and so forth. Second, they weave them into a new text, such as a clinical summary, newspaper article, personal narrative, or epidemiological report. Drawing on Bauman and Briggs's framework would suggest that this process of entextualization involves constructing a particular type of unit in which referents are related not only as products of knowledge-production practices but also as intrinsic features of the text itself.

Here the issue of genre, which emerged forcefully in Tirso's intervention, looms large. The way a report is written or a narrative is recounted opens up a set of expectations regarding how issues of symbolic capital, indexical calibration, and participation frameworks will play out and how they relate to particular sorts of sites. Clinical spaces in the delta are seldom receptive to performances of myths, even though healing songs can be heard there occasionally. In the epidemic, conflicts surfaced in precisely such settings when patients or relatives tried to tell narratives not invited by physicians or epidemiologists. Particular genres placed certain types of symbolic authority in the center: epidemiologists' reports incorporated sparse details provided by clinicians and parents but did not allow them to structure their explanations. The parents' narratives privileged entitlement, people's rights to tell stories that relate to their bodies and those of their children. *Notidiario* reporter Leo Romero created an "informative equilibrium" between the "sides" of government officials and residents. All of these types of accounts, including our own, attempted to achieve a degree of verisimilitude, to project their close iconic relationship to the bodies by focusing on points at which those bodies could produce knowledge: the child's symptoms or her last words, a parent's lament, lab results, a photograph, a quote from the MPPS minister. Different genres coded evidence in different sorts of ways.

This is not to say that each context permitted only one type of iconic relationship, indexical calibration, symbolic authority, or participation structure. Tirso instigated a conflict between genres by asking, in effect: Are epidemiological reports and tables the only way that knowledge can travel to Caracas? Why are they being privileged? What other perspectives are they displacing? If Mukoboina became the epidemiological ground zero, it also occasioned a conflict of genres. Our interviews indicated that the epidemiologists thought that they were providing powerful epidemiological techniques for turning fragments of uninformed lay experiences and behaviors into epidemiologically valuable information. Mukoboinans believed that epidemiologists had come to dialogue, expecting to perform their testimonios and to hear what the visitors' distinctive ontological position might yield. These conflicting generic expectations created resentment against RHS that perseveres in Mukoboina to this day, simultaneously prompting epidemiologists' accusation that "difficulty acquiring information due to the closed character of the community" foiled the epidemiological venture.

The issue of what we refer to as iconic transparency also played a central role in shaping these inequities. By this we mean shaping the features—visual and acoustic as well as textual—of an account in such a way that it seems to perfectly mirror that which it represents. A list of symptoms can thus purport to transparently and perfectly represent a patient's experience, just as the sequentiality of a parent's account can attempt to match the order in which events occurred. Different accounts of the same bodies and events, invoking different genres, make competing claims to iconic transparency. If an epidemiological table or a listing of laboratory results was able to make an account iconically transparent, clinical results were less effective in doing so. Clinicians and healers

demoted the status of parents' accounts to unreliable perceptions and problematic actions, even while appropriating crucial details for inclusion in their
own. Several questions arise: Who judges iconic transparency? What features
imbue an account with veracity? What enables an account to move between
sites and actors and to be considered credible in each? Genre is a crucial factor.
From our initial meeting in Muaina, Enrique decided that the team needed to
create words, numbers, and images that could travel to Caracas and be deemed
credible by national health officials and journalists. Laments and personal narratives would be very unlikely to gain standing in these locations, but numbers and diagnostic details—which Enrique and Charles carefully recorded in
their notebooks—could produce a formulation compatible with the reception
frameworks of public health officials and journalists in Caracas. Like genre,
language is important: none of the physicians, epidemiologists, journalists, or
national media audiences spoke more than a few words of Warao. Accounts in
Warao seldom made it out of the delta. Ruth Goldstein's (2014, 2015) meta-
phor of "traffic" captures all of these threads: the movement and the immobility, the channeling and the confusion, the competing desires to get things
moving and bring them to a halt, and the frustration of being caught up in the
middle of it all.

Speaking of capitalist production, Karl Marx ([1939] 1973, 517) wrote that
"circulation presupposes production at all points," and this statement is true of
accounts of the strange disease. John Urry (2007) argues that such things as bi-
cycles, cars, and airplanes are not intrinsically mobile but must be made to appear naturally mobile to their users. Anna Tsing (2005) argues that circulation
requires what she refers to as grooves or channels that facilitate movement but
also create "friction," limiting and shaping how things move. The Nabasanuka
clinic's two-way radio facilitated daily communication with officials in Tucupita, but static-filled messages from the clinic only reached particular institutional interlocutors and produced only silence and evasion. Urry indicates that
producing mobility also generates immobility, constraining the circulation of
subalterns and their discursive practices. The parents wanted their stories to
reach Chávez. Unlike discourse about diarrheas, however, RHS wanted talk
about the strange disease to circulate as little as possible; officials particularly
did not to want it to reach journalists, politicians, Tucupita's electorate, or officials in Caracas. They accordingly challenged assessments of the iconic veracity
of assertions by parents, Dr. Ricardo, the medical interns, the nurses, and the
team that a mysterious epidemic was afoot, the numbers used to track it, or any
diagnosis that departed from epidemiological "normality." Iconic transparency

of talk about the epidemic had to be undermined at all costs, even if it meant thwarting the clinical work undertaken by Dr. Cáceres and the nurses.

The accounts of the epidemic that claimed the highest degree of iconic transparency—and thus authority—were those written by epidemiologists. The preamble of the Mission Barrio Adentro epidemiologist Diego Escalante's report on Mukoboina is highly instructive. It describes the activities undertaken, thereby creating a model for the authoritative production of scientific knowledge about the epidemic. Its text and tables spell out the algorithm for systematically converting homes, lives, and deaths into numbers, the words of grieving parents into "data of hygienic-epidemiological interest." Mukoboinans only seemed to count when they were counted, when—to use Diane Nelson's (2009) play on the sense of *contar* in Spanish—when they told about their children through the authoritative technologies of enumeration provided by the visitors. The report embodied the complex relationship between collective and individual authorship explored by Matthew Hull (2012) for bureaucratic documents. The report states that all of the persons listed (including the nameless motorboat operators, school teachers, and community leaders) participated in all activities, including the "interviews with mothers, fathers, and other relatives of the deceased" and the observations and queries on which the report is based. Nevertheless, Dr. Diego, is listed as its author. Similarly, the 6 February 2008 report authored by regional epidemiologist Froilán Godoy relays material produced by Dr. Cáceres, the members of the 9 September 2007 epidemiological team that visited Mukoboina, laboratory personnel, and pediatricians and toxicologists ("specialists") and other personnel in hospitals in Tucupita, Maturín, and Puerto Ordaz. These reports thus powerfully take a range of dispersed documentary traces and voices that, like Dr. Cáceres and his superiors in RHS, were sometimes not in sync, and fashioned them into a single network that collectively produced both information and care. These documents thus embody what Hull (2012, 129) characterizes as a quintessential feature of bureaucratic organization as "a social form designed for collective action, a social technology for aligning efforts of a large number of people so that they act as one." Contrary to the parents' projection of RHS as often uncaring and incompetent, these documents project it as a single, unified network in which all professionals were acting in a caring and coordinated fashion to save the children's lives and figure out what was wrong.

Extending work on language and semiotic ideologies, Hull (2012, 12) suggests that documents can be analyzed in terms of the "graphic ideologies" espoused by persons who make, circulate, and use them. Writing against the common stereotype of bureaucratic documents as dull and purely instrumental, Riles (2006) and her collaborators suggest that bureaucrats get so excited about their documents that they can engender this same sense of admiration in ethnographers, leading them to appreciate the aesthetic properties and the power of documents' materiality as artifacts. Alissa Bernstein (2015) carefully documents how the makers and disseminators of health policies in Bolivia describe policies as "beautiful," elaborating an aesthetics they try to capture not only in official policy documents but also in PowerPoint files, pamphlets, notebooks, diagrams drawn on whiteboards, and oral presentations. Akhil Gupta (2012) suggests that even when bureaucratic writing circulates relatively little, it holds the power to create images of "the state" through the performance of acts of inscription. Scientific documents, according to Latour (1987), are imbued with a particular form of graphic ideology, one that projects them as a quintessential model of mobility, as comprising "immutable mobiles" that should be able to travel anywhere without changing meaning.

What particularly interests us about epidemiological reports on the strange epidemic is that they possessed *none* of these qualities. Their inscription was anything but a public, performative act. Their authors never seem to express pride in them or their creation or suggest that they bore any aesthetic qualities whatsoever. If documents have careers, as Richard Harper (1998) fruitfully suggests, great efforts were undertaken to contain and constrain their careers. Director Guillermo Rendón and other RHS officials used the epidemiological documents to discredit the numbers that Conrado presented in the Legislative Council in February and the ones we took to Caracas in August. Nevertheless, the documents themselves were not exhibited in press conferences or public meetings, their material and artifactual dimensions carefully hidden.

It might be presumed that rendering the most powerful representations of the epidemic invisible to everyone but a handful of officials was a product of controversy, given that the epidemic became a bone of contention starting in February 2008. These circulatory limitations are, however, fairly standard for RHS epidemiological reports. Why would the most authoritative documents be doomed to the least circulation? Arguing against Max Weber's (1978) projection of documents as indexes of bureaucratic authority, recent ethnographic work on documents suggests that they rather "precipitate the formation of shifting networks and groups of official and nonofficial people and things" (Hull 2012, 21). Marilyn Strathern (2006, 190) argues that "what gives systems in general their self-organizing properties is their capacity to define their own boundaries." Minister Serrano projected a graphic ideology that points to just this sort of boundary-work in the 13 August press conference in which he attacked the team's findings: "Normally, an epidemiological report is for my consumption. It is a paper for my work. We hope that epidemiologists will use it to help us, because this information—when used properly—is useful in guiding us; but it is susceptible to manipulation."[4] The quasi-military hierarchical structure of public health institutions is pictured here in Serrano's projection of epidemiological documents as being designed for one reader—the minister of health; other officials who read them would seem to be looking over his shoulder. Circulation beyond MPPS loses its status as forming part of knowledge production and becomes a political act that could undermine health.

If we were to stop our analysis at this point, however, we would share an analytic limitation of much recent work on bureaucratic documents: the way that they seem to retain the generalizing and abstracting a priori power of the categories of "bureaucratic" and "documents." While it is not inaccurate to refer to such officials as bureaucrats, given their employment by a state bureaucracy, they are also physicians and epidemiologists. Their documents are scientific reports. What would be most problematic, however, would be to allow this correspondence between scholarly and official perspectives to blind us to the way that the making and circulation of documents is also embedded in broader economies of circulation, which go beyond bureaucrats and their documents to include such forms as rumors and news stories. In chapter 8 we discuss how closely rumors, news stories, and epidemiological investigations and reports can be imbricated.

We thus might want to think more broadly about these epidemiological reports. On the one hand, these documents fused health and communication in claiming to be embodiments of iconic transparency. These reports defined health, without surpluses (Derrida) or leaks (Sapir). They similarly defined legitimate communication about health: only people who figuratively—but seldom literally—had these documents in hand could make accurate and authorized statements about the epidemic. MPPS enjoyed a monopoly over the production of knowledge about health and a virtual monopoly over its circulation and reception, which was limited to designated officials' summaries of their contents. They were, simultaneously, a powerful signe zéro, in Roman Jakobson's (1971) terms, a communicative function announced by the absence of a form. Unlike the festishism of documentary form studied by Riles (2000, 2006), it was the very inaccessibility of the form—even to most RHS employees—that made the reports powerful. Contributing to an epidemiological investigation did not, Mukoboinans learned, confer any rights to see it or even to request a summary of its contents. Health/communicative inequities were thus structured both by the positing of one type of account as the symbolic, indexical, and iconic embodiment of knowledge about health, thereby fusing health and communication, and denial of access to the forms, thereby severing this link. In a state in which public health institutions produce ill-health for 26,080 people[5] at the same time that they yield substantial capital and political power for party elites and their allies, this shell game of form and content, health and communication structured shifting alliances in an enduring racial economy faced with challenges from indigenous social movements and revolutionary ideologies.

Dilemmas of Knowledge Production and Circulation

Public health officials are not the only ones who face the complex dance that Bowker and Star (1999) point out between building complex indexical histories in the course of producing knowledge and rendering most of their features invisible in order to enable them to move. After Conrado and Enrique formed the team, the six of us were faced not just with analyzing the ways that others produced and circulated knowledge about the epidemic but with fashioning our own indexical histories and deciding what to erase in order to enable our findings to travel to Caracas. We invoked forms of symbolic authority (derived from Clara's and Norbelys's clinical training) and indexical calibrations of relationships between the diverse accounts and dying bodies (including our experience with Elbia). In addition, we had to build our own icons—from the report written to take to Caracas to statements to journalists to photographs to the book you are reading—and make thorny decisions about what we should circulate. Producing knowledge about the epidemic that was designed to circulate was both a powerful and a dangerous act: potential criminal prosecution provided an important reminder of these constraints.

The six of us faced a number of dilemmas, two of which were particularly challenging. First, numerous narratives, including the ones told in Mukoboina and Muaina, brought discussions of "bad medicine" (which anthropologists often refer to as "sorcery" and is known more broadly as "witchcraft") into efforts to figure out what was killing the children. While writing the report, Enrique stood up abruptly and declared, "After deep reflection, I reluctantly propose that all references to 'witchcraft' be erased from the final report—they shall remain with us." No one spoke; everyone understood all too well. Any allusion to bad medicine would result in our efforts being, to use anthropologist Arjun Appadurai's (1988) phrase, incarcerated by culture: our report would be dismissed as reflecting superstition, not science. Similarly, Tirso's point about the exclusion of nonhuman actors provided a powerful wakeup call, cautioning the other five listeners about the danger of erasing accounts not fashioned in epidemiological terms. Making explicit the inclusion of nonhuman participants in knowledge production, let alone including mythic evidence in a report, would have run the risk of rendering our investigation immobile, at least in terms of producing a report for health officials.

Second, we needed an epidemiological statement, such as "more than thirty-eight Warao have died from an unknown disease in Delta Amacuro State in 2007–2008," if our report was to attract the attention of health officials and reporters in Caracas, that is, a formulation that would embody Latour's notion of the "immutable mobile." However, the cost of creating mobility would be too high if the outcome was an abstract, decontextualized statement, severed from indexical links to bodies, laments, and narratives. For Enrique and Conrado, Tirso and Norbelys, as important as the specifics of the report was the meta-statement it made, showing that people classified as indigenous were not just failed receivers of knowledge about health but producers as well. The details that appeared in Muaina, which helped us to come up with a diagnosis, were overlaid with the acoustics of wailing. The challenge was to produce a statement that could travel to Caracas and be deemed credible by public health officials and journalists without erasing indexical links to how the team's knowledge-production process had sprung from the demand, "Tell me why my children died" and the parents' active participation. We were faced with a contradiction that followed us right through our landing on the marble floor of the lobby of the MPPS national headquarters and that will outlive the writing of this book.

Conclusion: Stratifying Knowledge, Multiplying Inequities

A deep irony of the search for a diagnosis is that everyone was trying to make sense of the situation, but all efforts were failing. Multiple forms of symbolic authority were deployed. As each failed, they also discredited the efforts of people guided by other modes of inquiry. Indexical calibrations abounded, all oriented toward charting how bodies could be turned into sites of knowledge production. Placing these points in locations that purportedly afforded the narrators a privileged perspective effectively displaced others. Just as their children's bodies provided the indexical point of origin and the parents' pain was represented as the affective ground zero, nearly all other actors relied on the parents' labor of care and narration while according their accounts little value as sources of knowledge. Structuring participation frameworks distributed knowledge-producing rights in unequal ways. Imbuing a particular account— whether a clinical description, epidemiological report, or mythically based analysis of water spirits, candles, or bats—with iconic transparency effectively denied iconicity to other accounts, which then could be read as reflecting only ignorance, superstition, or political interest. Imbuing some accounts with mobility impeded the circulation of other interpretations of the epidemic; some prominent participants claimed the right to determine what could circulate at all.

All of these dimensions were often used as means of establishing one ontological perspective as the viewpoint that could legitimately and accurately produce knowledge of the epidemic. To quite varying degrees, their use impeded people from establishing productive relationships to other perspectives and thereby building knowledge collaboratively and creating a sense of commitment to a common goal of stopping the epidemic. One group of participants did try to enter into indexical calibration, the enactment of participation frameworks, iconic transparency, and enhancing the circulation of accounts so as to bring in as many ontological perspectives as possible: the parents. They struggled to grasp the perspectives of others, to use them in making treatment decisions and in trying to keep their other children healthy, and to bring diverse ontologies into dialogue. Their potential contributions to facilitating more dialogue among everyone who was trying to save the children, were largely thwarted, however, by the low esteem in which their perspectives were held.

7

L A M E N T S ,

P S Y C H O A N A L Y S I S ,

A N D   T H E   W O R K

O F   M O U R N I N G

Enrique invited us to a meeting in Muaina on 28 July 2008. The team's collaboration had just begun, and the kickoff was to be an encounter in which people would speak one-by-one, each adding material in attempting to collectively unravel the epidemic. We would gather "facts" that could then be turned into a diagnosis and an epidemiological table, turning the deaths into cases to be plotted chronologically and geographically. We envisioned this formulation traveling into official declarations, public health policies, and media stories.

After climbing onto the dock from Tirso's boat, Charles, Clara, Norbelys, and Tirso walked past the open doorway of the first house on the eastern side of Muaina. The doorway, flooded with sunshine, led to a darkened interior that would confront us with our first direct encounter with a body claimed by the mysterious disease. On the right side of the house, we saw Basilio Estrella, the wisidatu who had treated both Eduardito and Dalvi, caring for a young man in a hammock; his song, which called on hebu pathogens to leave the body, was drowned out by the voices of five women and one adolescent, who became visible as we took another step forward along the dock. Standing directly opposite the doorway, we also saw Mamerto Pizarro's body lying in a coffin, bringing visual and auditory senses into disconcerting alignment. One of the mourners, her face transformed into a mask of grief and fatigue, was Florencia Macotera; Mamerto's grandmother, two of his aunts, a sister, and his brother, Melvi, all rocked back and forth beside Florencia as they collectively composed and performed laments. Each one sang verses that addressed Mamerto directly, giving the impression that they could bring him back to life by evoking—in the present tense—their most treasured memories of him and the ways their lives were intertwined, even as they announced the finality of his death.

We faced one of those scenes of unimaginable yet intimate horror where you feel propelled inexorably into a disquieting space from which you have the urge to turn and run. Needless to say, our expectations for the visit to Muaina—and at that point, for the team's collaboration—were abruptly upended. Enrique had known that the meeting's discussions would be permeated by the strident, disconcerting sounds of laments. Why had he staged it next to a dead body? Why had he wanted the sounds of lamentation to inflect every word spoken there?

Moving among myriad stories, reports, news articles, and other sources to navigate contrastive places, perspectives, and experiences and chart their routes of circulation and sources of immobility, chapter 6 explored their tremendous potential to reveal how health and health/communicative inequities are coproduced. Stories in particular are comfortable research objects—perhaps too much so. Easy to elicit, conveniently produced in encounters that grant considerable power to visiting researchers, it is too easy to reduce their meaning to reference, to the semantic content of their words, facilitating their transcription and translation. It is also too easy to edit and extract from them, to make slices of the stories circulate in academic texts, media settings, and policy proposals, rendering them mobile in ways that suit interests and discursive practices that may run counter to those of their narrators. Stories are sometimes too easy to position as boundary objects, held in common by actors occupying distinct social spheres but defined and used in different ways by each (Bowker and Star 1999). When stories are used as boundary objects, they are often taken as providing smooth, even automatic passages between sites and perspectives, making it too easy for "us" to think we understand "them."

Laments differ from stories along all of these dimensions, which is precisely why we found them so disruptive and so productive. Laments are terrible candidates for boundary objects. Laments cannot easily be inserted into clinical, epidemiological, or journalistic spaces, even along their borders. You cannot elicit the performance of a lament in the delta; only the immediacy of a death can do that.[1] Laments have rich referential content, powerfully invoking memories and images, but these come forward as fragments that are deeply woven into musical, poetic, and acoustic features and into relations between a lifeless body and the performers' bodies, which rock back and forth, grasp the corpse, and bathe it with tears. These dimensions resist transcription and extraction; they are even hard to summarize. Comprehending the words sung in laments requires fluency in Warao and immersion in the specificities of kinship relations, biographies, and histories of alignments and conflicts within and among settlements. Translating them is challenging.

In her widely influential "cosmopolitical proposal," Isabelle Stengers (2005, 994) urges us "to 'slow down' reasoning and create an opportunity to arouse a slightly different awareness of the problems and situations mobilizing us." Research should explore "multiple, divergent worlds," rejecting a position of certainty, the conceit associated with pretending to render them transparent, refusing to project voices as "master[ing] the situation they discuss" (996). Stengers sagely warns against the urge to encompass particular worlds, especially "to encompass those that refused to be encompassed by something else" (995). More than with narratives, rethinking the mysterious epidemic by starting with these laments invites a "cosmopolitical" project, given how laments demand to be heard at the same time that they cast listeners as overhearers in a conversation that is not for them, insisting that interpretive work be undertaken while simultaneously infusing words with multiple, complex meanings. The collective lament performance for Mamerto interlocked multiple voices, experiences, and perspectives intimately, simultaneously refusing to bring them into sync, to produce a singular, collective voice. The laments asserted their own power to demand particular actions even as they confessed their utter impotence, their inability to accomplish one overwhelming desire: to bring Mamerto back to life.

At the same time that these laments are eerily in sync with Stengers' cosmopolitical proposal, they challenge any unspoken rootedness in a privileged, distant, or liberal positionality, its construal as springing from a voluntary act of renouncing the illusion of certainty and omniscience and thinking up a new point of departure. A lament interpellates listeners. It reaches out and commands the bodies, ears, hearts, and minds of those in earshot. Responses are not fixed, predetermined, but are, to invoke Louis Althusser (1969), overdetermined, such that the affective and imaginative space that a response can occupy is shaped by the poetic and musical grip or traction of laments as well as the memories and explicit demands unfolding in their verbal content. Housed within the lament is the demand to circulate what is sung, but it is embedded in a cultural form that imposes barriers to circulation, that obstructs the stripping away of an acoustic materiality in order to yield a malleable and easily appropriated content. If responses to laments take the form of research, the inquiry will be powerfully locked in the dilemmas identified by the decolonizing methodology outlined by Linda Tuhiwai Smith (1999), tying the investigator to indelible visions of bodies torn apart by colonial violence and the political claims of competing and conflicting forms of knowledge. The laments' insistence on complex responses to an insoluble question—why did Mamerto, Dalvi, and Eduardito have to die?—demands a knowledge that academics would call theoretical or conceptual, one that scrutinizes assumptions and explores alternatives. The laments simultaneously demanded responses to the political claims lodged by the lamenters and the corpse, the challenge to take the words sung in the laments and spoken in the meeting "to Chávez," to national officials of the socialist government. Performing the lament for Mamerto hoarsely articulated residents' questions about health inequities and asserted health/communicative rights.

Responding to the unnerving demands made by these laments can thus unsettle conventional perspectives on health inequities, on the politics of knowledge, and on how anthropologists and other researchers relate to the worlds they document. Given the importance of poetic, musical, and acoustic features in how the lamenters interpellated the six of us, responding to their challenge requires looking closely at the work of mourning they structure.

Hypercathexis, Reality Testing, and the Work of Mourning

The phrase "the work of mourning" is, of course, Sigmund Freud's; his essay "Mourning and Melancholia" placed that work at the center of psychoanalytic thought, even as it suggests that mourning is not pathological and does not require therapeutic intervention ([1917] 1957, 244). Psychoanalysts now often read that essay less for what it can tell us about mourning per se than for how it illuminates object relations theory. We are interested here in object formation, but particularly in terms of how death shatters object relations and how the work of mourning reconfigures them. While Freud and later psychoanalysts provide crucial insights into mourning, keeping the poetics, acoustic materiality, and knowledge claims of laments in mind can extend psychoanalytic thinking about mourning.

Freud pinpointed the contradictory character of mourning. On the one hand, the work of mourning involves hypercathexis: recovering and reinternalizing the image of the dead person and imbuing it with such intense psychic energy "through the medium of a hallucinatory wish-psychosis" that "the existence of the lost object is psychically prolonged" (Freud [1917] 1957, 244, 245). Hypercathexis can create a fantasy world in which we allow ourselves to believe that the person never really died or will return. Nevertheless, reality testing requires that "each single one of the memories and situations of expectancy which demonstrate the libido's attachment to the lost object is met by the verdict of reality that the object no longer exists," leading to a struggle "so intense that a turning away from reality takes place" (255, 244). Crucially, he pointed out that this juxtaposition engenders both the "extraordinarily painful" character of mourning and the emergence of a "compromise" between the two processes (245).

Later readers of the essay have distanced themselves from how Freud projects the temporality of mourning. Judith Butler (2004, 21) suggests that the essay "implied a certain interchangeability of objects as a sign of hopefulness, as if the prospect of entering life anew made use of a kind of promiscuity of libidinal aim." She thinks that a linearity informs Freud's distinction between mourning and melancholia, which would equate mourning with forgetting; Butler argues that he later changed his mind, admitting in "The Ego and the Id" that reincorporation of the lost attachment "was essential to the task of mourning" (2004, 21). French psychoanalyst Jean Laplanche ([1992] 1999, 251–252) contends that "the Freudian theory of mourning" involves a unilinear process of stripping away memories.[2]

We would agree that casting mourning in linear and functionalist terms as a process that reestablishes a psychic status quo would be problematic, and some passages in Freud's essay do lend themselves to this interpretation. More careful attention to the temporalities projected in the German text lead us to conclude, however, that such interpretations may rest, in part, on problems of translation.[3] Freud called for attention to the specificities of relationships between *Erinnerungen* and *Erwartungen*, memories and expectations, between pasts and futures created through the work of mourning. His account invites a sense of open-endedness and indeterminacy and includes a stunning admission, in line with the sort of humility urged by Stengers: "Why this compromise . . .

should be so extraordinarily painful is not at all easy to explain" (Freud [1917] 1957, 245). Two features of his analysis, however, limit its power to illuminate object relations and mourning. First, in both *Jokes and Their Relationship to the Unconscious* and *The Interpretation of Dreams*, Freud is remarkably attentive to poetics, to creative ties opened up by partially freeing language forms from attachment to referential content in jokes, puns, and slips of the tongue, between formal and semantic dimensions of language, thereby affording remarkable insights into both memory and everyday life. Attention to poetics is, however, singularly lacking in "Mourning and Melancholia," somehow missing as a guide to the complex relations between hypercathexis and reality testing. Second, given his stress on specificities in the work of mourning, Freud's invocation of the general figures of "the mourner" and "the loved person" (*geliebte Person*) or "love object" (*Liebesobjekt*) and his neglect of the concreteness of relations between particular mourners and particular deaths is striking. With respect to both of these issues, we have much to learn from Mamerto's mourners and their lamentations.

Poetics, Musicality, and the Work of Mourning

In Delta Amacuro, lamentation centrally embodies and structures the work of mourning and how it is woven into everyday life. Lamentation is a powerful cultural form that claims ears, bodies, minds, hearts, and materialities through its distinctive poetic, musical, acoustic, and embodied features. These aspects also render the work of mourning reflexive, enabling words and sounds directed to the dead simultaneously to construct affective states, memories, bodily dispositions, and social relations, make political claims, and provide listeners with multiple channels—none transparent or unambiguous—through which to read them. The laments sung for Mamerto—like the ones for Elbia— can open up questions regarding the work of mourning that emerged from our discussion of psychoanalysis. This reflexive quality suggests that performers and listeners are actively scrutinizing both the significance and impact of Mamerto's death and how the work of mourning will reshape life.

The lamenters' words and voices highlighted the contradictory dimensions that Freud identified in the work of mourning. Each verse explored the specificities of the process of resurrecting Erinnerungen, memories, investing them with tremendous poetic, musical, and psychic energy. Mamerto's brother Melvi reflected on how they played together as children, traveled with their parents to Florencia's parents' home in Siawani to garden, and, shortly before Mamerto died, worked together for a contractor building houses in Muaina. Mamerto's grandmother remembered that he sometimes slept in her house and brought her fish. Florencia reflected with pride on his studies at the Indigenous University of Venezuela.

We suggest above that Freud did not simply view the work of mourning as a linear, gradual progression from hypercathexis to reality testing but emphasized the specifics of constructing memories and expectations; the question remains, however, of how these complex temporalities unfold, how opposing processes come together. The reflexive power of the poetic and musical features of the laments for Mamerto provide the means to tackle this question. Poetics, as Jakobson (1960) classically suggests, involves creative reuses of subtle grammatical and semantic properties of language. The poetic action in the laments drew primarily on the complex and elaborate verbal structure of Warao: mourners used what linguists refer to as tense and aspect forms to create poetic images and map their temporal contours.[4] Lamenters attached the present-tense marker *-ya* and the durative aspect form *-ha* to verb stems, sometimes both in the same word, to make images of the deceased appear to be unfolding at that moment and as if they would continue indefinitely into the future. Performers created tiny imagist poems that placed listeners in the middle of actions, as if they were currently sharing these experiences with the performers. At the same time, a struggle ensued within each voice through the inclusion of verb endings marked as past and punctual, particularly *-(n)ae*; here reality testing took each image and burst it apart, placing each memory definitively in an inaccessible past.

Melvi's lament suggests how finely the two temporalities were woven together.

1   Mano, oko daobasa serebu**ya** makina eku,
     My brother, we were making boards together in the sawmill,

2   ama ihi mamo**ae** diana.
     now you have left me.

3   Ihi yakerakore aniaokawitu karamu**yaha** hatanae,
     When you were well you used to get up right at dawn,

4   planta aida esoho**yaha** gasoi hatanae tatukamo,
     you were filling the large generator with diesel,

5   oko yaota**ya** yoriwere dao sepe**yaha**,
     we were working alongside one another planing the wood,

6   ihi mate yakerakore, wabanahakore,
     while you were still well, before you died.

7   Ama ihi momi wab**ae**.
     Now you died apart from me.

In lines 1 and 3–6 we stand alongside Melvi as he watches Mamerto get up at dawn and fill the generator and as the two brothers mill lumber. Melvi uses grammatical features that suspend time, placing himself, Mamerto, and listeners in the middle of these scenes.[5] Lines 2 and 7 contrastively place these memories and expectations in a past that has been sealed off from presents and futures. These features thus created the sort of struggle between multiple temporalities—lingering pasts, anticipated futures, and a harsh reality of temporal rupture—that Freud depicted. There is nothing gradual or linear here. The presents that each performer constructed were not bounded points in a linear trajectory but sites at which shifting, violent juxtapositions of multiple temporalities emerged. Struggles and compromises also became apparent in how these words were sung. In previous work, Charles referred to lines 1 and 3–6 as "textual phrases"; the focus is more textual than musical, consisting of rapid bursts of semispoken, semisung words that invite listeners—including other lamenters—to concentrate on their semantic content and poetic contours (Briggs 1992). Refrains (lines 2 and 7), on the other hand, are associated with reality testing; here speaking gives way to singing and narrative elaboration to bald statements about the finality of death. These moments of reality testing provided resting spaces that enabled lamenters to listen to other performers.

Having never met Mamerto, each poetic image presented us with one facet of his life, asking us to get to know him and to recognize the value of his life. Given that the textual phrases constructed Mamerto through his relationship with the performer, we were forced to confront how he was woven into that lamenter's being. Each refrain insisted that we confront the impact of his death, its devastating effect on the performer. The laments demanded that we see Mamerto not just as another patient, as case #37, or as a bundle of symptoms. He could not become for us just another rain forest resident, simply a subject who became knowable to us only by dying from the strange disease. Rather, he had to become a complex subject who bridged a heterogeneous range of places, times, activities, and relationships.

We had, of course, met Elbia. Although our friendship spanned only a few days, our encounters with her were intense, filled with pain, fear, the triumphal morning following her treatment by Avelino Campero, and the wrenching good-bye the morning of her death. We arrived the evening she died just as a brilliant sunset was consumed by the stillness of the encroaching darkness. As soon as Eumar cut the motor in the middle of the river and began a gentle arc toward the house, our hearts sank as we discerned the shrill voices of six women, including Elbia's mother and grandmother (figure 7.1). Displacing the hushed tones that had surrounded her makeshift hospital room for days,

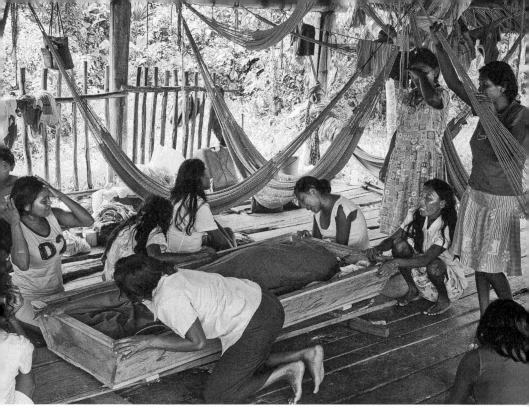

FIGURE 7.1. Singing laments for Elbia, Barranquita, 2008. Photograph by Charles L. Briggs.

the polyphonic expression of no-holds-barred emotions and high-pitched and high-volume wailing was overwhelming. As the whole team walked carefully into the house, avoiding gaps in the flooring and beams about to collapse, we saw that Elbia's hammock had been placed inside an open wooden coffin; she was shrouded in a dark green sheet. Elbia's two-year-old brother Romeliano was sometimes content playing in a hammock behind Anita, but he frequently came forward to utter his own cries at his mother's side. Rufina Gómez, another aunt, and Elbia's cousin Minia were positioned to the right of the coffin. On the left of the house were Arsenio Torres's sister Sinesia, Anita's sister Nilsa, and another of Elbia's cousins, Mirna, seated in hammocks. They were surrounded by a circle of women who watched and listened, then took their own turns by the coffin.

Anita's lament provided us with a crash course on Elbia's childhood and adolescence, education, her marriage to Mamerto, and her illness and death, an education that we expanded on later in conversations with Anita and Arsenio. When we entered, Anita was seated next to her younger sister, Rosaura, on the floor at her daughter's head (figure 7.2). She wore a clean white shirt and a white skirt with a rose pattern, the neat and orderly quality of her clothing contrasting with her unkempt hair, the distress evident in her face, and how she clutched the edge of the coffin, as if trying to hold onto her daughter's life. Anita wailed her song of farewell:

1 Manoboto, ihi mamoi narue diana.
   My child, you have already left without me.
2 Himinaha diana, tane takore ine onane hate.
   I will never see you again, so my tears will never cease.
3 Maukatida, tane takore ihi yakerakore, hohobuae,
   My daughter, when you were healthy, you used to dance and dance,
4 Hi minaha diana, tane takore ine onane hate, wabae tihi.
   I will never see you again, my tears will never cease, because you have died.
5 Bahinae akarata, alibro, acuaderno; hanoko eku, mikore onaya.
   You left behind your papers, your books, your notebooks in our home; when I see them I cry.
6 Manoboto, hake dauna eku hate, dau hikwarea idate.
   My child, tomorrow you will be in the forest, weeds will grow over your tomb.
7 Hiayamo obonobute are.
   I will always keep thinking about you.

Anita's lament focused on happy memories of Elbia; not surprisingly, she returned time and time again to the garden that Elbia and Mamerto had planted for her. She remembered, "You traveled with me to our garden. I went with you." Anita also stressed Elbia's generosity, how she often cooked and cut firewood for her mother. She emphasized Elbia's sense of humor, gracious disposition, and gregariousness, both with her own family ("at home you got along well with everyone") and others ("you were good to your relatives"). Anita remembered when they put on *ranchera*, *vallenato*, and *reggaeton* music videos: "In your grandmother's house you used to dance a lot, and I used to dance too. When you drank you danced. . . . In your grandmother's house, Rosaura, our sisters, and all the women danced. We drank beer, your father too. We all had fun. Mamerto also danced well. Nobody got jealous. I sang vallenato when you were just an adolescent. We sang when we drank a little, without even a guitar."

Elbia's mourners drew poetically on Warao grammar. Anita remembered in line 3, "My daughter, when you were healthy, you used to dance and dance." She also recalled, "*oko yakerakore hisiko hobibuae Hubasuhuru naruae*" (when we

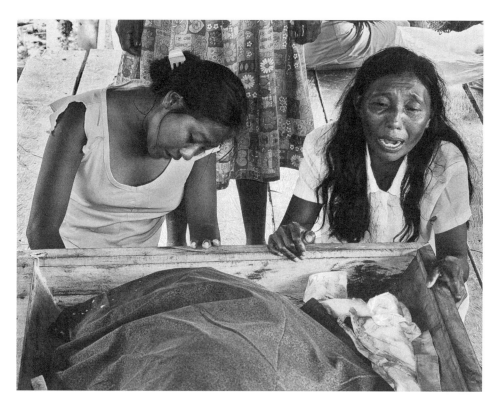

FIGURE 7.2. Anita Rivas (right) sings alongside her sister, Rosaura, 2008. Photograph by Charles L. Briggs.

were all well we went to Hubasuhuru and we would drink together), referring to New Year parties in the Rivas's ancestral home in Hubasuhuru. Here Anita used the aspect marker *-bu-* to convey the sense that these actions happened over and over, placing herself and her listeners in an imaginative space in which we can still picture Elbia alongside her mother and other relatives. *-Bu-* appeared again as Anita remembered Elbia's skill in telling jokes: "*tane takore tobo tia ihi, eno**bu**ya, yasa waraya*" (you were sitting there, laughing and laughing, telling jokes). Such grammatical features helped create small imagistic poems to bring Elbia back to life and project the pleasant memories indefinitely into the future, providing a powerful vehicle for hypercathexis. They enabled listeners who knew Elbia to enjoy the fleeting sense that she was alive and to draw them deeply into their own affective lifeworlds.

As Steven Feld ([1982] 2012, 1990) argues, based on decades of fieldwork in Papua New Guinea, laments often spatialize memories, lodging them in affectively charged places. Anita's affective landscape centered on the garden, her home, and Barranquita residents' ancestral settlement of Hubasuhuru on the one hand and the cemetery across the river that Elbia would soon be inhabiting. Laments similarly imbue material items with biographies. Elbia's gift of the canoe was made poignant by her mother's words: "You gave me your canoe, so that I could go cut taro and look for firewood." We learned that the gift of the garden came with a stipulation: "'Don't cut down the garden, Mama,' she said; she gave me her taro, Elbia said, 'so that my sister, my brother will have something to eat.'" Anita lamented, "You left behind your papers, your books, your notebooks in our home; when I see them I cry"; here she remembered not only her daughter's educational achievement but also the time they spent together in adult literacy classes in Barranquita—and Elbia's and Mamerto's patience in helping teach her parents to read.

Nevertheless, lamentation draws on Warao grammar just as deeply for reality testing. Each and every one of these images was cut off through the use of a tense-aspect form, -(n)ae, that placed the action in the past and signaled that it had ended. Reality testing was also effected through the referential content of lines. Lamenters stressed the finality of death with each refrain, punctuating statements of happy memories with "but now you have died," "you have left without me," or "now we will never see you again." Anita and other singers commented on the sudden, bizarre nature of Elbia's death. The grandmother remarked, "You had always been healthy, but then suddenly you collapsed." Her mother revealed the words they spoke in the intimate exchange that took place as she was dying (figure 1.19). In powerful passages, the singers combined durative aspect and future tense in projecting how their grief will dominate life after they make the trip across the river to bury Elbia. Anita intoned, "Tomorrow at this hour I will be in the forest. I will already be taking your corpse. I will walk behind, to watch them pile mud on top [of your coffin]." Anita added later, "Soon plants will be growing over you." Jacinta Gómez projected the point at which her grief will end definitively: "When I die, only then will I no longer grieve for you." The embedding of hypercathexis within reality testing emerges as the grandmother sings, "It will always be as if I were waiting for you."

In general, men participate in lamentation in the delta through attentive listening. As they prepare the coffin, place the body in it, and prepare for the trip to the cemetery, each action prompts an intensification of the lamentation. In some settlements, such as Muaina and Barranquita, very close male relatives also wail. Elbia's father, Arsenio, who had been watching from a nearby hammock, rose slowly during a lull (figure 7.3). He sat on the edge of the coffin, his abundant tears bathing Elbia's exposed face. He contributed no textual phrases

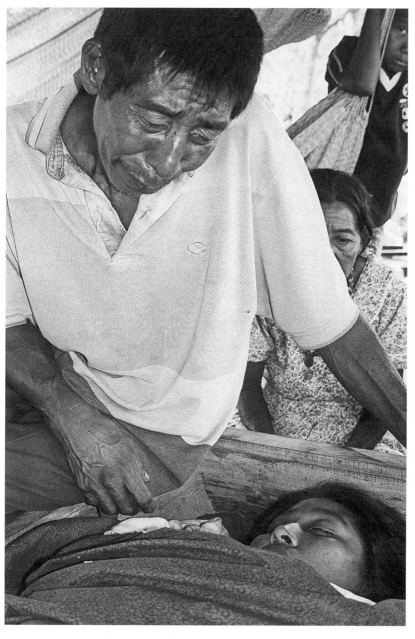

FIGURE 7.3. Arsenio Torres sings a lament, 2008. Photograph by Charles L. Briggs.

FIGURE 7.4.
Anita watches
her husband's
lament, holding
Romeliano,
2008. Photo-
graph by
Charles L.
Briggs.

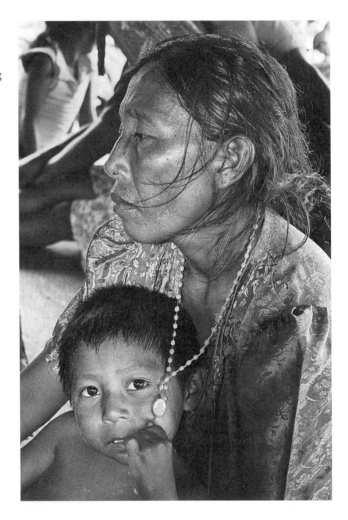

but intoned a refrain expressing the finality of her death: "My daughter, why did you leave without me? Now you have died and gone away." No elaborate road map for grief emerged here, nor did he participate in a poetic exchange with other mourners, but there were few dry eyes as he sang, and no one could miss the depth of a father's grief for his firstborn daughter. As she watched her husband wail, Anita was clearly moved (figure 7.4).

Juan-David Nasio, an Argentine-born student of Jacques Lacan, can help us illuminate the place of poetics in the work of mourning. Nasio follows Freud in tracing how love progressively dominates our internal world by taking in the image of someone we love in such a way as to "cover him or her over as ivy covers a stone wall." In grief we painfully retrace how our love for a person has attached itself "in very particular places of the wall, in its cracks and crevices," revealing how deeply and minutely our lives became intertwined (Nasio 2004, 29, 31). The laments' verses were indeed like vines, extending simultaneously into the performer and Mamerto, tracing how the experiences recounted linked them psychically, thereby resulting in intense pain and disorientation when these vines were suddenly severed. Going beyond individual and dyadic dimensions, Greg Urban (1988) argues that the acoustic features and poetic details of laments position them as crucial means of modeling affect and social relations in Amerindian central Brazil. The laments for Mamerto modeled the social fabric, the importance that one life and death can have, not just for one family and locality but, as we will see, for a broader social and political field.

Music, Acoustics, and the Politics of Listening

Listening to the laments helped the team members appreciate both how Mamerto's life was woven into those of his brother and mother and how Anita and Arsenio were discovering the multiple ways that Elbia reached into their psyches. However, as much as these poetic and musical features may tell us about the work of mourning, they do not account for how laments drew the six of us into the work of mourning and shaped how we would undertake the work of diagnosis and dissemination. Addressing this issue requires an exploration of other features of the laments. Erving Goffman's (1981) essay "Response Cries" is particularly suggestive. He argues that such utterances as "ouch" or "whoops," exclaimed suddenly after some kind of mishap, signal a temporary loss of control and provide what appear to be natural indexes of the emotional and/or physical state of the person who uttered them. They provide listeners, even strangers, access to our internal states. Although projected as involuntary and reflexive, response cries are conventional signals whose expression is shaped by our perception of those around us: children learn to emit different response cries depending on whether they are in the presence of peers, grandparents, or teachers. Goffman's formulation captures how such expressions project what is happening within individual bodies and simultaneously function to engage social relations, asking overhearers to interpret signs of internal distress as constructing both utterers and overhearers as particular types of social beings.

In the laments for Elbia and Mamerto, pain assumed the acoustic features of crying, of moans and wails, even as it was stylized. The lamenters used creaky voice, low pitch, high volume, and a special, affectively charged timbre, the suppression of the "singer's formant" (Sundberg 1974) between 1.8 and 3.8 kHz. The work of mourning did not frame these features as consciously stylized, as in storytelling, but as involuntary, transparent embodiments of internal, affective states. During the hours we listened to the lamentations, these acoustic features took us inside the people who were most deeply impacted by the deaths: their work of mourning resonated within us. This unavoidable act of listening did not determine what we felt or how we acted, but listening did overdetermine our responses, meaning that our feelings, thoughts, and actions would unfold within the parameters created by the laments.

Having widened the scope of psychoanalytic accounts of mourning by bringing in poetics and acoustics, we can also move beyond the assumption that the work of mourning is individual. Goffman argues that the projection of internal states is social and interactional, always more than an internal splitting of individual selves; if laments are perhaps the most elaborate response cries, they are also the most quintessentially interactional. Elbia's and Mamerto's relatives performed laments collectively. One person took the lead at any given moment, contributing themes that were then taken up by others. The remaining lamenters did not voice the same words or sing at precisely the same time or with identical pitch or voice quality; rather, other singers transposed the initial lines, reflecting their own relationships with Mamerto or Elbia and the most affectively charged aspects of their experiences. In musical terms, this texturing is called polyphony. Voices were coordinated in terms of pitch, volume, affective intensity, and timbre, as well as content, but these features never precisely coincided: voices never gave up their individuality. Composing, transposing, performing, and listening thus emerged together, with the emphasis shifting from one process to another from moment to moment.

In Barranquita and Muaina, houses generally lack walls; accordingly, we visitors, like other residents, were thrust into the acoustic space of mourning. The pain was inescapably inside all of us as our eardrums vibrated with the frequency of the affects generated by the performers. As Nadia Seremetakis (1991) argues for Greek laments, listening engages a broader sensorium and interpellates the body. Charles Hirschkind (2006) suggests with respect to Islamic sermons on cassettes that listening requires locating oneself in affective and ethical soundscapes. He argues that Islamic tradition locates performativity more squarely in listening than in speaking, pointing to listening as a locus for training minds, hearts, and bodies. Those within earshot of the laments could not avoid being interpellated by their sensory, ethical, affective, and bodily demands. These musical and acoustic features extended tendrils of ivy—albeit certainly not identical to those rooted inside their relatives—within us.

In Muaina, acoustic and musical features of the laments formed an over-lay for the poetics and referential content of the narratives being told at the meeting next door, shaping how we would perceive the complex knowledge-production process that was unfolding and rending it nearly impossible to think about severing epidemiological facts from the claims laments made on us. In particular, listening to Florencia's lamentation for Mamerto shaped how we subsequently heard her narrative, producing an involuntary doubling and an affective intensification. Dalvi's dying words provided Florencia with the words that she had sung for him in her lament: "Mama, I'm leaving without you now. I'm going now. My dead cousin Eduardito has come to get me. He's with me. I'm going now. We're going now." Lives and deaths, laments, narratives, and epidemiological details became intimately woven through textures and contents.

The laments for Elbia and Mamerto underline the importance of pushing concern with the specificities of the work of mourning well beyond a general-ized figure of an anonymous "loved one." Chapter 1 noted some of Muaina's history. It was established by Librado Moraleda as an experiment in organizing a revolutionary socialist project vis-à-vis forms of knowledge and agricultural and fishing techniques that formed quintessential embodiments of indigenous pasts and futures (see Clifford 2013). Librado sensed Mamerto's talent and lead-ership potential and sent him to the Indigenous University of Venezuela, a school that extended Librado's cosmopolitical vision of organizing life beyond formal definitions of "the political" and Eurocentric forms of knowledge. Elbia and Mamerto came to represent the future of the indigenous social move-ment for people in a wide area of the lower delta. They promised to usher in a new type of leader: young people who were not raised in large, bilingual, missionary-created towns but in small settlements. With their deaths, reality testing jumped scale: as the Macotera/Pizarro and Rivas/Torres familes were mourning their firstborn children, the lower delta was lamenting the death of its socialist dream yet again.

Circulation, Grievability, and the Scholarly Work of Mourning

Judith Butler (2004, 34) suggests that in the face of pronounced inequalities, "certain lives are not considered lives at all, they cannot be humanized," add-ing that "if a life is not grievable, it is not quite a life." In opening the Muaina meeting, Enrique projected how discrimination differentially values lives and deaths: "If this community was a criollo [nonindigenous] community, or of the upper class, I have no doubt that health authorities would have already taken charge of the situation. It seems as if the lives of us Warao . . . aren't worth anything to the criollo world." Freud ([1917] 1957, 244, 245) writes that what distinguishes melancholia from mourning is "a lowering of the self-regarding feelings," noting that "it is all the more reasonable to suppose that the patient cannot consciously perceive what he has lost." But can mourning and melancholia be neatly separated in the aftermath of Mamerto's death? If colonialism shapes which lives can become grievable, does it not affect daily life in ways that complicate both mourning and its difference from melancholia? Anne Cheng (2000, 24) suggests that melancholia structures racialized inequalities in such a way that it "conditions life for the disenfranchised and, indeed, constitutes their identity and shapes their subjectivity." A decade before Freud's essay appeared, W. E. B. Du Bois ([1903] 1990, 154) traced how racism complicated grieving for his infant son: "All that day and all that night there sat an awful gladness in my heart,—nay, blame me not if I see the world thus darkly through the Veil,—and my soul whispers ever to me, saying, 'not dead, not dead, but escaped; not bound, but free.'" Frantz Fanon (1963, 1967) famously stresses the individual and collective depersonalization that structures the violence and social death produced by colonialism. Enrique frequently disrupted epidemiologists' interpretations of the deaths by extending the time frame under consideration from July 2007 to the five hundred years of colonial violence in the delta following Columbus's arrival. In such a situation, is it possible to speak of "normal grief"?

Chapter 6 underlines the complexities of circulation, of the demand by the parents that knowledge about the epidemic be sufficiently mobile to travel to Caracas yet not so abstract and depersonalized as to sacrifice its connection to the collaborative process that produced it or the work of mourning in which it unfolded. Laments complicate these issues of grievability and circulation. Who is it that will hear about a life and death? What will be told and who will tell it? What effects should the circulation produce? Producing knowledge about the epidemic was embedded in complex, shifting relations among narratives, rumors, clinical encounters, news stories, and political rhetoric; we have explored how the six team members were embedded—each in a different way—within these complex circuits. All of these forms were structured, some much more directly than others, by the demand, "Tell me why my children died." The team, particularly Conrado and Enrique, helped create the context in which narratives were told. Laments, on the other hand, were entirely beyond the team's control. Lamenters not only instructed the team to circulate their words but modeled circulation by passing individual memories and questions about the death from performer to performer and then structuring

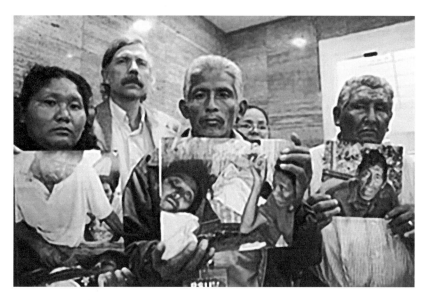

FIGURE 7.5. *El Nacional* photograph of team with pictures of Elbia Torres Rivas and her family, 2008.

how they would be received by listeners. Poetics, music, acoustics, and affects became inseparable: these were words that we could never turn into abstract, decontextualized numbers and epidemiological statements or sever from their contexts of production. The contradiction between indexical histories and forms of erasure, as articulated by Bowker and Star (1999), were built into each verse of lamentation and each word of the narratives that they overlaid. Words, numbers, and images produced in the investigation were shaped and their potential productivity conditioned on how they were inserted into the work of mourning.

One element of the tense encounter in the MPPS lobby in Caracas speaks with particular power and clarity to issues of grievability and circulation. From the beginning, Conrado and Enrique pushed Charles—sometimes literally—to take photographs of the parents; Anita and Arsenio's family asked him to document Elbia's illness, wake, and funeral. Selecting which photographs to take to Caracas was an important part of preparations for the trip. When a photographer for *El Nacional* appeared in the MPPS lobby, Enrique pulled out a manila envelope containing the eleven photographs and invited Tirso and Norbelys to select a print. When the photographer raised his camera, they each held up a photograph related to Elbia's death. Enrique chose one of Anita Rivas watching her daughter die (figure 1.19), Tirso a portrait of Elbia's grandfather (figure 1.18), and Norbelys one of Arsenio Torres performing a lament over his daughter's corpse (figure 7.3). The resulting *El Nacional* photograph brought the parents and their demand, "Tell me why my children died," into the MPPS lobby, etched on the bodies of the three team members who held up the photographs (figure 7.5). Their stated goal was to keep the images and laments attached to the account that the team transported to Caracas, thereby preventing our report from becoming abstract words and numbers or further "proof" of indigenous stereotypes. Tirso, Norbelys, Enrique, and Conrado viewed the juxtaposition of a story in a national newspaper with these photographs within a photograph as evidence that they had responded as fully as possible to the parents' demand to tell as many people as possible about their children's lives and deaths, to challenge what they saw as RHS's desire to stop circulation of the stories of their deaths and deny the grievability of their children's lives.

The *El Nacional* photograph embodies the media strategy that Enrique and Conrado put in place that first morning in Muaina when they launched a collective process of producing images, words, and numbers for transport to Caracas. It would be foolish to think, however, that this process unfolded in a linear fashion or that it simply fulfilled their vision. It involved a precarious relationship between heterogeneous sites, people, viruses, animals, technologies, and forms of knowledge production—ones that would not ordinarily intersect—amounting to what Bruno Latour (1987) might call an "actor network" or Kathleen Stewart (2007) might point to as one of those moments when heterogeneous phenomena come together in accidental juxtapositions that are particularly revealing. It involved a complex process that we call biomediatization, the coproduction of new objects (here, an epidemic) that have both biological and media components that arise through tense collaborations among actors with very different interests and perspectives. How the work of mourning shaped this biomediatization process and how collaboration between journalists and health officials eventually contained the work of mourning and imprisoned it anew in the lower delta is the focus of chapter 8.

_____

BIOMEDIATIZATION

Health/Communicative Inequities and Health News

One of the most revealing episodes during the meeting in Muaina came when Conrado opened a dog-eared file folder during a lull in the proceedings. The laments had ended and the funeral procession had left for the cemetery. Muaina residents' heated accusations against a healer had been suspended while a commission went to the neighboring island to subpoena Francisco Pérez. Those left behind were milling about in Olga Pizarro's house, taking turns sitting in the hammock or one of the three white chairs. Conrado had carried the folder under his left arm all morning, but only then began to reveal its contents to groups of four or five people at a time, holding the extracted papers as if they were sacred objects. Ordinarily soft-spoken, unassuming, and low-key, Conrado's kind face hardened and his voice acquired an angry edge.

The contents were two articles that had been torn—literally—out of *Notidiario*; they provided our first glimpse of the stories that appeared in February 2008 in the wake of Conrado's and Alonzo Moraleda's confrontation with RHS officials in the Legislative Council: "Cases of Diarrhea Are Brought under Control in Antonio Díaz" (20 February) and "Wisidatus Are Not Causing the Deaths of Indigenous Children" (22 February). Our circle included Norbelys, Olga Pizarro, and several other Muaina residents. Conrado's commentary outlined the confrontation in the Legislative Council, the rumors spread by health officials that blamed parents and healers for the deaths, the February 2008 epidemiological investigation, and the events surrounding Vice Minister Martinelli's visit. The ensuing discussion focused squarely on the looming divide between the articles and what the parents had done to save their children, the efforts by residents in Mukoboina, Muaina, and elsewhere to figure out what was going on, and the repeated demands by Conrado and others that RHS act swiftly and decisively to diagnose the epidemic.

Conrado was actively initiating a collaborative process of creating pasts, presents, and futures. The folder became a prompt for configuring memory, not just of the events of the previous February or the epidemic as a whole but of how health had been experienced as violence for decades. He used the articles to cast the meeting in Muaina as a turning point in which indigenous leaders, healers, and parents could join in diagnosing and stopping the epidemic and assuming a transformative role on health issues. The articles also formed the basis for projecting a future that would not mirror the bitter past, one in which delta residents would not bear the brunt of acute health inequities and health/communicative inequities. Throughout our investigation, Conrado took the folder with him everywhere.

The way Enrique opened the meeting suddenly fell into place. Gesturing at Mamerto's body and the laments performed next door, Enrique characterized the epidemic as the product of class and ethnic inequities, noting how an epidemic among nonindigenous children in an elite neighborhood of Caracas would have received an immediate, overwhelming response. At that juncture Enrique continued, "That's why I ask the people of Muaina, with all my respect and consideration, we want to record from beginning to end. This record can provide a base, a support, a force to enable us to convey this painful situation that is taking place." Then he drew us more deeply into the revolution the brothers were plotting: "I count on you, Dokomuru, if you will excuse me, and

Dr. Clara here—you must commit yourselves if this case needs to be brought to the central government."

Even before the team had an inkling of what might be causing the epidemic, Conrado and Enrique conceived a media strategy. They knew that forcing the government to take more forceful steps to end the epidemic, improve health conditions in general, and replace health-based stereotypes of delta residents would require transforming media coverage of health issues. Reducing their intervention into the history of health news coverage of indigeneity to a media strategy would, however, fail to capture the complexity of biomediatization. Rather than focus in this chapter on how diseases are projected in "the media" per se, we develop an approach to biomediatization itself, challenging binary oppositions between "the media" and medicine by examining how diseases, epidemics, drugs, and medical subjectivities (such as those of doctors and patients) are coproduced through collaborations between health and media professionals. The commonsense view of health news is that journalists take knowledge produced in biomedical sectors, translate it into nontechnical terms, and transmit it to lay audiences. We reflect on press coverage of the epidemic in analyzing how this view can fuel a lethal status quo by reproducing health/communicative inequities, naturalizing biomedical authority, and impeding efforts to address health problems. In outlining how deeply media representations of health are embedded in everyday life, we build on insights that emerged in Conrado's critical analysis of the *Notidiario* coverage and the team's efforts to work with journalists in generating coverage that would challenge health and health/communicative inequities.

Normalizing the Power of Health News

Existing perspectives on science, medicine, and media—shared by scholars as much as by scientists, doctors, and journalists—trivialize one of the most pervasive features of contemporary life. Received wisdom characterizes media and medicine as separate spheres, dominated by contrasting and often opposing professional cultures (Seale 2002). Knowledge about diseases, risk factors, and treatments is fashioned in laboratories, hospitals, and public health agencies and then circulated to "the public" by clinicians, journalists, health educators, and, increasingly, the Internet and social media. The brown folder challenged this perception. In February 2008, Conrado and Enrique saw that rumors, politics, racial/ethnic stereotypes, epidemiology, journalism, and lay voices got all mixed up in complicated and undemocratic ways as they shaped not just news stories but the very objects they reported, including epidemics, populations, and public health policies. Accordingly, just as the team's mediatization strategy would shake up both Venezuelan officials and stereotypes of indigenous people, the critique that unfolded as Conrado opened his brown folder can help us unsettle received scholarly wisdom about health and media.

News coverage of health issues is marked by a striking contradiction. On the one hand, it is of huge importance to media, medical, and public health organizations, both public and private. Health news has grown in media markets worldwide, even as other news beats have shrunk. Hardly a day goes by that the *New York Times* does not publish a health-related story; it is not uncommon for three to six to appear in a single day. U.S. national network television news bureaus and CNN have all hired physicians as medical editors, and medical talk shows and medical-drama TV series have large audiences. As we were writing in 2014, the largest Ebola outbreak in history was unfolding in Africa and beginning to spark cases in Europe and the United States; as Ebola prompted widespread concern among public health officials and publics, Ebola stories often appeared on the front page of newspapers worldwide, led national and cable network news reports, and peppered social media and the Internet. For their part, clinics, hospitals, health maintenance organizations, and public health officials hire journalists to help them "get their message" into media sources. The Internet and social media are saturated with health content; news stories, information requests, and other such digital communications produce "big data" that epidemiologists use to track disease outbreaks. In Venezuela, health reporting is prominent in such opposition newspapers as *El Nacional* and *El Universal*, and a health page appears most days in the pro-government *Diario VEA*. Delta Amacuro's regional paper, *Notidiario*, publishes health stories nearly every day. Ratings in various other countries indicate that health stories are close to the top in terms of audience interest.

Nevertheless, scholars have, by and large, been uninterested in investigating health news. Journalism researchers have generally seen it as a specialized topic, less important than politics, violence, crime, or economics (see Seale 2002). Medical anthropologists and STS scholars often use media objects, mainly newspaper articles, as sources of information without documenting and analyzing how these objects are produced, circulated, and received; even as they argue in favor of the virtues of ethnography, news coverage of health receives virtually none. The anthropology of media has become a vibrant subfield, but its practitioners seldom look at health. Accordingly, health news falls through the scholarly cracks.

There is, however, a scholarly literature on health news, particularly in health communication and studies of the public understanding of science. Researchers have identified processes by which coverage of epidemics moves from an initial sense of alarm to strategies for "containing" threats and distancing readers/viewers from them (see Ungar 1998). Some work, such as that by Martin Bauer (1998), investigates how the proliferation of health news has come to medicalize society itself, reshaping conceptions of bodies, social relations, and science through projections of biomedicine. Scholars, nonetheless, commonly focus on a single diagnostic category, particularly HIV/AIDS, Ebola, and influenza, and they privilege biomedical categories (see Bowker and Star 1999; Conrad 1992). Articles often begin with a summary of the biomedical "facts" of the disease, thereby reproducing commonsense understandings of biomedicine and public health as generating authoritative knowledge that precedes mediatization. Joffe and Haarhoff's (2002) study of Ebola coverage in Great Britain begins, for example, with a background section that provides the history of Ebola outbreaks, its virology, symptoms, and transmission. A common concern of scholars is with what Briggs and Hallin (2016) refer to as a linear-reflectionist perspective that envisions health news as transforming biomedical facts into popular discourse; journalists are then evaluated with respect to the extent they "distort" clinical, genetic, or epidemiological knowledge. Challenging the medical versus media opposition can enable us to examine how new medical objects that frighten audiences turn out to be biological-cum-media mixtures, fashioned through interactions between health and media professionals and reflecting complex entanglements of professional logics, practices, and institutions. Similarly, during the mysterious epidemic, the relationship between epidemiology and news coverage did not involve reporting preexisting facts but constituted a dynamic and productive process in which reporters, epidemiologists, and health officials coproduced new biological-media objects.

For example, the cholera epidemic that began in 1991 was one of the most important health news stories in Latin America's history. From the time that early cases appeared in Peru in January, Venezuela's health minister, Pedro Páez Camargo, and health reporters collaborated in producing a plethora of stories that appeared daily in newspapers and on television. As they tracked the epidemic from country to country, stories examined the history of the disease and its symptoms, modes of transmission, available treatments, and prevention measures. In Venezuela, public health officials and reporters projected that three "high-risk populations" would be responsible for creating an epidemic, should one emerge: the poor living in urban barrios (about half of Venezuela's population), street vendors of food and drink, and indigenous people. Photographs, largely archival, created powerful visuals connecting biomedical information with frightening visions of dehydrated patients and scenes

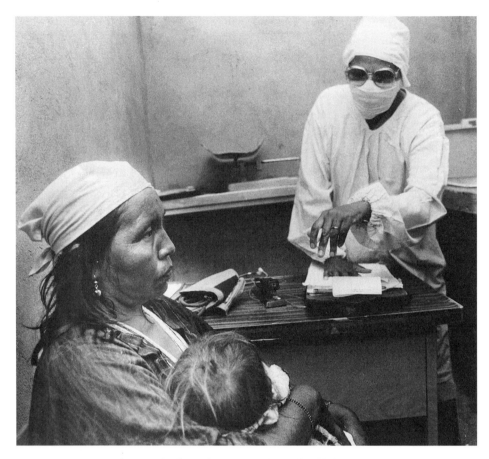

FIGURE 8.1. Photograph of an indigenous mother and child that appeared in *El Nacional* during the cholera epidemic, 1991. From *El Nacional* archives.

of barrios, street vendors, and indigenous people (figure 8.1). This process was quite successful in meeting health officials' goals—disseminating biomedical information on cholera and creating the anxiety they saw as necessary in order to prompt people to adopt hygienic measures.

Public health officials and reporters shared what Briggs (2005a) refers to as a biocommunicable model, a cultural model of the creation, circulation, and reception of health-related knowledge. They assumed that the process of communicating about a health issue begins when professionals use clinical and epidemiological techniques to produce biomedical knowledge, which is then passed along to reporters through press releases, press conferences, and responses to journalists' questions. Journalists were then responsible for translating information from medical registers—medical ways of speaking and writing—into lay language and transporting the knowledge to laypersons. The latter were charged with replacing their ignorance of the disease with the knowledge they were receiving and turning ministry recommendations into behavioral changes.

Biocommunicable models assume that medical objects exist before communicative processes begin. Careful analysis of the coverage of the cholera epidemic suggests, however, that such objects and their media forms are coproduced simultaneously. A fairly stable narrative of "the cholera epidemic" and its model of transmission was evident by March 1991, even though there were no cholera cases in Venezuela until December; in other words, media and biological components were fused even before the bacteria had came to the country. Once *Vibrio cholerae* arrived, it had already been wedded to the racial, spatial, and class characteristics projected in health stories; how people perceived and reacted to the epidemic was shaped by this mediatized image of *Vibrio cholerae*, social inequality, and fear. Middle-class and wealthy Venezuelans felt that they had to take few prevention measures, given that they were not members of the three high-risk populations, while low-income Venezuelans often felt—given their lack of adequate access to potable water and waste disposal infrastructures, fuel, soap, and other resources presented as crucial prevention measures—that they could do little to prevent infection. The "story" was so firmly in place by December 1991 that it—rather than actual epidemiological research—largely became the basis for official policies and practices.

When cholera cases emerged in Delta Amacuro in July 1992, the urban barrio and street vendor components of the narrative dropped out; stereotypes of indigenous Venezuelans as unhygienic, superstitious, passive, and ignorant of biomedicine became the focus of a flood of local and national coverage. Regional health officials told stories to reporters that drew on anthropological accounts of indigenous rituals associated with the consumption of crabs, thereby weaving "Warao culture" into an outbreak of a waterborne disease in an area lacking facilities for potable water and sewage disposal and where clinics were few and far between. Turning apocryphal stories about crabs, rituals, spirits, and shamans into epidemiological explanations, they did not recount the heroic efforts of local leaders and ordinary citizens in the delta working around the clock with physicians and nurses to bring boatloads of patients to clinics, scenes that they had actually witnessed over and over. A narrative about the cultural and medical otherness of "the Warao ethnic group" became a national discourse. Slowly losing its direct connection to cholera, it formed a mainstay of indigenous stereotypes. It was available to Health Minister Serrano in 2008 in explaining a new epidemic: "Please don't forget that the indigenous people have different customs."[1] This narrative of disease and culture helped shape what Carmen Buenaventura saw when she visited the delta and listened to Lourdes Rodríguez, MPPPI's Delta Amacuro representative, retell the Mukoboina story as a case in which "ancestral knowledge" turned into witchcraft.

Conrado and Enrique had not forgotten the crab story. When the February 2008 stories recycled the 1992 images of an unhygienic, superstitious, and ignorant indigenous population, their anger was rekindled. Conrado and his interlocutors X-rayed how health and media professionals had once again collaborated in coproducing a new medical/mediatized object—and had once again turned acute health inequities into a cultural pathology. The discussions in Muaina analyzed how the biomediatization process reproduced RHS's monopoly on the production of legitimate knowledge—even when little knowledge was being produced and RHS failed to persevere until it produced a diagnosis, meanwhile deflecting possible political consequences. Conrado's and Enrique's anger sparked an analysis of biomediatization and its crucial effects in shaping health practices and policies, an analysis that we extend here.

The Revolution, Media, Health, and a Kidnapping

To be sure, many things had changed since the cholera epidemic. Chávez gained the presidency and championed popular participation in governance and health care for low-income Venezuelans. Things had also changed in media institutions. The new epidemic emerged in the middle of a *guerra mediática* (media war) that pitted the socialist government against commercial media, most of which were vehemently anti-Chavista. Media during the Chávez period has been the subject of much scholarly attention, which itself has often embraced political polarization. A widely disseminated story asserts that Chávez exercised dictatorial control over the media landscape.[2] During his presidency, government television stations increased from one (VTV) to seven; pro-government and largely state-financed *Diario VEA* was joined by two other newspapers. Claims that government media displaced private institutions are contradicted, however, by the findings of Nielsen affiliates' estimates that the audience share of government channels only grew from 2 percent in 2000 to 4.4 percent in 2008.[3] Observers do agree on one point: news coverage in anti-Chávez commercial media versus pro-government media differs radically. In an ethnography of news coverage of crime, Robert Samet (2012, 20, 22–23) argues that a looming gap between pro- and anti-Chávez journalistic camps was apparent not only in perspective and content but also in the emergence of "two separate professional tracks," which rendered collegial relations nearly impossible; employment in one sector excluded subsequent work in the other.

Health, as a news topic, contradicts these generalizations. Given the visibility of both health and media in the acrimonious conflict between the government and political opposition, one would think that health news would be doubly polarized. Charles and Clara wrapped up an extensive study of health news in July 2008, just days before leaving for Delta Amacuro and encountering the epidemic. It included content analysis, ethnography, and interviews with health officials, journalists and editors, clinicians, and lay audiences, and it focused on the extent to which revolutionary epistemologies had been incorporated into health journalism in pro-government media and how much this coverage differed from that in the opposition media. In the end, it was hard to distinguish whether a story came from a pro- or antigovernment source.

In interviews and stories, Chavista and opposition journalists alike reproduced health/communicative inequities. Take the private tabloid *2001* and pro-government *Diario VEA*. Both feature full-page health sections in most daily editions, and they have reporters who exclusively report health. Their health reporters both rely primarily on their lists of "experts" in developing stories. Journalists representing both camps responded with the same look of surprise and skepticism when we asked if they used laypersons as sources. The *Diario VEA* reporter described Venezuelans as self-medicators; she disqualified laypersons as sources because they rely more on "witchcraft" than doctors. An editor at *Diario VEA* noted that "the paper's directors don't see health as an important part of its mission," joining the health reporter in casting this "beat" as apolitical. She discounted readers as potential sources of information—they had too many "errors" in their biomedical knowledge to contribute knowledge about health. Leo Casagrande of ViVe TV, who occasionally covered health, was the only reporter who saw *el pueblo*, particularly indigenous and other "socially excluded sectors," as producing valuable perspectives and practices.[4] Venezuela is not alone in failing to revolutionize the common practice of privileging health professionals' perspectives over those of laypersons. In Cuba, health journalists similarly have their lists of specialists and see themselves as conveying medical knowledge to "the people," who they often accuse of self-medication and other failures to heed their physicians' advice (Briggs 2011a).

In February 2008, Conrado and nurse Alonzo tried to create revolutionary press, to use lay perspectives derived from "socially excluded sectors" (in Chávez's lexicon) to expand the scope of the "fundamental social right to health." Aided by Dr. Ricardo's letter, extensive discussions with the parents, and his observations of what had taken place in the Nabasanuka clinic, Conrado appeared in Tucupita and attempted to create a public debate. The results were mixed. Conrado was indeed pictured on *Notidiario*'s front page; although the reporter noted that he had presented information on the epidemic in the meeting, Conrado only appeared as an incidental element in a battle between camps of nonindigenous politicians. The event, however, challenged RHS's efforts to silence the epidemic and its monopoly on the biomediatization of health. The diarrheal investigation by RHS constituted an elaborate biomediatization campaign, one oriented toward invoking another object—not a strange new undiagnosed disease but the familiar, politically unproblematic category of diarrheas.

In subsequent weeks, epidemiology and news coverage did not occupy separate realms but were coproduced in three ways. First, the diarrheal investigation responded to news coverage of the council's attention to the epidemic. Second, the diarrheal investigation was designed to produce news coverage, to provide a context in which Vice Minister Martinelli could visit the lower delta with RHS's director, demonstrate MPPS's concern with the health of residents, and call attention to the diarrheal investigation. In a newspaper photograph, Vice Minister Martinelli, her body draped in revolutionary red, is shown approaching one of the "small patients affected by water-borne diseases"; the caption suggests that the photo documents her observation of the clinical phase of the investigation. A third dimension emerged in Conrado's voice as he pointed to how epidemiology can be designed as a means of preventing media representations.

Conrado reported that the diarrheal investigation was accompanied by an around-the-clock effort to paint the Nabasanuka clinic and fill it with medicines and furniture that was not rusted and antiquated. Nurses suggested that the makeover anticipated an impending visit by a national official; residents were determined to use the occasion to talk about the mysterious epidemic. Then deputy regional epidemiologist Benjamín López arrived in Nabasanuka one night and summoned Conrado out of bed saying, "Moraleda, early tomorrow morning, at 4:00 AM, you have to get up and bathe, because at 6:00 we are going to form a commission and leave for Orinanoko. It's important. We need to work on the case of the children who are dying. . . . We need to create an epidemiological barrier and distribute medicines." Conrado added, "He gave a thousand details, made up a thousand things—and I believed him." Conrado was surprised the next day to find that López made only fleeting visits to several settlements that had never reported cases of the strange disease and asked only superficial questions. Returning in the afternoon, they passed a boat containing RHS director Dr. Guillermo Rendón and other passengers. López asked, "How are you, Guillermo?" "How are the people around here?" asked Dr. Guillermo in return. "Everything is fine, no fevers or anything, absolutely nothing," responded López.

When Conrado arrived back at Nabasanuka, fellow residents scolded him. Dr. Guillermo had arrived with Vice Minister Martinelli that morning, "and they just stayed a short time, like tourists." Nabasanuka residents, famous in Delta Amacuro for in-your-face confrontations with visiting authorities, would have demanded a meeting; because Dr. Guillermo didn't introduce her, they didn't realize who the vice minister was until later. Conrado observed, "Now I see that those people *kidnapped me* so that I wouldn't talk to anyone." Framing it as a human rights violation, he pointed to how health/communicative inequities are individual and collective simultaneously. "I was the president of the health committee, and they silenced me." Reporters and the vice minister got only RHS's perspective, and the *Notidiario* article lauded the "very ambitious" anti-diarrheal campaign without even mentioning the strange epidemic.

The cholera epidemic and the events of February 2008 convinced Conrado and Enrique that biomediatization is a crucial factor in producing health and health/communicative inequities. In order to transform both health conditions and news coverage, they realized that they needed the sort of detailed epidemiological data that would enable them to tell their story to the press. At the same time, they wanted to create an archive that would also, as we suggest in chapter 7, remained tied to the parents, the children, and the capacity of delta residents to produce valuable knowledge about health. It was precisely their analysis of the role of biomediatization in the larger economy of health and social justice that fired interest in generating a new type of press coverage.

Given the nonrevolutionary cast of health news, it was notable that in Caracas in August 2008 a brief revolutionary moment in media coverage emerged, one in which health journalists for elite newspapers treated four indigenous, working-class Venezuelans as credible producers of health knowledge. *El Nacional*'s Carmen Buenaventura noted in her first article on the epidemic that "the community decided to create a commission" after RHS failed to act. Her lead was a quote from Conrado. Citing the number of deaths, Carmen characterized Conrado's goal of putting the epidemic "on record" (*dejar registro*). Stereotypes of politically passive, easily duped indigenous actors who cannot assimilate biomedical knowledge seemed to vanish. When the team reviewed the press coverage the day after the confrontation, Enrique realized with satisfaction that he had accomplished his goal, announced that morning during the meeting in Muaina, of turning knowledge production into "a base, a support, a force to enable us to convey this painful situation." Conrado, still clutching the brown folder that was his archive, realized that it would now include the sort of coverage he had dreamed of: stories and images that drew attention to the dead children, the parents, their demands, and the right of people classified as indigenous to contribute knowledge about acute health inequities and to confront them.

To be sure, there had been costs along the way. Chapter 6 discusses the decision to erase discussions of "bad medicine" from the report and statements to officials and reporters. This deletion shaped news coverage and policy debates while we were in Caracas, but Carmen's interview with MPPPI's Delta Amacuro representative transposed the figure of malevolent "ancestral knowledge" from the background of available stereotypes into the foreground, thus countering the positive story of indigenous people confronting an epidemic. Recall that *Diario VEA*'s health reporter asserted that trusting "witchcraft" more than doctors disqualified lay Venezuelans as health news sources. The old stereotypes were there, just waiting to be recycled; biomediatization became, once again, a mechanism for casting indigenous people into the realm of Otherness and superstition. This sort of backtracking undermined the story that Carmen had carried for several weeks about how people classified as indigenous had produced health knowledge.

The epidemic offered a major opportunity to reporters for opposition media. *El Nacional* and *El Universal* reporters had lost their cozy relationship to health officials; given political polarization, the newspapers' antigovernment stance, and the central role of health in governmental policies and opposition attacks, MPPS officials seldom made themselves available to opposition journalists. Spokespersons for the vehemently anti-Chávez Venezuelan Medical Federation accordingly gained greater importance as sources. In a pre-epidemic interview, *El Universal*'s Ramona Herrera complained that ministry officials "don't talk to us, don't give us information." Suddenly, government officials were now anxious to talk to opposition reporters, giving press conferences, requesting interviews, and providing comments nearly every day.

Remarkably, it was how the opposition press framed the story that helped lead to its demise. We called ourselves a team (*un equipo*) rather than a commission, and we did not call our work a denuncia. We believed that claiming to be a commission would leave us open to attack by government agencies as making false claims to official authorization and suggest that only governmental institutions had the right to investigate health issues. The denuncia interpretation would have positioned us as attacking the Chávez government, clearly not our goal. Nonetheless, reporters imposed these labels on us, no matter how often we told them that neither applied. In her first article, Carmen suggested that Conrado, Enrique, Norbelys, and Tirso "decided to create a commission," thereby providing an opening for the RHS director to declare that "at no point had he authorized any commission whatsoever to investigate." The term "denuncia" appeared in the title of articles beginning with Ramona's first story in *El Universal*; Minister Serrano used it in referring to our report and to us as well ("the ones who made the denuncia"). Referring to the team as a commission facilitated our demotion to the status of illegitimate and unreliable interlopers once official commissions visited the delta.

According to the story journalists told from the start—which team members helped coproduce—our work was prompted by RHS's failure to investigate the epidemic adequately, produce a diagnosis, and inform national officials. Accordingly, our report could remain newsworthy only for as long as credible official investigations were absent. From the beginning, however, Conrado and Enrique also sought to challenge long-standing health inequities and health/communicative inequities. Because journalists respected indigenous leadership and knowledge only insofar as it was framed as filling gaps in official information, MPPS could undermine the team's visibility by sending commissions and announcing results, effectively consolidating MPPS's position as the sole authorized locus of epidemiological knowledge producers and highlighting its vast resources for producing, validating, and circulating health knowledge.

Reporters accepted without question the officials' framing of the debate as revolving around epidemiological information that MPPS health professionals produced and controlled. To counter the reporters' projections of the team as having status as researchers, RHS director Dr. Guillermo attempted to discredit us in *Notidiario* as "self-proclaimed scientists." Vicente Medina, a physician who self-identifies as Warao, accused Clara in *Ultimas Noticias* of confusing the symptoms of diarrheal and respiratory diseases with those of rabies, arguing that she placed deaths from "a variety of causes" within a single diagnostic category. He deemed it "irresponsible" to present a diagnosis based on clinical evidence, given that "other diseases can generate the same symptoms," without, however, specifying which others he had in mind. For his part, regional epidemiologist Froilán Godoy asserted, "It can only be known with certainty, based on the studies that have been conducted, that levels of lead in the blood of Warao are highly elevated," thus resurrecting the lead-intoxication hypothesis, which had already been rejected. At the same time that this statement jumped scale to turn a few blood samples into an epidemic, Dr. Froilán did not suggest any treatment or prevention measures for the implied public health crisis of widespread lead poisoning.

The brunt of the officials' reassertion of control rested on the statistical attack, the war of numbers, that MPPPI minister Taller started: "I don't think
there could have been so many deaths." Reporters recognized that large discrepancies were apparent in the statistics that officials used to counter the team's
results, but they never grasped the point that MPPS's numbers reflected acute
health inequities: the only patients counted were those seen by physicians. Our
interviews indicate that twenty-one of the patients were seen in Nabasanuka
and/or Tucupita; complications surrounding diagnosing rabies probably led
to eliminating some of these from the official count. Ten patients were not seen
in either of these facilities, and seven more were examined in nursing stations,
enabling MPPS to declare its official ignorance of these seventeen deaths; journalists did not challenge them on it. Given that MPPS never undertook a case-
by-case investigation and that the commissions did not visit most of the places
where deaths occurred, MPPS could keep most of the cases—as in the cholera
epidemic and the count of "normal" infant mortality—off the books. The team
was, however, complicit in this process. After we finished our work in Santa
Rosa de Guayo, we concluded that documenting other deaths in that area was
less important than taking detailed documentation of thirty-eight deaths to
Caracas and pressing for action, including a rabies vaccination program: other
people might already have been exposed. This decision deprived other parents,
however, of the opportunity to tell their stories, and it erased them from the
statistics that we carried to Caracas.

The way that the press closed down the story after MPPS declared on its
website that "there is no rabies in Delta Amacuro" is telling. Once the government's commissions announced their conclusion—even without providing evidence or responding to reporters' questions—they could reclaim their rightful
monopoly over the production and transmission of epidemiological knowledge.
We learned in conversations with commission members that the scientific basis
was collecting bats, which turned out to be negative for rabies. Nevertheless,
their research was limited to less than two dozen bats collected in a single night
in Santa Rosa de Guayo, hardly an adequate sample to determine that rabies
was not and had not been present in the delta. More broadly, the entire biomediatization process was predicated on the emergence of consensus regarding a
single pathogen and its human effects in terms of symptoms and deaths; simply
by denying the hypothesis that best explained the clinical evidence, MPPS shut
down biomediatization.

By framing the story as a war of numbers and then granting legitimacy
to MPPS's statistics, journalists had reinstated a biomediatization process in
which they collaborated with government officials in producing understand-

ings of what constituted health, disease, and knowledge of them and restricted access to the shaping and debating of policies. In the end, opposition reporters helped restore the very monopoly over health knowledge that had generally shut them out of its circulation; they helped restore the legitimacy of a government they despised. Paradoxically, it was the government's own television channels—VTV and ViVe TV, which have so often been slammed by opposition politicians and international commentators as sources of government propaganda—that sustained the idea that uncommissioned actors could legitimately talk about an epidemic.

Biomediatization, the Archive, and the Repertoire

This chapter began by looking over Conrado's shoulder at his archive of *Notidiario* articles and how it prompted him to look for alternative ways to get the story out. As performance studies scholar Diana Taylor argues, archives are generally envisioned as sites containing stable sets of enduring materials, fixing them in ways that render them "supposedly resistant to change" and organized with an eye to reproducing social power. Archives accordingly stand in contrast with performance, "the so-called ephemeral repertoire of embodied practice/ knowledge" (Taylor 2003, 19). Taylor examines the place of photographs, records, and other artifacts used by the Argentine dictatorship (1976–1983) in exerting control over the lives and deaths of the "subversives" they tortured and disappeared, showing how these documents were reused by the Mothers and Grandmothers of the Plaza de Mayo in performing memory and political resistance. The striking contrast between archives and repertoires, seemingly matching an indigenous versus nonindigenous divide, is well illustrated by the gulf between epidemiological documents destined to become part of Delta Amacuro's official health archive and performances of narratives, laments, and healing.

Conrado's brown folder, however, presents a challenge to static, binary oppositions between archives and repertoires. In what she refers to as "the DNA of performance," Taylor (2003, 168) argues that relatives of the disappeared used photos "to bring together the science (DNA testing) and the performative claims in transmitting traumatic memory." However, placing science in the realm of the archive and politics in that of performance would prevent us from thinking through the way that the brown folder critically examined how scientific objects were constructed in the first place. Conrado's performance of knowledge about the epidemic in the Legislative Council, the rumors about fruit, fish, and malpracticing healers, the diarrheal investigation, instructing reporters on how to see dying patients, Conrado's "kidnapping," and a disappearing act that hid a vice minister from residents were all part of the production of a quintessentially scientific object, an epidemic. An epidemiological archive that was not meant to be read, official performances that embodied visual and statistical archives, and portable dog-eared archives that provided antiscripts for collaborative performances of old injuries and new beginnings pointed to how the epidemic challenged any scientific/political or archival/performative binary.

Jesús Martín Barbero (1987) claims that a significant scholarly limitation springs from basing research on commonsense assumptions about "the media," thereby participating in the boundary-work (Gieryn 1983) that seems to separate "the media" from other cultural and institutional spheres. Medicalization (Conrad 1992) performs a similar sort of boundary-work on phenomena whose definition and understanding are dominated by health professionals. Health news is built on both these powerful forms of boundary-work, positing the separate existence of scientific facts emerging from biomedical sectors that enter into media institutions for packaging and sale to laypersons. If analysts implicitly believe that they know in advance what media and medicine are and then restrict themselves to examining only the areas where the two seem to overlap, they will overlook the power of biomediatization and how only particular phenomena, voices, and perspectives come to form public archives of medicine in the first place. Biomediatization thus enjoins not merely an additive but an exponential effect between fields associated with medicalization and mediatization, even as the boundary-work that seems to keep them separate blinds us all to the performative power of these intersections.

Wherein lies a new point of departure? Telling a simple story of instrumental collusion, of a crass alignment of self-interests, would not help us think through the mysteries that emerged in the epidemic. Why did opposition newspapers like *El Nacional* help the government officials contain a serious threat to their control over biomediatization? And why did the government's television channels, VTV and ViVe TV, provide revolutionary health news, challenging MPPS's position and threatening the reporters' professional security? What is most significant here is not the specifics of the rabies epidemic but how biomediatization largely served to close off the threat that emerged when laypersons were recognized as producing and circulating knowledge about an epidemic, particularly laypersons whose lives have been shaped by the stereotype that they cannot even understand medical statements, let alone produce them.

Conclusion

This complicated and potentially productive story of the role of biomediatization in reproducing health inequities highlights both what it takes to open up more egalitarian spaces and how quickly the status quo can be restored. Press coverage of the cholera epidemic and of the fruit, shaman, and diarrhea stories of 2008, on the one hand, and the Legislative Council and Caracas stories on the other point to the need to rethink health news, to see it not just as a place where medical facts are problematically popularized but where collaborations across sites and across professional and lay perspectives and practices coproduce what we take to be medical facts about epidemics and other medical objects. Who gets ratified as producers of health knowledge and who become its designated reproducers and receivers helps to shape tangibly real outcomes, like dead bodies and unrecognized demands for justice. However, if the rethinking does not go beyond questions of which health issues get published, broadcast, or tweeted, then the impact on how health is defined and who gets to shape health policies and practices will be minimal. The epidemic demonstrates that what is framed as media coverage of health forms part of the production of crucial central boundary objects, phenomena that are of significance to persons occupying distinct positions and that appear in different terms for each. Ironically, everyone—even the journalists who wrote the stories and the photojournalists who shot the pictures—took the media stories with a grain of salt. Everyone knows that *El Nacional* is an opposition newspaper and that *Notidiario* responds, if not consistently, to caudillo interests. Yet at the same time, articles on the epidemic could prompt massive epidemiological investigations, augment the emotional, social, and political effects of an epidemic, confront health-based constructions of indigeneity, and circulate worldwide. In short, they mattered.

In Delta Amacuro, the creation of indigenous-controlled media has not become a significant site of struggle, but elsewhere it forms a key locus for building new indexical histories and modes of circulation. A robust literature has emerged on how indigenous activists have used media, in Faye Ginsburg's (2008, 139) words, in "attempting to reverse processes through which aspects of their societies have been objectified, commodified, and appropriated."[5] In Latin America, indigenous peoples have created what scholars have identified as a distinct field of cultural production using indigenous film, video, and other media productions (Salazar and Córdova 2008). In the lower delta, nongovernmental organizations (NGOs) have provided a few residents with video equipment and training. In Delta Amacuro, however, there is little media production, nearly all of it controlled by NGOs funded by petroleum companies interested in extracting oil in an ecologically complex region; rocking the political boat is not on the agenda.

Conrado's and Enrique's interest was not in an indigenously controlled sphere of media production but in gaining access to dominant media. Enrique is a news junkie. He pays for multiple DirecTV connections so that he can spend several hours nightly watching television news while other family members view soap operas and cartoons. He and Conrado were also painfully aware that the local newspaper, *Notidiario*, plays a dominant role in defining public discourse in Delta Amacuro State. They had identified both health and media as principal sites for inflicting violence on Warao people and then naturalizing it as unavoidable collateral damage caused by "Warao culture." They also recognized that in both arenas, people classified as indigenous enjoyed little agency—even less than in politics, education, or religion. Health and media also provided important loci of double consciousness, to use W. E. B. Du Bois's ([1903] 1990) powerful phrase, for gauging what criollos in Tucupita were saying about "the Warao."

Conrado's and Enrique's intervention confirmed what emerges from community-based media monitoring groups working in places where inequalities loom large, though health news seldom forms the focus of such efforts. Biomediatization is based in shifting collaborations among multiple professional practices and institutional sites. Here we have tried to extend Conrado's efforts to open up this black box, recognizing that people who have felt the stigmatizing power of biomediatization are best positioned to deconstruct the naturalization that generally blinds us all to its effects. Given that biomediatization reproduces commonsense constructions of "medicine" and "the media," critical interventions—including scholarly ones—require challenging both of these cultural constructs and seeing how their borders are continually remade.

Conrado's and Enrique's biomediatization strategy—into which we were suddenly interpellated—was not born of abstract discussions held in air-conditioned rooms and sponsored by NGOs and international agencies. It emerged next to dying bodies and proliferating anxieties, accompanied by the disconcerting sounds of laments and parents' recitations of their children's dying words. In Caracas, four working-class people from the rain forest who experience discrimination every time they set foot in Tucupita became national figures. The stereotype that people classified as indigenous—regardless of their class or professional standing—are incapable of assimilating biomedical discourse, of comprehending physicians' words, was challenged when both opposition and pro-government print, radio, and television media confirmed their status as producers of biomedical discourse. Try to imagine the shock emerging when this recognition was granted simultaneously by the government's own media, the opposition newspapers and television stations, and media outlets around the world.

We could argue that what Menéndez refers to as the hegemonic medical model (HMM) both depends upon and gives rise to a communicative medical model (CMM). Nevertheless, we think that such a proposal would be counter-productive for two primary reasons. First, like biomedical models, constructions of health communication are always multiple and often competing. Second, proposing parallel communicative and medical models would reproduce the boundary-work that sustains commonsense constructions of both health and communication. It would rather be more productive to think about how the complex interactions of forms of care performed by healers, biomedical professionals, and laypersons are imbricated with complex, interlocking health/communicative practices—and how some get exalted and others denigrated. Menéndez (2005, 2009) calls for an epidemiology of diverse forms of medical knowledge, for systematically documenting all perspectives and practices that bear on health, disease, and health care. What is equally necessary is an epidemiology of health/communicative ideologies and practices. This book suggests why such an epidemiology is necessary and how fruitful it can be for efforts to create new ways of tackling global health problems.

Epilogue

The intensive interaction between team members and journalists ended late Friday night, 8 August 2008. Dawn found Conrado, Enrique, Norbelys, and Tirso at the bus terminal on the eastern edge of Caracas. Elated from the sense that encounters with journalists had enabled them to fulfill their promise to the parents, they purchased tickets to Tucupita on the government's bus line. As they climbed the metallic circular staircase to the departures floor and sipped small cups of strong coffee, they noticed two men in black leather jackets following them. After boarding the bus, two women, similarly dressed in black leather jackets, watched them menacingly. At the first stop the two women descended, never seeming to take their eyes off Conrado, Enrique, Norbelys, and Tirso, and two more passengers ascended; similarly attired in black leather jackets, they took the same seats. It was if the bodies had changed but the eyes remained the same, identically focused on the four. This same pattern was repeated at the rest stop beyond Barcelona and station calls in Maturín and Temblador. Each pair exchanged whispered comments. There seemed to be bulges under their jackets, suggesting the presence of a *hierro*, a pistol. Two hours shy of Tucupita, two young men with black jackets and sunglasses raised their voices. One announced, staring straight at them, "When we reach Tucupita there will be more corpses. We'll be celebrating a funeral." By the time the bus entered the Tucupita terminal, the sense of hope, the "what if the world could be different and ethnic discrimination might end" feeling that blossomed in Caracas had given way to recognition of the price of challenging dominant practices of biomediatization.

Threats continued upon returning to the lower delta. Conrado and Enrique in particular became edgy. One evening, BBC reporter Ben Rampton unexpectedly appeared in Hubasuhuru during our return to the delta. As he slept peacefully in a hammock at Tirso's house, Conrado and Enrique arrived suddenly—and uncharacteristically late at night. Enrique was livid—at that point, a journalist was the last person he wanted to see. In the end, the team's spontaneous challenge to biomediatization practices had been swept away by the tense, inadvertent collaboration between opposition journalists and government officials. Media professionals stayed within accepted bounds of critique during the epidemic. Official anger and threats of penal sanctions were leveled at the team, not at the journalists who participated actively with politicians, health officials, and team members in biomediatizing the epidemic.

9

———

TOWARD

HEALTH/COMMUNICATIVE

EQUITIES

AND JUSTICE

Listening to so many parents talk about the experience of losing children, it became clear that the places where their anger consistently outweighed fear, hope, and pain were those where the connections between health inequities and health/communicative inequities were most intimate, productive, and uncertain. In the preceding pages, we have explored multiple sites in which health inequities and health/communicative inequities came together. Here we wish to build these observations into more general ways of thinking about health/communicative inequities and to help us imagine the contours of health/communicative justice.

The concept of syndemics, developed by medical anthropologists Hans Bauer and Merrill Singer (Singer 2009; Singer and Clair 2003) can help us conceptualize how health inequities and health/communicative inequities connect. Their term refers to situations in which multiple diseases combine with limited access to health care, environmental degradation, discrimination, and poverty to compound susceptibility to and the adverse effects of diseases in an exponential rather than simply additive fashion. What would happen if we placed health/communicative inequities in this mix? Delta Amacuro provides powerful evidence of how crucially health/communicative inequities structure syndemics, including epidemics and "normal" deaths from diarrheal diseases, respiratory infections, tuberculosis, and untreated cancers as well as the underlying political-economic inequities associated with environmental degradation, lack of sanitary infrastructures, and everyday discrimination.

What is particularly useful about the concept of syndemics for our purposes is how it connects diseases, sites, environmental factors, and forms of inequality. The acrimonious encounters between Mukoboinan residents and epidemiologists provide just one indication of how health/communicative inequities thwart identification of the underlying factors that produce health problems and health inequities. Health/communicative inequities that emerge in clinical and epidemiological settings, public health policy debates, and mediatized projections of medical difference produce a deep, pervasive, and ongoing assault on the resilience of individuals, families, and settlements. This is the syndemic effect of health/communicative inequities: they are the glue that connects heterogeneous and dispersed health inequities in the experience of those who are affected by them, in the perceptions of practitioners and policy makers, and in everyday practices of care. In connecting all these elements, health/communicative inequities become a multiplying factor, exponentially augmenting the negative effects of other factors.

Cholera, Health/Communicative Inequities, and the Epidemiological Apparatus

The roots and implications of health/communicative inequities run deep in Delta Amacuro. Prior to 1992, health conditions were terrible in the lower delta. Child mortality was even greater than the 26 percent documented in 2011 (Villalba et al. 2013). Tuberculosis was widespread. Malaria was endemic near the border with Guyana, sometimes becoming epidemic. But health was not yet invested with special power to define the pervasive Warao versus criollo divide and shape bureaucratic and political structures; the domains of education, religion, development, and politics were at least as important. The bureaucratic office that most visibly shaped the lives of delta residents was the Regional Office of Indigenous Affairs, not RHS.

This situation changed dramatically with the 1992–1993 cholera epidemic. Health/communicative dimensions were central to how that epidemic unfolded. News of the first cases in the lower delta reached RHS on 2 August; by 14 August, RHS officials had reported forty deaths and 1,000 cases to *Notidiario* and national newspapers.[1] Then the national epidemiologist reprimanded regional epidemiologist Daniel Rodríguez, reminding him that the ministry had, in an internal directive, ordered that only cases that had been "confirmed" by laboratory results would be included in official counts. There was no laboratory in Delta Amacuro at the time that could process cholera samples; even after the Tucupita Hospital was able to process samples, only a small fraction of the patients treated at rural clinics were ever tested. Note that these health/communicative inequities were imposed first on the regional epidemiologist; one of the chief and quite explicit aims of this strict case definition (which violated WHO guidelines) was to limit biomediatization of the epidemic. By turning hundreds of lower delta cholera deaths into the official figure of thirteen, the imposition of health/communicative inequities helped to hide the epidemic from international scrutiny.[2]

Health/communicative inequities were also deeply inscribed in how residents themselves experienced cholera. Clara witnessed a striking example during her work as one of the key RHS officials charged with ending the epidemic. Scores of patients arrived late one night at the Pedernales clinic in the northwestern corner of Delta Amacuro State. Some patients had only Warao, not Spanish, names, so the intake nurse simply assigned them names. The next morning, she called patients to receive their medications using these names. Having heard them only once, while weak, dehydrated, and disoriented, many did not remember them. Their failure to appear when called was interpreted as ignorance, noncompliance, and resistance, prompting the nurse to remark aloud, "You see how stupid these Warao are. They don't even know their own names!" Magdalena Benavides, the RHS director at the time, explained both child mortality and the epidemic in the following terms: "The Indians—they're people who accept death as a normal, natural event in their lives. . . . They will think that when a disease comes along that decimates them, it's because one of those evil spirits is getting even with them. . . . In their case, we have to teach them to take care of their lives, because they don't love their lives."[3] Reporters for *Notidiario* and national newspapers collaborated with public health officials in producing stories that consolidated a narrative of an indigenous population whose members were incarcerated by an irrational, premodern culture, believing in spirits and healers rather than doctors.

At all of these sites, health inequities were woven together tightly and explicitly with health/communicative inequities, tying morbidity and mortality to perceived failures of learning, listening, thinking, and acting about health. As it entered into clinical practice, epidemiology, and health policies, this stereotype became an "immodest claim of causality," to use Paul Farmer's (1999, 23) apt phrase, used in explaining why cholera was spreading and people were dying. Photographs of cholera refugees camped in squalid conditions were used to bring these stereotypes of passivity and filth to life. Cast as unsanitary subjects, "the Warao" seemed to require paternal intervention due to their members' irrationality, inability to control their own bodies, and incapacity to care for themselves and their children, thereby disqualifying themselves from full participation as citizens.

Cholera came during a time when the caudillo's hold on political power was threatened on two fronts. First, the Movement toward Socialism Party (MAS), of which Enrique and Librado Moraleda were members, was challenging the two parties that had shared power since 1958 and the dominance of Delta Amacuro's caudillo, Emeri Mata Millán; in 1994, MAS's Armando Salazar was elected governor. Second, Librado helped organize and lead the Union of Indigenous Warao Communities in 1990, which took as central goals the demarcation of land in the lower delta for indigenous residents and ending the labor exploitation and ecological damage associated with the lumber and palm heart industries; both issues threatened the political and economic hold of the caudillo and its business allies. In Tucupita in November 1992, the union staged a massive protest, linked to the global indigenous social movement's "500 Years of Resistance to Columbus." Even though this insurrection emerged in the middle of the cholera epidemic, its leaders, including Librado, medicalized the disease: the epidemic never appeared on the union's agenda. The union thus inadvertently assisted the caudillo and RHS in depoliticizing health inequities and health/communicative inequities, placing them outside of the inequalities they were challenging; the result, ironically, was to turn them into more powerful political tools.

Millán used his leverage with the two nationally dominant political parties to end Salazar's MAS administration after only a year and crippled the indigenous social movement, countering its decolonial ideology by reasserting paternalistic projections of a politically naive and passive population requiring supervision and instruction. Just as the British used cholera, plague, and smallpox to justify colonialism in India as benevolent and necessary following the Great

Rebellion of 1857 (Arnold 1993), the narrative that emerged from the cholera epidemic became the ideological charter for reestablishing control. The relegation of delta residents to what Chakrabarty (2000, 8) refers to as "an imaginary waiting room of history," as never quite ready to enter fully into modernity, was articulated in medicalized terms, as reflecting cultural forms of medical incompetence that had been proven by medical facts on the ground. These purported facts were, however, neither epidemiological statistics—which had been largely erased under national orders—nor observations by the physicians and nurses who treated the patients but biomediatized images generated through collaborations between RHS officials and both regional and national journalists. They magically transformed a pervasive and fatal intersection between health inequities and health/communicative inequities into a portrait that fused medical pathologies and health/communicative disorders in such a way that the latter purportedly explained the former. Characterized as a product of a historically distant cultural past rather than of the dynamic and unstable political present of the early 1990s, this image was temporalized in such a way as to ensure its stability and mobility. Even as it implicitly retained its indexical roots in the cholera epidemic, it became available whenever and wherever needed. It could be projected forward in such a way as to make other sorts of futures— specifically the ones conjured by the indigenous social movement—simply unthinkable.

Given the medical locus of this projected lack of agency and rationality, RHS itself became the key institution of ideological domination over areas considered indigenous, even as political parties, missionaries, and the ministries responsible for education and development also continued to shape daily life materially. By the mid-1990s, RHS could reinscribe this narrative daily in clinical settings, epidemiology, policy statements, and news stories, constantly generating proof of the health and health/communicative failure of "the Warao." Being a failed health subject could be read as performing one's self-exclusion from full participation in modernity, citizenship, and politics.[4]

This situation is similar in some ways to what Loïc Wacquant (2002) refers to as the "carceral apparatus" in the United States. He points to the massive and disproportionate numbers of African Americans who have been convicted and sent to U.S. prisons as structuring the extreme inequality sparked by a deregulated labor market through both class and racial segregation. Three of Wacquant's points are particularly relevant to our discussion. First, the carceral apparatus, he argues, becomes the central "race-making institution" for refashioning both the material and ideological dimensions of the categories of African Americans and whites. Second, that apparatus also has "extra-penological" functions that mark African Americans with stigma, constrain their lives both inside and outside the prison, impose a territorial segregation even beyond the concentration of poor African Americans in the ghetto, and turn schools, public housing, and social welfare agencies into means of extending the reach of the carceral apparatus. Third, Wacquant suggests that one of the crucial effects of the carceral apparatus has been to locate African American acts of protest within the prison, where they are largely invisible to media professionals.

In Delta Amacuro, a new racial hypervisibility similarly emerged, but it was centered not on "criminality and devious violence" but on an image of biomedical failure, and it was produced in public health rather than penal institutions.[5] Consolidating the cholera narrative thus permitted a form of governance that centered on what we will call the *epidemiological apparatus*. The perceived characteristics of epidemiology as a locus for producing distanced, objective, and comprehensive facts positioned it as continually charting the features of an "ethnic group" that was defined in medical terms. Rather than being rooted in epidemiological facts, which it largely failed to produce, the epidemiological apparatus relied mainly on cartographies of biocommunicability, maps of how medical knowledge should travel in linear fashion from nonindigenous medical professions to indigenous laypersons—and the failure of these projected recipients. The power of this new apparatus was experienced through its seemingly magical ability to turn a massive public health failure into a cultural failure that was indelibly inscribed on the interiors—minds and bodies—of all individuals classified as Warao. Conrado's dog-eared brown folder was an archive that documented this transformation of health/communicative inequities into an image of health/communicative incompetence, inaugurated in the aftermath of the cholera epidemic but reinscribed on a daily basis since. When a new epidemic began, he knew that unless this transformative power was exposed and rendered ineffective, more deaths would be turned into even more ideological cover for political subjugation.

Glimpses of Revolutionary Health Communication

Notably, the mysterious epidemic did not emerge during the dominance of the traditional political parties but in the eighth year of Chávez's socialist revolution. Health care and media organizations were both already being transformed globally, in tandem with new forms of market domination, and they soon became battlegrounds for conflict between the Chávez government and the opposition. How did the intimate dance between health inequities and health/communicative inequities move across this new political stage?

Articles 83 and 84 of the 1999 Constitution defined health as "a fundamental social right, and obligation of the State" and required the public health system to be "participatory" and guided by principles of "social integration" and "solidarity." Both in his weekly television program and on official broadcasts carried on national holidays, President Chávez frequently pulled a small copy of the Bolivarian Constitution out of his pocket and exhorted citizens to read it and to demand that government employees implement its principles, citing Articles 83 and 84 frequently. Both the Constitution and the socialist government's health programs countered decades of privatization and commodification and turned health into a primary site for constructing "the State" rather than the market.[6] Turning health care delivery into a key test of the revolution's success sparked massive infusions of capital from national oil income as well as attempts by the anti-Chávez opposition to discredit and disrupt public health programs. But as health care became a revolutionary praxis, did health/communicative inequities similarly receive critical scrutiny? Did health communication become revolutionary? The answers are mixed and complex.

Our research on Mission Barrio Adentro suggests that it initially presented a major breakthrough in tackling health inequities and by innovatively joining them, initially, to efforts to circumvent health/communicative inequities.[7] Highlighting how Barrio Adentro had uprooted a crucial site of health/communicative inequities, an enthusiastic resident of a huge Caracas barrio contrasted the demeaning way Venezuelan medical personnel had often treated him with his treatment by Cuban physicians at the Barrio Adentro *consultorio* in his neighborhood: "[The Cuban doctors] treat you marvelously well: 'Come over here. Have a seat. What's wrong?' 'Look, I have this.' 'Aha, you need an X-ray, right away. Please step over here. We're going to help you. We're going to give you the medicines that you need.' . . . That's the way we should be treated, because we are human beings. It makes you want to go to the clinic." In this example, health/communicative rights were conveyed by Cuban physicians' use of the formal pronoun, *usted*, in addressing patients, rather than the familiar *tu* and condescending tone that, he states, are often used by Venezuelan physicians and nurses with working-class patients.

Barrio Adentro also transformed problematic connections between health inequities and health/communicative inequities through the constant participation of barrio residents as members of health committees in the mission's daily work, including collaboration in clinical settings, designing treatment and prevention activities for their neighborhood, and accompanying physicians on afternoon visits to homes (see Feinsilver 1993). Notions of equality and solidarity organized Barrio Adentro across social scales, from doctor/patient/

health committee interactions to neighborhood-level planning to the overall administration of the program.[8]

We would not for a second want to claim that efforts to confront both health and health/communicative inequities can be attributed solely to Cuban health professionals. Barrio Adentro first emerged in Caracas's Libertador Municipality when a sociologist, planners, and community workers conducted research and held extensive, creative conversations in the barrio with barrio residents. These interactions were shaped by the informal social movement of the poor that had developed critical perspectives on health. In these discussions, working-class Venezuelans—many of whom had never previously taken on leadership roles—pinpointed connections between health inequities and health/communicative inequities as a central locus for critical reflection and intervention (Briggs and Mantini-Briggs 2009).

Unfortunately, few bureaucrats got the message. This failure—along with the socialization of health professionals through highly inegalitarian notions of doctor/patient interaction and public health professional/target population relations—largely condemned revolutionary models of health care to a bad marriage with health/communicative inequalities. An encounter in June 2006 with an old friend brought this point home. A dedicated proponent of the revolutionary transformation of health, he had become the director of the National Office of Health Committees at the Ministry of Health. Committee members, many of whom quintessentially embodied the revolutionary vision of "popular participation" that Chávez celebrated, were constant visitors to his office. He asked us one afternoon to help him prepare a PowerPoint presentation for the First National Meeting of Health Committees. One slide boldly declared, "It is the mission of this Office to teach *el pueblo* how to exercise popular power over the health of their communities." Charles gently pointed out that this formulation reproduced a prerevolutionary biocommunicable cartography, a cultural map of how knowledge about health is produced and circulates, and is or at least should be received. This cartography constructed a monolithic state as possessing knowledge that must be instilled in the people. We gently suggested that this top-down, linear view contradicted his office's charge of supporting health committees in taking an active role in shaping health care in their neighborhoods, in promoting horizontally organized exchanges of knowledge and collaboration. "Oh, you're right!" And yet, each of his slides assumed biocommunicable models that projected revolutionary health perspectives as being generated on the upper floors of the ministry building, traveling to regional offices, then requiring the mediation of MPPS clinicians for dispersal to "the people."

Even health professionals like our friend, who believe deeply in the Bolivarian Revolution, seemed to be so deeply attached to the notion of themselves as the knowledge producers that they were generally unable to see the transformation in health and health communication taking place around them. Eventually forgetting how important creative, horizontally organized exchanges of knowledge had been to its creation and daily operation, Barrio Adentro focused increasingly on top-down planning, its work centering on building large facilities with fancy medical technologies. The role of health committees was increasingly eclipsed starting in 2006, and it became less common for Cuban doctors, who grew scarcer, to live in the neighborhoods they served.

Small experiments in transforming health/communicative inequities did occasionally emerge from MPPS offices. As coordinator of the National Dengue Fever Program from July 2002 to October 2003, Clara shifted the focus away from fumigating adult *Aedes aegypti* mosquitoes, an orientation that had favored biomedicalized perspectives with their heavy reliance on capital and technology, not to mention lucrative contracts for purchasing massive quantities of insecticides. Instead, she placed health communication at the center. Dengue education pamphlets that sexualized both the mosquito's proboscis (drawn as a phallic appendage) and the target audience (drawn as naive, defenseless, and buxom housewives) were replaced by materials stressing people's knowledge of the spaces in which they live, study, and work and their ability to transform them. Such activities as D-Day (where the D stood for dengue) invited health professionals, politicians, manufacturers, children, teachers, and workers to participate in egalitarian exchanges of ideas about dengue control and efforts to eliminate the standing water in which mosquitoes proliferate. Chávez himself became a dengue health educator as he announced these efforts on his weekly television program, *Aló, Presidente*, and urged all Venezuelans to participate, from cabinet ministers to elementary school students (see Briggs and Mantini-Briggs 2005). Placing health communication at the center and stressing an egalitarian dispersal of knowledge production and circulation fostered widespread participation. This example also illustrates, however, the precariousness of revolutionary transformations of health communication. After the national coordinator position shifted to another ministry official, biomedicalized models and technological solutions soon dominated once more, and laypersons were once again constructed as needing to overcome their ignorance by assimilating expert knowledge—lest they be responsible for infecting themselves, their families, and their neighbors.

We have argued throughout that intersections between health inequities and health/communicative inequities helped produce the mysterious epidemic, thwarted diagnosis, and intensified its negative effects. A turn to scholarly frameworks can help deepen our understanding of the relationship between health inequities and health/communicative inequities and assist us in developing a language for analyzing and transforming them, a task we take up toward the end of the chapter.

Aspects of Latin American social medicine (LASM) and critical epidemiology are particularly relevant to this discussion, given how they helped shape socialist health policies in Venezuela and other countries in the Americas that have elected left-leaning governments.[9] We focus here on Eduardo Menéndez and Jaime Breilh, whose work has informed our discussion at numerous points. Menéndez argues that biomedicine on the one hand and indigenous and vernacular healing on the other are not autonomous spheres but are relationally defined. Central to this relational process, according to Menéndez (2009, 41), is what he calls the hegemonic medical model (*modelo médico hegemónico* or HMM).[10] The model's focus is not on health but on disease, which is viewed as being caused by pathologies that correspond to delimited, specific diagnostic or nosological categories identified by medical science. The hegemonic medical model views human beings in individual, apolitical, asocial, and ahistorical terms, meaning that historical, social, cultural, and political dimensions are deemed irrelevant to its causal, mechanistic view of linear relationships between specific pathogens and associated diseases. Medical knowledge is monopolized by health professionals, as defined and enacted in institutional settings and focused on pharmaceutical, surgical, and other biomedical interventions. Menéndez argues that this model reduces a multiplicity of subjectivities and forms of knowledge to the singularity of the scientific rationality of professionals, thereby overlooking the subjectivities of patients, their relatives, and others and their contributions to knowledge.

Breilh, for his part, rejects perspectives that simply describe "directly observable health conditions." He is particularly interested in the historical shaping of the fundamental political-economic and social dimensions of the distribution of resources and power and emphasizes "the effects of the triple inequity in shaping health: inequities of social class, gender inequities, and ethnic inequities" (Breilh 2010, 36). These are precisely the crucial dimensions that escaped clinicians' and epidemiologists' work on the strange epidemic, as they were unable to think beyond proximal causes—the ingestion of poisonous fruit or fish, mercury, lead, adenoviruses or enteroviruses—to explore the underlying factors that piled the epidemic on top of the daily toll of "normal" deaths.

LASM and critical epidemiology are particularly important for connecting health inequities with knowledge production. Menéndez explores how care is deeply entwined with issues of knowledge: "each group produces and reproduces (or not) each form of knowledge through its own daily labor" (Menéndez and Di Pardo 1996, 20). Even as LASM and critical epidemiology scholars deconstruct such categories as medicine, disease, health care, and risk, however, they leave largely unexamined the central role of ideologies and practices of communication and media in reproducing hegemonic epidemiologies and associated clinical and public health practices and policies. Menéndez and Di Pardo (2010) scrutinize how print media in Mexico portray health, disease, and medicine, revealing how biomediatization constructs public health programs as a "catastrophe" and recruiting left and right, journalists, officials, and scholars alike in projecting their failure. Their argument largely rests on identifying discrepancies between media content and epidemiological statistics, thereby reproducing media and medicine as distinct, bounded domains. While Breilh (2010) incorporates indigenous health knowledge into his critical epidemiological framework, thereby expanding definitions of health and the perspectives that inform them, he does not, however, consider either the range of communicative practices surrounding health used by people classified as indigenous or the effects of forms of communicative discrimination in producing health inequities. By implicitly embracing an ideological construction of communication that separates it from and subordinates it to health, medicine, disease, and health care, Breilh and Menéndez are less attuned to the pervasive and often perverse sites and processes in which health inequities and health/communicative inequities are coproduced.

In North America, work in social epidemiology similarly offers insights and produces blind spots. Nancy Krieger has taken major steps toward deconstructing epidemiology, viewing its social and political location, and exploring alternative formulations. She examines how epidemiological research and analysis are constructed in textbooks, exploring assumptions that limit its scope and reify dominant methods. Krieger (2011, 27) does not, however, investigate how scientists' location as "part of the societies in which they are raised and work" might lead them to reproduce not just "the ideas and beliefs of their times" but also dominant communicative practices. She acknowledges that her work is limited by her "fluency only in English, coupled with [her] passable ability to read scientific texts in Spanish and French." Krieger observes that "English currently is, for good or for bad, the dominant language of scientific texts on epidemiologic theory and research" (2011, ix). What happened in the delta indicates, however, that epidemiologically relevant knowledge is produced not only in other dominant national languages but also in those spoken by people whose health is shaped by the very political, social, environmental, and material factors she analyzes and whose knowledge production is excluded from scientific texts. The distribution of symbolic capital, as Bourdieu (1991) refers to it, enables some people to use scientific registers to fashion their statements about health as authoritative, thereby producing the inequities and assumptions she questions. If we are to rethink epidemiology in such a way that the contributions of people who live in Mukoboina can gain traction, placing health/communicative inequities at the center will be crucial.

Paul Farmer's (1991) celebrated research on Haiti links health inequities and health/communicative inequities in important ways. His work points, like Barrio Adentro, to the importance of egalitarian, respectful interactions between physicians and patients in confronting health inequities. Farmer's decades-long clinical and ethnographic work began as the HIV/AIDS epidemic emerged and became a two-pronged mode of documenting and intervening into an emerging fatal link between health inequities and health/communicative inequities. His analysis skillfully crosses scales, moving from Haitian cases and narratives to examine the effects of the CDC's projection of homosexuals, Haitians, hemophiliacs, and heroin users as high-risk populations. His exploration of HIV/AIDS conspiracy theories points to their role in critically engaging these connections. Scrutinizing the role of health/communicative inequities in producing health inequities would, however, enable him to juxtapose his tremendous capacity as a storyteller with efforts to challenge factors that restrict access on the part of the populations he champions to egalitarian roles in communicating about health.

Based in her long engagement with both medical anthropology and the philosophy of language, Veena Das (1995, 2007, 2015) has produced some of the deepest ethnographic explorations of links between health inequities and health/communicative inequities. She traces how the voices of survivors of the chemical "accident" at Bhopal were silenced in court proceedings and international debates, the way that the violence of the partition of India has remained inscribed on the bodies of raped and widowed women for decades, the anti-Sikh violence that followed the 1984 assassination of Indira Gandhi, and the quandaries that shape everyday experiences of health and health care for the poor in India. Rather than extracting narratives and fashioning them into linear, coherent wholes, Das examines how both violent and healing effects emerge through stories inscribed on bodies and domestic spaces or told only through silences or in fragments. Das (1985) documents how Sikh women whose husbands and male children had been burned alive faced violence at the hands of neighbors and officials alike for telling their stories, providing remarkable insight into how the effects of communicative and physical violence intersect.

The field of health communication models how health inequities and health/communicative inequities intersect. Critical approaches point to the way hegemonic or mainstream health communication scholarship and practice envision hypodermic-like injections of knowledge as being what is required to turn ignorant laypersons into biomedically literate and behaviorally compliant subjects (Seale 2002; Dutta 2008). Such pathbreakers as Deborah Lupton (1994a, b) and Paula Treichler (1999) forged critical perspectives that captured the central role of representations of diseases—and of epidemics in particular—in shaping social life. Lupton pinpoints the need to critique the assumptions that structure dominant frameworks and practices in public health, and she advocates for developing alternatives. Mohan Dutta (2008; Dutta and Basu 2011) uses a "culture-centered critical health communication" approach that draws on subaltern, postcolonial, and decolonial studies in criticizing how the Eurocentric bias of dominant approaches excludes the health knowledge produced by the populations they target. Dutta uses ethnography in challenging assumptions that masquerade as empirical reflections of communicative processes, how interventions are designed, and the measures of effectiveness used to evaluate them, stressing the centrality of ideological projections, political and economic contexts, and material inequities. Dutta and Dutta (2013, 14, 24) stress the need to replace "top-down, West-centric models of expert-driven messaging" with participatory projects that focus on "listening to the voices of local communities," thereby locating alternative rationalities and building new approaches to health communication from the bottom up.

Our reflections on the epidemic point to ways of extending these scholars' valuable contributions into a broader framework for opening up questions of health/communicative inequities and envisioning health/communicative justice. Given the heterogeneous and shifting character of the voices we have examined, we would be hard pressed to identify the voice of the community that Dutta identifies as a point of departure. Would it include healers, who often distance themselves from the perspectives of people they see as uninformed noninitiates? Finding subaltern voices not tainted by dominant rationalities is difficult in settlements where DirecTV subscriptions beam in soap operas, news broadcasts, and *Aló, Presidente*, and people bring newspapers, news, political gossip, and DVDs from Tucupita. Taking an ethnoracial category, "the Warao," as a starting point might be equally problematic. It would reproduce the indigenous versus nonindigenous chasm that structures the epidemiological apparatus. Additionally, accounts of the epidemic were not contained by such boundaries but circulated among doctors, nurses, healers, epidemiologists, and parents through clinical encounters, Warao Radio, and Tucupita's media. Further, using an opposition between top-down and bottom-up perspectives to frame either interventions or scholarly perspectives would position one or the other of these oversimplified biocommunicable models at the center of efforts to sort through complex and shifting politics. We have traced how a crucial way that health/communicative inequities were structured and made to seem natural rested precisely on the biomedical authority biocommunicable model, which pictures a linear, hierarchically organized transfer of knowledge produced by health professionals to laypersons via health communicators, clinicians, and journalists. As Briggs and Hallin (2016) suggest, this is the model that is generally invoked when the health of a racialized population is targeted, providing a central mechanism for blaming health inequities on the projected communicative failure of its members. The complex, contradictory details of how accounts of the epidemic emerged and moved were never contained by such linearities and binaries: everyone relied on the parents' accounts, even as healers and health professionals relegated them to the status of failures to heed medical advice. Finally, locating research within the sphere of health communication—and thus potentially reproducing the categories of medicine and communication—can leave intact the foundational separation that fuels health/communicative inequities and renders them largely invisible.

Our goal here—which is certainly not to minimize the contributions of a number of our most esteemed interlocutors—is twofold. The first is to suggest that the critical reflections on the epidemic that took place in the delta in 2007–2008 cut to the heart of debates on health, communication, and inequality that scholars have identified. Second, building on the insights that emerged from the mysterious epidemic can extend how scholars have conceptualized these issues and identify the outlines of a new framework for identifying health/communicative inequities and justice.

Epilogue

Health/communicative inequities get woven into the fabric of care and power in such a way that they can exert ironic effects. The director of RHS, Guillermo Rendón, bore primary responsibility for turning health/communicative inequities into a means of suppressing knowledge of the mysterious epidemic and maintaining the status quo when delta residents challenged the epidemiological apparatus. In the end, Dr. Guillermo was not immune from health/communicative inequities. He died in a public hospital in November 2008, several months after the debate over the strange epidemic was silenced, following an automobile accident on the road to Caracas. He called out from the gurney where they had placed him in the hallway, "I am a doctor! Listen to me! I can tell you what you need to do to save my life!" But his own bodily and geographical position at the time transformed him into just another patient; his health/communicative rights did not include exercising a voice in his own care. When no one around him would listen, Dr. Guillermo picked up the cell phone that had enabled him to rein in his subordinates in Delta Amacuro to appeal to Governor Montoro; hearing the fading voice of her political ally, within seconds Montoro called Anzoátegui's governor, who immediately phoned the director of Anzoátegui's RHS, who without delay found in his cell phone's address book the hospital's director, who ran across the short distance from his office to the emergency room. However, before he could redirect priorities to suggest that the man in the hallway was not just a patient, that he was Delta Amacuro's highest public health official, it was too late: health/communicative inequities had led to Dr. Guillermo's demise.[11]

On 21 August 2008, a stroke of the pen—actually a keystroke by a subordinate that updated the MPPS website—rendered the epidemic invisible once again. Attacking the team's report, declaring its presumptive diagnosis officially null and void, and reclaiming a monopoly over epidemic knowledge extracted MPPS from any accountability for the deaths and of the obligation to respond to the parents' demand, "Tell me why my children died." Even as MPPS ministers, RHS directors, and regional epidemiologists come and go, new physicians arrive to work with Nabasanuka's nurses and patients, and "normal" deaths continue, the mysterious epidemic has entered into the melancholic registers of daily life for the children's parents, stories that circulate across the lower delta and the fragile borders of stereotypical conceptions of indigenous and other politically subordinated Venezuelans.

Epidemics are not the only contexts in which structural factors strip lives of value so deeply that their termination seems to require no official response, generate no accountability, and restrict their grievability. In the face of the grim toll of state-sanctioned political violence in South Africa, Guatemala, Spain, and elsewhere, stories that had long been officially disappeared have gained new lives. As bodies are disinterred, forensic specialists and relatives render their causes of death legible in political as well as scientific terms. We would not want to romanticize truth and reconciliation commissions, which can turn televised narrative encounters into what are touted as national acts of cleansing, displacing the need to transform structural inequalities. Nor would we want to equate racial regimes of political violence with an epidemiological apparatus; to do so would appropriate other bodies to draw attention to the people who died in the mysterious epidemic. But we cannot stop wondering why "Tell me why my children died" seemed to require no response, whether from epidemiologists arriving with high hopes of figuring out what killed them, clinicians squirming as new Mukoboinan children arrived, or politicians who cry revolution, popular participation, and solidarity when asking for votes. Will the bodies of Jesús and Lizandro, Gabriel and Yuri, Yordi, Yomelis, and Henry never rise from their muddy graves to demand a response, not just to the question of why they died but of how their lives became officially ungrievable? The parents demanded a public explanation and public accountability for the deaths, for a dialogue. If deep structural inequities resulting from state or corporate policies and practices sometimes provide the basis for epidemics and thwart their visibility, would it be unthinkable to hold something like a truth and reconciliation commission as part of a collective process of creating accountability and countering social death for this and perhaps other epidemics?

Pathbreaking work in medical anthropology has alerted us to the power of geographies of blame (Farmer 1992). The performance of a diagnosis of a stigmatizing disease—whether it be cholera, HIV/AIDS, tuberculosis, Ebola, or schizophrenia—invokes powerful categories of subjects, diseased bodies, pathological environments, and therapeutic objects. At least from the time that Mary Mallon (who came to be known as "Typhoid Mary") became the first highly mediatized "healthy carrier" (Leavitt 1996), the performative utterance of stigmatizing diagnoses became an important way that powerful fictions like "society" and the "state," along with categories of race, gender, sexuality, and nation, are imbued with life, meaning, and political force. Rabies, of course, has one of the longest and most dreaded histories along these lines, defining a perceived divide between governments that conscientiously protect citizens against potentially treacherous pets versus disorderly regimes that seem to leave people vulnerable to attacks by drooling and mangy dogs, if not vampires and other horrors that come in the night.

The story of the mysterious epidemic was shaped, however, not by the utterance of a highly charged diagnostic label, like cholera or Ebola, but by a taboo on the official utterance of a word that might implicate a socialist government. The epidemic is not exactly a case of what Michael Taussig (1999) calls the "public secret," what everyone knows but that cannot be spoken, nor did it develop as a conspiracy theory—a singular occult truth that reveals all when whispered to those in the know. Epidemiologists hinted to us years later that they had suspected rabies and looked for bats, but the word was not echoed in every professional corner and yet mischievously concealed from patients, parents, reporters, and national authorities. Our goal here has not been to deconstruct the emperor's invisible clothing, to unmask illusions that seem to fool everyone—except omniscient researchers.

Such arguments are now familiar, and they would appear to have already accomplished much of what they are likely to achieve. Our path here has been much more mundane, humble, and, ironically, innovative, identifying a ubiquitous dimension that, to use Ralph Ellison's (1972, 152) powerful phrase, is "hidden right out in the open." We do not claim clairvoyance: our entanglements in the epidemic—from the time Conrado recruited us through the writing of this book—are no less precarious than anyone else's. We are similarly hardly immune to failure. Despite ways that the epidemic opened up questions of health/communicative inequities and temporarily disrupted them, hardly anyone in the delta was vaccinated against rabies; the epidemic was officially disappeared; and calls for a far greater role for lower delta residents in shaping health policies and practices were rebuffed. The epidemiological apparatus remains firmly in place.

Perhaps all we can claim is to have been present when these events unfolded and to have learned to listen, after decades of collaboration, to people whose proximity to unconscionable deaths is paralleled only by their ability to turn them into insights. They have no secret laboratories or statistical formulas, only decades of close observations regarding why people die from preventable and treatable diseases and why their deaths seldom seem to engender public debate and never accountability. What we might call the Chávez effect—ordinary people inspired to think differently and explore new possibilities for achieving equity—was crucial, although in unexpected ways, as a political system that blithely embraced poverty and inequality gave way to one committed to solidarity with poor and indigenous Venezuelans. Hearing Chávez's televised calls each week for a collective dreaming about a more equitable and just world and the central place that he accorded health in this process—and for holding bureaucrats accountable for blocking social transformation—helped inspire Conrado and Enrique to convert their long-standing commitment to ethnoracial justice into an epidemiological investigation. The figure of the Comandante prompted the parents to turn their demand, "Tell me why my children died" into the imperative, "Take our words to Chávez." But witnessing a new proliferation of death and a new regime of ungrievability in the middle of the Bolivarian revolution sparked anger, critical engagement, and a demand for change that resounded globally.

If the situation was less one of a smoking gun than of a finger in the wound, to invoke the phrase with which Diane Nelson (1999) poignantly unsettles stories of political violence in Guatemala, wherein lies the wound? The epidemic revealed not just unique features of health and politics in the delta but dimensions of much broader health-scapes. Menéndez argues that the labor of care is relationally distributed in such a way that family members do a great deal of it, even as health professionals largely get the credit, constituting what we might call a relational distribution of the labor of care. Miriam Ticktin (2011) argues that extending care to diseased but morally worthy immigrants helps justify new moral orders, global inequalities, and security regimes; we would add that reducing care to medicalized interventions provided by health professionals and overlooking forms afforded by family members, friends, and neighbors is crucial for sustaining what Ticktin terms "regimes of care." The mysterious epidemic pointed to an equally pervasive relational division of the labor of producing and circulating health knowledge. Rendering health/communicative inequities and forms of labor invisible similarly lies at the heart of new global, national, and local orders of care and domination.

Four features are particularly noteworthy. First, this relational division unfolds in a vast range of sites, from homes to healers' houses to nursing stations to clinics and hospitals to laboratories to epidemiologists' offices to newsrooms to places where public health policies are produced, debated, and disseminated. Second, the production, circulation, and reception of health knowledge is structured in many of these sites in such a way as to turn differences of ontology, training, and practice into health/communicative inequalities. Third, the labor of producing and circulating health knowledge assumes different forms in these locations; nevertheless, some of the most significant overlaps lie in recurrent health/communicative inequities, particularly as they are embodied in such seemingly stable binaries as indigenous/nonindigenous, black/white, poor/middle class, female/male, LGBT/straight, immigrant/citizen, disabled/able bodied, and layperson/health professional. In an important sense, we could say that health/communicative inequities provide the glue that enables heterogeneous sets of people, places, practices, technologies, and material relations to be perceived as health systems. Finally, the relational division of health knowledge is not a smoothly working mechanism that centralizes discourse and power but rather creates obstacles to the production and circulation of the very knowledge that generates the evidence it requires to constitute itself as evidence-based medicine and public health (Adams 2013a). In short, by demeaning and containing the work of key participants and thwarting possibilities for dialogue, health/communicative inequities structure health systems in such a way as to produce nonknowledge as systematically as they produce knowledge.

How health/communicative inequities structure care thus extends beyond such social binaries to embrace status differentials within the ranks of physicians, nurses, and other health care workers. Mohan Dutta analyzes how asymmetries of power and knowledge model health communication as a linear knowledge transfer at different scales, from hierarchical relations between health professionals and laypersons in local contexts to the production of health knowledge in dominant geopolitical centers and its transport to "marginalized peripheries in the Third World" (Dutta and Dutta 2013). Health care professionals in Delta Amacuro are, more broadly, seen as lowly receivers of knowledge in relation to professionals occupying prestigious positions in MPPS and clinical institutions in Caracas, who in turn look up to their colleagues in the CDC, the Pan-American Health Organization, and WHO, and leading researchers in "the global north" (even as they sometimes deride them as capitalist and imperialist agents).

In the days before the Internet digitized the circulation of health knowledge, the status of public health professionals in Venezuela was symbolized by the type of manuals in their possession. The most prestige was accorded to those boasting WHO documents in English; employees possessing Pan-American Health Organization documents in Spanish came next; they were followed by those bearing materials produced by the ministry for professionals, all the way down to laypersons who could claim only a health education pamphlet. In a politics of the copy (Hayden 2010), possessing a photocopy of a manual on which someone else had inscribed his or her name conferred a status inferior to that of the original owner. Health/communicative inequalities, in short, create their own forms of materiality, even as they help structure other material relations.

A number of anthropologists have argued that the emergence of a "new humanitarianism" (Ticktin 2011) or "humanitarian reason" (Fassin 2012) turns social suffering associated with epidemics, emergencies, and gender violence into supposedly apolitical appeals to a moral order based on a medicalized universal model of bodies and, in this way, provides rationales for maintaining European and American geopolitical dominance (see also Redfield 2013b). Such organizations as Médecins Sans Frontières distribute press releases and e-mails that call for empathy—and contributions—in response to stories of acute suffering and deprivation. These organizations, like other global health programs, position themselves as needed to circulate personnel, technologies, forms of treatment, and knowledge from what Latour (1987) refers to as centers of calculation to populations in which health burdens but not health resources are concentrated. Specialists in global health produce knowledge about these loci of suffering and bring it back to more privileged populations. Humanitarian regimes thus reproduce health/communicative inequities globally even as they project a humanitarian role in reducing health inequities. Delta Amacuro is hardly the only place where health inequities and health/communicative inequities are coproduced; we are dealing here with a global problem, one that limits global health agendas and can extend unequal geopolitical relations.

We noted in the introduction that scholars have lauded inclusion of the Quechua phrase *sumak kawsay* (translated as *buen vivir* or "good living") in the Bolivian and Ecuadorian constitutions. From the perspective of critical epidemiology, Breilh (2010, 97) points to this concept "as a potent idea, one of those ideas that are indispensable in epochs of unrest and social transformation for guiding collective struggles." At the same time that we are similarly convinced of the transformative power of indigenous perspectives, we worry that romantic projections of indigenous conceptions of buen vivir, as currently proliferating in scholarly, media, and policy realms, can risk the sorts of appropriations of dominant constructions of indigenous healing for curing the ills of modernity that Michael Taussig (1987) identifies with the fetishization of the figure of "the shaman." Catherine Walsh (2010a) distinguishes between modes of incorporating buen vivir through what she calls "functional interculturality," meaning assimilations of the concept that reproduce the power of dominant structures, rather than "critical interculturality," using indigenous concepts to question existing structures and advance social, political, and epistemic change. If the incorporation of indigenous perspectives centers on decontextualized phrases that seem to sum up some sort of homogeneous "indigenous" cosmovision, it will amount to little more than functional interculturality. Walsh (2010b) cautions that sumak kawsay is not a free-floating cosmovision that suddenly entered politics with the writing of new Bolivian and Ecuadoran constitutions, but forms part of a long history of efforts by indigenous social movements to decolonize and transform natureculture worlds for the benefit of all. Such efforts to incorporate indigenous perspectives must rather go hand in hand with challenging the health/communicative inequities that generally thrust indigenous contributions into wastebaskets labeled ignorance, superstition, and premodernity.

Giving elites a powerful new phrase that supposedly came from the poor is likely to extend health/communicative inequities. Learning to listen to indigenous ways of producing knowledge about health fundamentally involves unlearning dominant, essentialist portrayals of indigenous knowledge as autonomous, as existing independently of nonindigenous knowledge production; we have documented how this assumption often constructs racialized populations as being incapable of grasping, let alone critiquing or guiding, biomedicine. This process entails, in Linda Tuhiwai Smith's (2008) terms, "decolonizing methodologies," a critical epistemological practice that "is attentive to how . . . knowledge is produced" (Blackwell 2011, 24). We have argued that it also requires decolonizing health/communicative ideologies and practices. Inequalities are apparent not just in which principles are celebrated but in the distribution of the everyday structures and practices that shape how they are valued, where they can travel, and who is authorized to circulate them. Addressing health/communicative inequities forms a crucial dividing line between liberal appropriations of the mantle of "the indigenous" versus efforts to identify and transform sources of inequities.

Any effort to construct health through romantic and empathic tropes now encounters the hard realities of the world of biosecurity. In the United States, calls to transform health infrastructures into biosecurity apparatuses and dire warnings that public health resources were insufficient to counter possible attacks, even before the events of 9/11, prompted a securitization of public health in the United States (Collier, Lakoff, and Rabinow 2004). Andrew Lakoff (2008) argues that repositioning emerging infectious diseases in the domain of national security involves a broader shift from specific threats against national populations to imagining a "catastrophic disease threat" and modeling uncertainty through scenario-based projections. Briggs (2011b) documents the restructuring of health/communicative infrastructures and practices both before and after 9/11 and how they formed part of a transition from the "medicalization" (Conrad 1992) to the "biomedicalization" of social life (Clarke et al. 2003). Declaring a state monopoly on the production and circulation of knowledge about epidemics and threatening to criminalize whistleblowers now fits into these new modes of defining "the state" in terms of biosecurity; disorderly and unauthorized ways of responding to news of a bioterrorist attack might, we are told, have more catastrophic effects than the biological impact itself: a panicked public might require military suppression (Schoch-Spana 2004).

The biosecuritization of the Venezuelan state is dwarfed in comparison with U.S. post-9/11 legal and institutional measures. There the Department of Homeland Security is now ultimately responsible for organizing communication in the event of an "emergency." We are not convinced that Giorgio Agamben's (1998) notion of "states of exception" is terribly helpful in analyzing governance and political subjectivity in general, but the term seems to neatly capture how the "threat" of an epidemic, a bioterrorist attack, or other public health emergency rationalizes restrictions on health/communicative rights as normal and necessary. If biocommunicable business as usual leaves little room for perceiving the value of lay contributions to knowledge about health in clinical, epidemiological, health communication, and media venues, the securitization of health threatens to widen the scope of health/communicative gaps between health and media professionals on the one hand and laypersons on the other and between people designated as specialists versus the vast ranks of health workers.

Toward Health/Communicative Justice

The insights that emerged in the epidemic can, we think, contribute much to developing a novel approach to health issues by placing health/communicative dimensions at the center. We present below a preliminary outline of health/communicative inequities and the sites where they commonly emerge and how the contours of health/communicative justice might be imagined.

Doctor-patient encounters certainly provide a key site in which health/communicative inequities emerge, but it is important to keep in mind the roles of other health workers, such as nurses, epidemiologists, receptionists, guards, and lab technicians. The epidemic pointed to how these participants can either ameliorate or deepen health/communicative inequities. For example, it is problematic to assume that practitioners of complementary and alternative medicine will necessarily respect the health/communicative labor of their patients or that health/communicative inequities necessarily or inevitably structure clinical encounters, given the Barrio Adentro experiences with Cuban doctors.

Linguistic difference augments differential access to languages of symbolic authority. Lack of fluency in dominant languages and/or professional registers can prompt stereotypes of patients' perceived incapacities to participate in health communication and clinical medicine. Patients' trajectories from Nabasanuka to Tucupita to Puerto Ordaz brought home the importance of linguistic inequities as patients and their relatives were routed along itineraries that provided more specialized care and forced them more and more into silence. The need for translation augments health/communicative inequities when it further limits interaction to providing answers to professionals' questions, erasing what seem to be medically irrelevant or resistant interventions by participants and their relatives. The recruitment of spouses, children, nurses, motorboat operators, or even passersby as unpaid translators reveals how institutions fail to recognize the importance of translation, as based on language ideologies that envision translation as simple and mechanical. Perceiving translation as unimportant and embodying this perspective in clinical interactions provides one of the clearest manifestations of the boundary-work that continues to police the borders between health and communication.

The question of which modes of producing knowledge are privileged is crucial. If the participation of patients and family members is recognized only when they are responding to queries by health care professionals, then metacommunicative understandings of whose knowledge matters are made absolutely clear. Genre is one of the most pervasive and least explored arenas of health/communicative inequities; if the only narratives accorded value are those associated with biomedical case presentations—or that provide the data for electronic medical records and reimbursement forms—then everyone's health/communicative rights are severely limited, including those of physicians. Excluding songs (Barz 2006) or poetic and other creative self-expressions (Biehl 2005) diminishes possibilities for novel perspectives and collaborations even as it makes health/communicative inequities clear.

When the complex ontological calibrations and shifts performed by patients and their relatives and neighbors go unacknowledged or are stigmatized, health/communicative inequalities abound and diagnosis, prevention, treatment, and social relations are impacted. Given that definitions of health professional and patient are relational, failing to perceive and value the health/communicative labor and care that laypeople do deprives physicians, nurses, and other health workers of crucial insights into how they can better structure their own health/communicative labor and attempt conceptual border crossing. It is simply more productive to construct yourself in relation to complex, heterogeneous, actually existing people who themselves move between multiple positions and offer complex practices of care and health/communicative labor rather than vis-à-vis impoverished stereotypes and caricatures.

When the burden of health/communicative labor falls too heavily on patients and their relatives, they frequently get chastised for self-diagnosis, for trying to take away the physician's control over how worlds intersect. As we mentioned in the introduction, the Institute of Medicine's eye-opening study of racial inequities in the quality of care received by African Americans and Latinos/as in the United States was absolutely clear in tying how clinicians project their patients as failed health communicators to the delivery of inferior care. These sorts of projections are themselves sources of health/communicative failure, violations of health rights, and obstacles to everyone's efforts to grasp and grapple with health problems.

Menéndez's insight that the everyday work done by laypersons is crucial to clinical medicine bears extension into epidemiology. A fundamental theme of this book has been that clinical medicine is not the only site where health/communicative inequalities help produce health inequities and render them less visible. Although the Delta Amacuro epidemiological apparatus may provide an extreme case, public health, epidemiology, and medical research shape social categories elsewhere—as work by Thurka Sangaramoorthy (2014) on

Haitians and HIV/AIDS in Miami and Michael Montoya (2011) on Mexicans and diabetes demonstrates, to cite just two examples. Research by medical historians on how colonial differences get constructed through health suggests that these connections run deep in historical and political terms.[1] Epidemiologists' efforts also depend—perhaps even more invisibly—on the labors of laypersons, of people like Mukoboinan parents.

With regard to health communication, Dutta (2008) points to the role of "experts" in shaping evaluation metrics as a key means by which health/communicative inequities are reproduced: people targeted by health communication efforts seldom get to determine how their own success or failure will be measured, let alone assess the work of professionals. Mukoboinans provided their own set of metrics: How well were epidemiologists able to listen to them? How willing were they to share their results or even their hypotheses? Parents challenged pathologists for failing to obtain consent for the autopsies and provide the results. At the forefront of both death and epidemiological visibility, Mukoboinans asserted their health/communicative rights in the interests of stopping the health inequities that were decimating their children. Their reward was receiving disparaging comments about their communicative conduct, not dialogue. In revolutionary Venezuela, things didn't have to turn out this way: in the early days of Barrio Adentro, health policies were shaped by dialogues between professionals and residents that took place in the spaces they served, exchanges that continued on a daily basis. The categories of doctor, patient, and neighbor continued to be relationally defined, but the distinctions between them were constructed through horizontally organized dialogues that afforded real knowledge of similarities and differences and identification of common goals. Nevertheless, it was MPPS health bureaucrats who didn't get it, who failed to see that health/communicative *equities* had helped give rise to Barrio Adentro. Rather than turning the elimination of health/communicative inequities into a major goal of MPPS health policies and practices more broadly, officials progressively undermined these lateral exchanges by reducing the role of health committees and placing greater emphasis on building impressive clinics and hospitals, in which laypersons entered as patients, not collaborators. It might be easy to see how unhealthy health policies (Castro and Singer 2004), those that lead to ill health through the very way they are designed, are structured around health/communicative inequities at multiple scales, but Barrio Adentro points to how innovative policies can be organized around multi-scalar efforts to achieve health/communicative justice as well.

What about "the media"? Representations of health are prominent globally; wherever health inequities are evident, they enter—sometimes explicitly—into news coverage.[2] Here is a primary site where health/communicative inequities jump scale between clinical interactions, health education and prevention programs, and ways that populations are constructed in epidemiological terms as reporters juxtapose sources, sites, and perspectives in the same story. These collaborations also produce gaps between different scales, places, and perspectives as journalists make decisions about what to cover, whom to quote, and how to frame stories and as health professionals open or close doors, forbid their subordinates to speak to reporters, or simply say, "No comment." Individuals classified as indigenous in Venezuela or as African American or Latino/a in the United States are often pictured on camera, on mic, in newspaper stories and photos, or on Internet sites and in social media as speaking and acting in ways that represent them as failed communicators, as not getting it or being out of the loop. For example, a Latina nurse in a *San Diego Union-Tribune* column on the proliferation and intractability of diabetes among Lationos/as states, "Latinos go to doctors just when they feel sick." The article continues, "She says that there is a tendency to define a disease as 'God's will, that there is nothing they can do.' "[3] Such projections of cultural reasoning construct Latinos/as as a vast, homogeneous population of failed health communicators and health problems as resulting, in part, from the behavioral effects of these cultural and communicative shortcomings.

We have argued consistently that what is at stake here is not simply "the media," that such problems do not emerge exclusively from a domain dominated by journalists, a sphere that exists apart from those in which health knowledge is produced. Clinicians, epidemiologists, and policy makers are affected by health news and participate actively in making it. Health inequities are biomediatized objects, created through complex interactions in which media and medical professionals, politicians, patients, pathogens, and infrastructures dispersed in multiple sites are involved. These intersections matter, both ideologically and materially, in terms of how health/communicative capacities are assessed and the consequences they generate. When a story constructs its intended audience in ways that exclude the population it describes, journalists, health professionals, and readers or viewers form a "we" that is observing a "them" from a safe distance. Coverage of the 2014 Ebola epidemic shifted when health workers were infected while caring for patients in Spain and the United States. Calls for epidemiologically ill-advised measures like quarantines and travel bans, particularly on Fox News and conservative social media sites, shored up the borders between a Global North "us" and a West African "them" that suddenly appeared dangerously close and frighteningly precarious. Presented as intrinsic features of medical processes, the models of biocommunicability that shape health news stories—and their profound capacity to arrange individuals and populations hierarchically—are seldom opened up for debate, and the people they stigmatize are rarely invited to respond.

And then there are the whistleblowers, like the delta parents, people who challenge health/communicative inequities. They can be patients and their relatives who continue with their stories when the doctor or nurse tries to cut them off, who bring a printout from a website to support their queries or requests, or who get labeled as resistant or noncompliant because they question their diagnosis or treatment plan. They can also be groups of people with signs and petitions who demand a new clinic or changes in official practices. And, of course, they can be people who show up with documentation of a disease that doesn't exist officially and demand an investigation. The parents, Dr. Ricardo, some of the nurses, and the six team members all stepped into this position. Such disruptive strategies have much to teach us about health inequities, health/communicative inequities, how they are connected, and demands for health/communicative justice.[4]

It would be tempting to match each element on our partial list of health/communicative inequities and sites where they commonly emerge with an inventory of corresponding strategies for achieving health/communicative justice. Such a move would, however, reproduce many of the problems that emerge when health inequities are framed as issues of human rights: turning them into universal schemas that project ahistorical, decontextualized individuals and circumscribed, bounded social practices.[5] Moreover, given that in these pages we have only begun to lay out the problem of health/communicative inequities, it is too early to offer an agenda for achieving health/communicative justice. Moreover, it is neither our job nor our goal to shape—and thus limit—the scope of discussions of health/communicative justice in advance. Rather than attempting to dictate an agenda, we have tried to play the part that we were assigned: helping to bring the approach to health/communicative inequities devised by Conrado, Enrique, Norbelys, Tirso, and the parents "to a lot of people" and thinking through their vision of health/communicative justice. Mapping health/communicative rights involves history, context, technologies, political alignments, and the need to confront particular health/communicative inequities and health problems; a single, universalistic declaration drawn up in comfortable meeting rooms by experts is, we think, not a good place to begin.[6]

Nevertheless, we would like to draw attention to some of the connections between health inequities and health/communicative inequities that delta residents made in the course of the strange epidemic; they provide some basic principles that warrant broader discussion:

- No one should have their contributions to care or to the production of health knowledge erased or pathologized.
- What counts as the knowledge relevant to shaping health policies and practices should not be monopolized by any social sector, such as physicians or epidemiologists.
- An individual's classification in terms of gender and sexual orientation, race, class, disability, or professional standing should never provide grounds for dismissing his or her health/communicative labor.
- Biocommunicable models that project who produces health knowledge, how it circulates, and who receives it should be identified and debated, not taken as reflections of facts in the world. Collective efforts to create alternatives, particularly ones revolving around the insight that all of us produce valuable knowledge about health, are crucial.
- Defining populations as health/communicative failures violates health rights and thwarts health/communicative justice. When epidemiologists, public health officials, or journalists do so, people identified with such groups or populations have the right to challenge them.

One of the key dimensions of the Declaration of Alma Ata of 1978 was that laypersons, particularly those facing large disease burdens, should be able to participate in the design and implementation of health programs. As Lynn Morgan (1993, 5) suggests, however, national governments and international agencies imposed definitions and forms of "participation" in such a way that they often became "compulsory, manipulated and contrived." Nevertheless, efforts to promote participation as a means of contributing to social equity have continued in many forms. Researchers have explored ways of transforming epidemiology (Breilh 2003; Brown 1997) and health research (Minkler and Wallerstein 2008) in order to place the perspectives, needs, and goals of disease-burdened populations at the center. In Venezuela, Ecuador, and Bolivia, "popular participation" has been framed in the new millennium as a central means of transforming society in such a way as to counter market-based logics and achieve greater equity.

Among the many constraints that impede efforts to democratize health and health care, we have stressed the fundamentally undemocratic character of how health/communicative labor is simultaneously broadly distributed and hierarchically organized. Despite initiatives that promote intercultural health practices or efforts, such as Dutta's (2008), to transform health communication programs into means of advancing social justice, we are not convinced that health/communicative inequities are receding. The role of industrialized states and powerful nongovernmental organizations in imposing health solutions in the name of humanitarianism may be oriented toward ameliorating health inequities, but its top-down character deepens health/communicative inequities on multiple scales. As Vincanne Adams (2013a) argues, global health has increasingly embraced the "evidence-based" reliance on statistical analysis and the relegation of other forms of knowledge to the status of unreliable "anecdotal" evidence that organizes contemporary clinical medicine, thereby further marginalizing knowledge produced by people who do not possess the training or infrastructures needed to generate supposedly objective forms of statistical truth.

Even if someone could wave a magic wand, we are not so naive as to think that achieving health/communicative equity would automatically end health inequities and resolve persistent and debilitating health problems. Nevertheless, exploring—and participating in—a remarkable effort to democratize discourse about health leads us to suggest that attempts to achieve greater equity cannot succeed if they do not also identify and respect health/communicative rights. There are complexities and pitfalls here, to be sure, as in any call for democratization. As Nancy Krieger (2011) insists, however, radically reducing health inequities will require more radical forms of democracy. We have used the term health/communicative justice rather than health/communicative rights in order to circumvent premising this effort on universalistic models of autonomous individuals who enjoy the liberty to pursue their self-interest. Our goal is certainly not to reproduce the market-oriented or neoliberal reconfigurations of medicine that emerge as pharmaceutical advertisements that exhort viewers to make their voices heard by telling their physicians to prescribe the medication on the screen.[7]

Respecting health/communicative rights cannot be framed as a liberal or humanitarian gesture extended by those in power to people who are deemed to be powerless. We did not initiate these efforts to expose and confront health/communicative inequities, nor did they begin in a conference hall or an academic or governmental office. Emerging in the middle of a devastating epidemic, these efforts always had a much broader goal: that of decolonizing health, of turning health into a site in which people experience justice and respect. Our collaborators always saw what they were doing as opening up new possibilities for everyone, for other indigenous populations as well as people whose lives are not pervasively structured by ethnoracial asymmetries. They demonstrated that confronting health/communicative inequities is not something that we can afford to put aside until after we finish the hard work of confronting health inequities or fixing health systems, nor can the two be usefully detached from one another.

The parents' demand, "Tell me why my children died," can still be heard in the Delta Amacuro rain forest, their children having become the ghosts who haunt the racialized borders of a politico-sanitary system.[8] The parents are not alone: there are myriad people around the world offering to share what they know about health, who want answers to their questions about health problems and inequities. The takeaway, for us, is clear. Joining this dialogue holds the key to new beginnings that can fix broken health systems as much as broken hearts.

ACKNOWLEDGMENTS

Writing an acknowledgments section is generally something of an afterthought, a last bit of text inscribed as the manuscript is about to be sent to the publisher. For us, this section has been one of the most difficult to write. Acknowledgments generally look back from the bounded and secure position of "the author." But what do you say when the book was occasioned by unconscionable and undiagnosed deaths? How do you thank the people whose reactions to the loss of their children gave rise to the demand, "Tell me why my children died," thrusting you into a project that you had never anticipated or desired, whose parameters were so innovative and complex that you can only hope that your response is adequate? It is in this spirit that we offer the following acknowledgments.

To the families in Barranquita, El Cocal, Hanahoana, Hokorinoko, Hominisebe, Horobuhu, Mukoboina, Muaina, Sakoinoko, Santa Rosa de Guayo, Siawani, and the others where children died in the epidemic: We thank you for asking the six of us to collaborate with you in finding out what was killing your children, for your efforts to articulate the value of their lives and the grievability of their deaths, as well as for the charge to "take our words to Chávez"—in short, for making us part of your work of mourning. We also salute the local representatives who helped their settlements face death and fear and who worked with the team in organizing the meetings that enabled parents to tell their stories and make our work of epidemiology and documentation possible.

To Conrado, Enrique, Norbelys, and Tirso: We have never faced a more difficult challenge, nor received a greater honor than your call to join the efforts you organized to stop the epidemic and to transform health in the delta. We thank you for your friendship and trust, and also for the many ways your insights have enabled us to grow as persons, scholars, and practitioners. We hope that this book will help provide the recognition that you deserve for your brave efforts to take on a mysterious disease and a health system.

To the physician, nurses, and medical interns: Working with you during the epidemic and, in the case of the nurses, during myriad subsequent conversations provided us with a deeper appreciation of the complexity of the seemingly impossible situation you faced with your patients in 2007–2008 and the professionalism you demonstrated in attempting to diagnose and treat them. Given the difficult and bitter memories that the epidemic engendered, we hope that this book will help complement them with a renewed sense that your efforts have come to form an important chapter in the history of health care in the delta.

To the epidemiologists and public health officials charged with investigating the epidemic and formulating health policies for the delta: The mysterious epidemic challenged epidemiological models and political sensibilities alike. We appreciate your willingness, once tempers had cooled and the political fallout had dissipated, to reflect with us on the uncertainties and complexities you faced in tracking the disease.

To the scores of healers who treated patients with the strange disease: Next to cholera, which killed so many of your colleagues, the mysterious epidemic was perhaps the most disconcerting health problem you faced. We deeply appreciate your willingness to speak openly about your most troubling cases and the dreams that sustained your efforts to make sense of what had occurred.

To the journalists who spoke with us about covering the mysterious epidemic and other health stories: We thank you for your candor, for your willingness to step behind the coverage and explain the constraints under which you were operating, as well as the times when you responded to our questions by telling us to go back to your stories to find answers.

We thank the many people who facilitated our work. The residents of Hubasuhuru, especially the Gómez family, provided our home in the lower delta. In Nabanasanka, the families of Conrado and Enrique Moraleda as well as Fathers K'Okal Josiah and Zachariah Kariuki and Sisters Carla Pianca and Luigina Goffi of the Consolata Mission extended generous hospitality and provided spaces where the team met for extended periods to reflect on what had taken place. In Tucupita, we thank Belkis Ruiz Valderey and Hector Romero for their hospitality, friendship, and revolutionary critique. Pedro Martínez opened up issues of education in the delta. Francisco Moraleda and Rosalino Fernández in Nabasanuka and San Francisco de Guayo and, in Valencia, Sol Alegría Mantini de Castillo and Orietta Castillo Mantini transcribed some two hundred hours of recordings; they were assisted by Leopoldo Pajoi

Mantini, Carla Alegría Castillo Mantini, Fiorela Jirón Mantini, and Pierina Jirón Mantini. Carla Castillo Mantini and Hernán Jirón Mantini helped us in compiling an archive of news stories. We are deeply indebted to Dr. Stefan Erasmi and Christopher Jung of the Cartography GIS and Remote Sensing Section of the Institute of Geography at the Georg-August University of Göttingen for creating detailed maps.

Financial support for the team's work was drawn from funds provided by the J. I. Staley Prize from the School for Advanced Research (SAR) and the Bryce Woods Prize from the Latin American Studies Associations, along with royalties for *Stories in the Time of Cholera*; delta residents decided that these funds could best be devoted to diagnosing the epidemic and taking the results to Caracas. Also, SAR granted Charles a Weatherhead Fellowship in 2009–2010 that provided a delightful space for writing a first draft of this book; our stay in Santa Fe was generously extended through Steve Feld's kindness. Conversations at SAR with Lynn Morgan, Jim Trostle, Chris Teuton, and Sherry Farrell Racette, which included tenacious readings of preliminary chapters, were invaluable. The Cultural Logic of Facts and Figures project at the Norwegian University of Science and Technology provided research and publication support. Sergio Recuenco read several parts of the manuscript. Alissa Bernstein, Ruth Goldstein, Cole Hansen, Nancy Scheper-Hughes, and Rosalynn Vega consulted on the subtitle. Maureen Katz and Jed Sekoff helped illuminate issues of psychoanalysis and mourning. The Lichtenberg-Kolleg of the Georg-August University of Göttingen provided a snowy and extremely collegial six months in 2013, part of which was devoted to yet another rewrite of the manuscript, as well as a sustained interrogation of Freud's "Trauer und Melancholie." Thanks to many friends and readers there, including Bill Bell, Jyotirmaya Sharma, William Uricchio, Martin van Gelderen, and particularly Regina Bendix. Miguel Gandert, Gert Schwab, Antoinette Saxer, and John Vokoun generously lent their expertise to curating the photographs and video footage; Miguel and Kalim Smith returned with us to the delta in 2009, continuing the work of documentation. Jill Hannum lent invaluable assistance in reorganizing the manuscript, and Liz Kelley proofread expertly. At Duke University Press, Ken Wissoker supported our work, and Danielle Szulczewski and Karen Fisher provided careful editing. Nicholas Behney kindly assisted on the bibliography and index. João Biehl's generous readings provided gracious support and challenged us to push our thinking on a number of crucial points. Audiences around the world have provided invaluable critiques of the ideas discussed here in the course of lectures, conferences, and exhibitions of the photographs.

NOTES

Introduction

1 World Health Organization, "Ebola Situation Report," 6 May 2015, http://apps.who
   .int/ebola/en/current-situation/ebola-situation-report-6-may-2015, accessed 8 May
   2015.
2 Adam Nossiter, "Fear of Ebola Breeds a Terror of Physicians," the *New York Times*,
   27 July 2014, http://www.nytimes.com/2014/07/28/world/africa/ebola-epidemic
   -west-africa-guinea.html?_r=0, accessed 15 February 2015.
3 See Paul Farmer and Rajesh Panjabi, "Ebola Does Not Need to Be a Death
   Sentence," *Huffington Post*, 16 October 2014, http://www.huffingtonpost.com
   /paulfarmer/ebola-does-not-need-to-be_b_5996652.html, accessed 8 May 2015.
4 We document this epidemic in our book *Stories in the Time of Cholera* (Briggs and
   Mantini-Briggs 2003).
5 A study conducted during the 1950s–1970s by Miguel Layrisse, Johannes Wilbert,
   and their colleagues placed prepubescent mortality at 50 percent (Wilbert 1980).
   Research in the northwestern delta in the late 1990s, led by Jacobus De Waard,
   calculated that 36 percent of children die in their first year of life (Servicio de Apoyo
   Local 1998). A study of 200 delta mothers by anthropologists Werner Wilbert
   and Cecilia Ayala Lafée-Wilbert (2007) determined that nearly 39 percent of their
   children had died; 78 percent of these deaths occurred before the age of four. The
   latest and most comprehensive findings, compiled from quite a number of regions
   of the delta, are by Villalba et al. (2013). They found that in 2011, child mortality was
   approximately 26 percent.
6 We use the term "settlement" rather "community," given the way that the latter term
   has evoked notions of a bounded, homogeneous, cohesive social body. Such a projection would be at odds with our efforts to explore the heterogeneity and shifting
   definitions that emerged in static and reified constructions of indigenous people and
   "the Warao" specifically.
7 In Delta Amacuro State, nursing stations are often referred to as *dispensarios*, while
   facilities with resident physicians are called *ambulatorios* or *medicaturas*. The term
   clínica is generally used in reference to one of the privately owned facilities located

in Tucupita. We use the terms "nursing station" for dispensarios and "clinics" for public facilities with resident physicians, thereby distinguishing them from the hospitals located in Tucupita and elsewhere and the Center for Integrative Diagnosis in Curiapo, which provided a higher level of care and is affiliated with the Mission Barrio Adentro.

8   The idea of slowing down the analysis comes from Isabelle Stengers (2005).

9   For references relating to nonknowledge, see Riles (1998, 2006), Strathern (1999), Taussig (1999), and Wagner (1984). Geissler (2013) explores the production of nonknowledge in the context of public health.

10 For examples, see Dumit (2012) and Healey (2004).

11 Research on biomediatization also emerged in Charles's collaboration with Daniel C. Hallin on news coverage of health in the United States and Latin America (Briggs and Hallin 2007, 2016).

1. Reliving the Epidemic

1   Population figures are taken from the Indigenous Census conducted in 2001 (Instituto Nacional de Estadística 2003). The census lists Mukoboina's population at seventy-five. Community representative Inocencio Torres told us that a census conducted by residents in early 2007, in support of a petition for a nursing station, placed the population at eighty-six.

2   Our use of the present tense in some sections throughout part I is not intended to invoke what is called an "ethnographic present," which seems to render time irrelevant in favor of producing the illusion of unchanging social worlds. Indeed, time lies at the heart of each individual's story as people face new challenges and changing perceptions over shifting temporal contours of life and death. We rather adopt here a "narrative present" as a means of highlighting the time of narration and the narrators' efforts to draw their audiences into the immediacy of the worlds they were relating.

3   We discuss in chapter 3 an epidemiological investigation in Mukoboina and nearby settlements that was carried out by a team led by a Cuban epidemiologist. Their data present slightly different names and ages in a few cases. Gabriel, for example, is Angel Javier in their records, and they list Yuri's age as three. Mukoboina parents only had a national identification card for one child, Ángel Gabriel, enabling us to check how his name is officially recorded. In the remaining cases, we have used the names as given by the parents on several occasions in Mukoboina and verified by Inocencio, Conrado, and Enrique.

4   The Cuban epidemiologist's data list 30 August as the date of death; Venezuelan epidemiologists, using clinical records, report 31 August.

5   This information was provided in an *Informe* (Report) dated 6 February 2008 by the regional epidemiologist, p. 1, the first document in a compilation of reports dating from 2007 and 2008, based on work by the Office of the Regional Epidemiologist, Delta Amacuro State, about health conditions in Manuel Renaud Parish.

6   The Cuban epidemiologist's data list Yordi's younger brother as Robert and give his age as two; they give Yordi's age as six.

7   There is clearly a disagreement in this account regarding ethical conduct at the moment of and following Yomelis's death between the Torreses and medical personnel. Without attempting to resolve it, we do think it worthwhile to note that it is common practice in most hospitals to separate family members from patients upon death. In other words, the doctor's intervention with the parents may have reflected hospital policy as much as the specifics of the case and/or differential treatment of patients classified as indigenous.

8   See Moraleda (1979), Moraleda and López (1982), and Escalante and Moraleda (1992a, 1992b).

9   See Briggs (1996a) for a fuller description.

10 The spelling of the names is taken from an examination completed by Mamerto in conjunction with a literacy and adult education program sponsored by Fe y Alegría.

11 This representation of Elbia's experience is a composite drawn from a wide range of sources, including accounts by her mother and other relatives (given on several occasions), Macotera's and Indalesio's testimony, and conversations with cousins and other relatives in Hubasuhuru. A crucial information source that is lacking is Elbia herself, and this limitation should be borne in mind.

12 Testing for the Babinski response is done by rubbing the lateral side of the sole of the foot with a blunt instrument from the heel to the toes. If the big toe moves upward and other toes fan out, this is referred to as the Babinski response or sign. It is normal for infants under two, but, for adults, it suggests the presence of a serious neurological problem.

13 Most medical textbooks have a section on rabies. Jackson (2000) and Plotkin (2000) provide useful reviews of the literature, and Gilbert et al. (2012) report a study of rabies exposure in the Peruvian Amazon.

14 "Since elimination of rabies virus at the site of infection by chemical or physical means is the most effective mechanism of protection, immediate washing and flushing with soap and water, detergent or water alone are imperative (this procedure is recommended for all bite wounds, including those unrelated to possible exposure to rabies). Then apply either ethanol (700 ml/l) or tincture or aqueous solution of iodine" (see World Health Organization, "Guide for Post-Exposure Prophylaxis," http://www.who.int/rabies/human/firstaid/en/, no date, accessed 17 September 2015).

2. When Caregivers Fail

1   The 2001 Indigenous Census puts Nabasanuka's population at 453.

2   One or two walls are frequently built on the sides through which rain frequently enters; the other sides are left open for ventilation.

3   Following common usage in the delta, we use the term "nurse." It should be borne in mind, however, that these practitioners were trained through the Program of Simplified Medicine rather than in courses of study in schools of nursing.

4 Here we use the common form of address and reference for physicians in the delta, title and first name.

5 In the delta, medical interns are generally addressed as either *pasante* (intern) or doctor. These interns were months away from graduation, and patients and nurses generally referred to them as Dr. [first name]; we accordingly follow this usage here.

6 We use first names for nurses, as is common practice in the delta.

7 While lower-ranking healers are generally addressed by their first names, using first names is considered disrespectful for prominent ones. A title of respect, often *daomata* (which can be roughly translated as "sir"), is often used. We accordingly follow local preferences by referring to higher-ranking healers by Mr. [first name].

8 In Warao, these terms are singular; the plural of wisidatu, for example, is *wisimo*. For simplicity, we use the same term in both singular and plural senses.

9 Johannes Wilbert (1987, 1993) provides the most extensive discussion of Warao healing. Dale Olsen (1996) analyzes the healer's musical repertoire. And see Briggs (2008).

10 For a detailed ethnography of herbal knowledge and practice, see Werner Wilbert (1996).

11 Spirits purportedly detest menstrual blood.

12 Spirit-possession healing has been amply documented in Venezuela, such as by Pollak-Eltz (1972) and Ferrándiz (2004).

13 Mr. Francisco chose to use a pseudonym.

14 Johannes Wilbert worked in Morichito for decades, and his students—including anthropologist H. Dieter Heinen and ethnomusicologist Dale Olsen—along with his son, medical anthropologist Werner Wilbert, have also worked in the area.

15 These narratives emerged in Charles's work on Warao narrative over the years. They are included in an extensive collection of myths by British colonial folklorist Walter Roth (1915).

16 See, for example, Salas de Lecuna (1985: 255–260).

17 Some stories cast her as the daughter of a conquering Spaniard, others as that of a vanquished indigenous leader, but they converge on her metamorphosis through water, generally that she was captured by water spirits or raped by a water serpent. Like the Warao nabarao, she represents beauty, desire, danger, and death associated with water.

3. Explaining the Inexplicable in Mukoboina

1 Literary scholar Patricia Wald (2008) brings these different accounts together admirably.

2 Coronil (1997) elucidates the centrality of oil to shaping perceptions of what he characterizes as Venezuela's social and natural bodies.

3 The first two doses were administered in Caracas.

4 This information comes from a report (*informe*) dated 6 February 2008 by regional epidemiologist Froilán Godoy (a pseudonym).

5 Ibid.

6　We spoke with Froilán Godoy in Tucupita in July 2011.

7　These quotations are taken from a ministry summary of Mukoboina-related epidemiology.

8　We spoke with Wilfredo Sosa in March 2010.

9　We spoke with Yolanda Othegui in Tucupita in July 2011.

10　In the 1990s, small placer mines extracted gold and silver from an area in the southeastern part of the delta, and mercury was employed in the process. As a part of our cholera research, we visited them—real Wild West, disordered and unregulated spaces, in 1995.

11　We interviewed Antonio Peña and Ronaldo Domínguez in Tucupita in July 2011.

12　Our account is based on this report and details provided by people who met with Dr. Diego's team.

13　Coordinación de Epidemiología, Estado Delta Amacuro, "Informe preliminar de visita a la Comunidad de Mukoboina," 20 September 2007.

14　In other words, the stethoscope revealed a succession of short, sharp noises rather than an unobstructed flow of air.

15　The first, indicating that nerves in the neck are irritated, is usually performed with the patient supine, with a hip flexed at 90 degrees. The Kernig sign emerges if pain is registered when the lower leg is extended. In testing for the Brudzinski sign, the clinician places one hand behind the supine patient's head and another on the chest, then raises the head while holding the chest in place, to see if the hips and knees flex when the head is raised.

16　Septicemia is an immunological response to the widespread presence of pathogens in the bloodstream.

17　We document this visit, news coverage, and the media-epidemiology connection in subsequent chapters.

18　The first is reported in a document listed as "Informe" (Report), without date or author, and the second, by Benjamín López, is titled "Informe de actividades realizadas en la parroquia Manuel Renault," Municipio Antonio Díaz, 13 March 2008.

19　Sakoinoko is listed as having been visited twice on 14 February 2008; if this is not a mistake, it was thus visited six times.

20　The report is titled "Muertes de Origen Desconocido: Resumen de Situación."

4. Heroes, Bureaucrats, and Ancient Wisdom

1　Throughout, we have tried to use ways that the people we feature are generally addressed. The case of journalists is more complex. People who know them generally use first names. We have accordingly have used first names for journalists we have interviewed.

2　This description is based on the paper's position in 2008.

3　"Niños indígenas no mueren por comer frutas," *Notidiario*, 15 February 2008, 5.

4　In keeping with common usage, we refer to her as Vice Minister Martinelli.

5　Neither the reporter nor the officials mention that the rumor's source is another RHS professional.

6 We discuss this coverage in Briggs and Mantini-Briggs (2003).
7 "Es verdad que están muriendo nuestros hermanos warao," *El Nacional*, 9 August 2008.
8 The Spanish reads: "Llama a la reflexión que quienes explotaron a los indígenas por más de 500 años y los esclavizaron vengan a tomar como bandera algo que ocurrió hace algunos meses y en lo que el Presidente y el Ministerio ya habían tomado cartas."
9 The Spanish, ¡Me montaron cachos!, is even stronger, the metaphorical reference to sexual infidelity being particularly clear.

5. Narratives, Communicative Monopolies, and Acute Health Inequities

1 See Briggs and Mantini-Briggs (2003). For parallels in Brazil and Peru, see Nations and Monte (1996) and Cueto (1997).
2 See Briggs (1986), Cicourel (1982), and Mishler (1986) on research interviews.
3 Freud ([1900] 1965) provided a classic account of these processes in *Dreams and Their Interpretation*, but they have been greatly elaborated upon since by psychoanalysts.
4 A vast literature documents relationships between multilingualism and social identity; for examples, see Hill (2008), Urciuoli (1996), Woolard (1989), and Zentella (2002).

6. Knowledge Production and Circulation

1 One such case is discussed in detail in Briggs (1998).
2 Many scholars have extended Goffman's work on participation frameworks. For examples, see Levinson (1988) and Irvine (1996).
3 Dr. Vicente Medina, widely recognized as "the first Warao doctor," was working for Antonio Díaz Municipality at the time, but as a political, not health, official.
4 Laura Weffer Cifuentes, "Reconocen muerte de waraos por causas desconocidas," *El Nacional* 14 August 2008, 8.
5 See Instituto Nacional de Estadística (2003).

7. Laments, Psychoanalysis, and the Work of Mourning

1 It is, however, quite possible to ask people to repeat verses of laments that they have sung previously; in Hymes's (1981) terms, however, such acts are reports of performances past.
2 Julia Kristeva (1989) extended Freud's thinking about the pervasiveness and persistence of melancholia, depicting it less as pathology than as a painful but productive force. Anne Cheng (2000), Angela Garcia (2010), and other writers have reflected on the complex ways that melancholia gets woven into the fabric of racial inequalities and vice versa.
3 Charles discusses these issues in a letter to Dr. Freud (Briggs 2014).

4   Osborn (1967) presents a valuable analysis of Warao verbal morphology.

5   Lines 3 and 6 use a different form, *-kore*, which similarly places the utterances in the middle of an unfolding time before illness and death gripped Mamerto.

8. Biomediatization

1   "Reconocen muerte de waraos por causas desconocidas," *El Nacional*, 14 August 2008, Ciudadanos section, 8.

2   Even some anti-Chávez media analysts contest this view. Cañizález (2010) suggests that the private media not only helped Chávez become an influential public figure after his release from prison in 1994 (following the coup attempt he led in 1992) but also played an important role in his first electoral victory in December 1998 and remained largely supportive until the middle of 2001. A period of "confrontation without truce" marked 2002–2004, followed by a period of accommodation—still carried out under the banner of a media war—between the anti-Chávez private press and government and pro-Chávez media. See also Bisbal (2009).

3   These figures are taken from data compiled by AGB Panamericana de Venezuela Medición, S.A., and published in Weisbrot and Ruttenberg (2010).

4   Our samples included all health news in a selection of national and regional newspapers in 2002, the April–July 2009 coverage of H1N1 (or "swine flu"), and one-week periods taken at random between 2002 and 2008. They yielded few exceptions to linear, hierarchically ordered perspectives. Casagrande was the only reporter we encountered among the twenty-five journalists we interviewed who challenged the linear transmission model of biocommunicability.

5   See also Wilson and Stewart (2008) and Fisher (2013).

9. Toward Health/Communicative Equities and Justice

1   "El cólera está matando a los waraos del Delta," *Notidiario*, 14 August 1992, 12.

2   The two of us visited every part of the lower delta in 1994–1995 and asked residents about their experiences during the cholera epidemic. On the basis of these conversations, we estimated that approximately 500 people had died in the epidemic. See Briggs and Mantini-Briggs (2003) for documentation of both this research and the official count.

3   Interviewed by Charles on 31 March 1995.

4   While working as an RHS administrator in 1993–1994, Clara witnessed how this narrative was used to socialize newly graduated physicians who had just arrived to begin their obligatory year of service. They would be ushered from office to office to meet with the directors of each RHS division, all of whom would recount the story of the cholera epidemic. These introductions portrayed deplorable health conditions in the rain forest in such a way as to systematically convert structural factors into a pervasive cultural incapacity to understand the very biomedical knowledge that idealistic young doctors had hoped to impart.

5   Wacquant (2002, 56), emphasis in original.

6 See Jaén (2001), Armada (2002), Briggs and Mantini-Briggs (2003, 2009).

7 We conducted fieldwork in 2005–2006 in low-income neighborhoods, clinical sites, and government offices in Caracas and other parts of Venezuela (see Briggs and Mantini-Briggs 2009).

8 Christina Getrich et al. (2007) suggest that "noise," the emergence of discrepant models with different actors and at different organizational levels, can thwart the success of health programs. The remarkable consistency of articulations of Mission Barrio Adentro's basic philosophy by Cuban physicians, patients, health committee members, and Chávez's media presentations is thus interesting.

9 See Laurell (2003) and Waitzkin (2011) for discussions.

10 See also Gordon (1988).

11 Here we must clearly state the limitations of our research. This is the account that circulates among his former colleagues in the RHS in Delta Amacuro State.

Conclusion

1 See Anderson (2006), Arnold (1993), Hunt (1999), and Vaughan (1991).

2 We draw here on work that Charles conducted with Daniel C. Hallin (see Briggs and Hallin 2016).

3 Denise Nelesen, "Programs Tell Latinos about Diabetes," *San Diego Union-Tribune,* 7 June 2003, E5.

4 We do not want to romanticize all resistance to health/communicative inequities. Some of it is mobilized these days in the United States by pharmaceutical corporations—in collaboration with the patient advocacy organizations that they fund—in order to sell more drugs. Doctors' rights to diagnose their patients in keeping with the professional practices and ethical principles can come into conflict with demands by patients for prescribing a drug they saw on television as well as insurers' and government officials' demands to curtail care in keeping with fiscal or politico-religious mandates.

5 For a basic source on health and human rights, see Mann et al. (1999).

6 There are other valuable precedents where people have asserted calls for health/communicative justice. For example, in the 1980s, HIV/AIDS activists in the United States and elsewhere stormed meetings, pored over scientific publications, confronted officials, and worked with physicians and journalists (Epstein 1996).

7 See Clarke et al. (2003) and Rose (2007) on the centrality of the figure of the empowered and self-interested individual in contemporary reconfigurations of health. Dumit (2012) documents the role of pharmaceutical advertisers in creating "expert patients" who systematically seek out health knowledge and rationally deploy it to their advantage. Briggs and Hallin (2016) trace the emergence of the self-interested individual patient-consumer in news coverage of health and how it is contradicted and complicated by other projections of health subjects.

8 See Gordon (1997) on haunting and the way that ghostly absences form a constitutive outside (Butler 1993; Laclau and Mouffe 1985) that structures systems of inequality.

REFERENCES

Adams, Vincanne. 2013a. "Evidence-Based Global Public Health: Subjects, Profits, Erasures." In *When People Come First: Critical Studies in Global Health*, edited by João Biehl and Adriana Petryna, 54–90. Princeton, NJ: Princeton University Press.
———. 2013b. *Markets of Sorrows, Labors of Faith: New Orleans in the Wake of Katrina*. Durham, NC: Duke University Press.
Agamben, Giorgio. 1998. *Homo Sacer: Sovereign Power and Bare Life*. Translated by Daniel Heller-Roazen. Stanford: Stanford University Press.
Agha, Asif. 2007. *Language and Social Relations*. Cambridge: Cambridge University Press.
Althusser, Louis. 1969. *For Marx*. Translated by Ben Brewster. London: Allen Lane.
———. 1971. "Ideology and Ideological State Apparatuses." In *Lenin and Philosophy and Other Essays*, translated by B. Brewster, 127–186. New York: Monthly Review Press.
Anderson, Benedict. (1983) 1991. *Imagined Communities: Reflections on the Origin and Spread of Nationalism*. London: Verso.
Anderson, Warwick. 2006. *Colonial Pathologies: American Tropical Medicine, Race, and Hygiene in the Philippines*. Durham, NC: Duke University Press.
Appadurai, Arjun. 1986. "Introduction: Commodities and the Politics of Value." In *The Social Life of Things*, edited by Arjun Appadurai, 3–63. Cambridge: Cambridge University Press.
———. 1988. "Putting Hierarchy in Its Place." *Cultural Anthropology* 3(1): 36–49.
Armada, Francisco. 2002. "Neoliberalism and Population Health in Latin America and the Caribbean." Ph.D. dissertation, Health Policy and Management, Johns Hopkins University.
Arnold, David. 1993. *Colonizing the Body: State Medicine and Epidemic Disease in Nineteenth Century India*. Berkeley: University of California Press.
Asad, Talal. 2007. *On Suicide Bombing*. New York: Columbia University Press.
Austin, J. L. 1962. *How to Do Things with Words*. Cambridge, MA: Harvard University Press.
Ayala Lafée-Wilbert, Cecilia, and Werner Wilbert. 2008. *La mujer warao: De recolectora deltana a recolectora urbana*. Caracas: Instituto Caribe de Antropología y Sociología.

Bakhtin, Mikhail Mikhailovich. 1981. *The Dialogic Imagination: Four Essays.* Edited by Michael Holquist. Translated by Caryl Emerson and Michael Holquist. Austin: University of Texas Press.

Barz, Gregory. 2006. *Singing for Life: HIV/AIDS and Music in Uganda.* New York: Routledge.

Bauer, Martin. 1998. "The Medicalization of Science News: From the 'Rocket-Scalpel' to the 'Gene Meteorite' Complex." *Information sur les Sciences Sociales* 37: 731–751.

Bauman, Richard. 1977. *Verbal Art as Performance.* Prospect Heights, IL: Waveland.

———. 1986. *Story, Performance, and Event: Contextual Studies of Oral Narrative.* Cambridge: Cambridge University Press.

Bauman, Richard, and Charles L. Briggs. 1990. "Poetics and Performance as Critical Perspectives on Language and Social Life." *Annual Review of Anthropology* 19: 59–88.

———. 2003. *Voices of Modernity: Language Ideologies and the Politics of Inequality.* Cambridge: Cambridge University Press.

Benjamin, Walter. 1969. "The Storyteller." In *Illuminations*, edited by Hannah Arendt, translated by Harry Zohn, 83–109. New York: Schocken.

Bernstein, Alissa Shira. 2015. "The Making and Circulation of Health Reform Policy in Bolivia." Ph.D. dissertation, Medical Anthropology, University of California, Berkeley.

Beverly, John. 2004. *Testimonio: On the Politics of Truth.* Minneapolis: University of Minnesota Press.

———. 2005. "Testimonio, Subalternity, and Narrative Authority." In *The Sage Handbook of Qualitative Research*, 3rd ed., edited by Norman K. Denzin and Yvonna S. Lincoln, 547–558. Thousand Oaks, CA: Sage.

Biehl, João. 2005. *Vita: Life in a Zone of Abandonment.* Berkeley: University of California Press.

Biehl, João, and Adriana Petryna, eds. 2013. *When People Come First: Critical Studies in Global Health.* Princeton, NJ: Princeton University Press.

Bisbal, Marcelino, ed. 2009. *Hegemonía y control comunicacional.* Caracas: Editorial Alfa.

Blackwell, Maylei. 2011. *¡Chicana Power! Contested Histories of Feminism in the Chicano Movement.* Austin: University of Texas Press.

Bolivarian Republic of Venezuela. 2006. *Constitution of the Bolivarian Republic of Venezuela*, 3rd ed. Caracas: Ministerio de Comunicación e Información.

Bourdieu, Pierre. 1991. *Language and Symbolic Power.* Translated by Gino Raymond and Matthew Adamson. Cambridge, MA: Harvard University Press.

Bowker, Geoffrey C., and Susan Leigh Star. 1999. *Sorting Things Out: Classification and Its Consequences.* Cambridge, MA: MIT Press.

Breilh, Jaime. 1979. "Community Medicine under Imperialism: A New Medical Police." *International Journal of the Health Services* 9(1): 5–24.

———. 2003. *Epidemiología Crítica: Ciencia Emancipadora e interculturalidad.* Buenos Aires: Lugar Editorial.

———. 2010. "La epidemiología crítica: Una nueva forma de mirar la salud en el espacio urbano." *Salud Colectiva* 6(1): 83–101.

Brenneis, Don. 2006. "Reforming Promise." In *Documents: Artifacts of Modern Knowledge*, edited by Annelise Riles, 41–70. Ann Arbor: University of Michigan Press.

Briggs, Charles L. 1986. *Learning How to Ask: A Sociolinguistic Appraisal of the Role of the Interview in Social Science Research*. Cambridge: Cambridge University Press.

———. 1988. *Competence in Performance: The Creativity of Tradition in Mexicano Verbal Art*. Philadelphia: University of Pennsylvania Press.

———. 1992. " 'Since I Am a Woman, I Will Chastise My Relatives': Gender, Reported Speech, and the (Re)production of Social Relations in Warao Ritual Wailing." *American Ethnologist* 19(2): 337–361.

———. 1993. "Personal Sentiments and Polyphonic Voices in Warao Women's Ritual Wailing: Music and Poetics in a Critical and Collective Discourse." *American Anthropologist* 95(4): 929–957.

———. 1996a. "Conflict, Language Ideologies, and Privileged Arenas of Discursive Authority in Warao Dispute Mediation." In *Disorderly Discourse: Narrative, Conflict, and Inequality*, edited by Charles L. Briggs, 204–242. New York: Oxford University Press.

———. 1996b. "The Meaning of Nonsense, the Poetics of Embodiment, and the Production of Power in Warao Shamanistic Healing." In *The Performance of Healing*, edited by Carol Laderman and Marina Roseman, 185–232. New York: Routledge.

———. 1998. " 'You're a Liar—You're Just Like a Woman!' Constructing Dominant Ideologies of Language in Warao Men's Gossip." In *Language Ideologies: Practice and Theory*, edited by Bambi Schieffelin, Kathryn A. Woolard, and Paul V. Kroskrity, 229–255. New York: Oxford University Press.

———. 2000. "Emergence of the Non-Indigenous Peoples: A Warao Narrative." In *Translating Native Latin American Verbal Art: Ethnopoetics and Ethnography of Speaking*, edited by Kay Sammons and Joel Sherzer, 174–196. Washington, DC: Smithsonian Institution Press.

———. 2003. "Why Nation-States Can't Teach People to Be Healthy: Power and Pragmatic Miscalculation in Public Discourses on Health." *Medical Anthropology Quarterly* 17(3): 287–321.

———. 2005a. "Communicability, Racial Discourse, and Disease." *Annual Review of Anthropology* 34: 269–291.

———. 2005b. "Perspectivas críticas de salud y hegemonía comunicativa: Aperturas progresistas, enlaces letales." *Revista de Antropología Social* 14: 101–124.

———. 2008. *Poéticas de vida en espacios de muerte: Género, poder y el estado en la cotidianeidad Warao*. Quito, Ecuador: Editorial Abya-Yala.

———. 2011a. " 'All Cubans Are Doctors!' News Coverage of Health and Bioexceptionalism in Cuba." *Social Science and Medicine* 73: 1037–1044.

———. 2011b. "Communicating Biosecurity." *Medical Anthropology* 30(1): 6–29.

———. 2014. "Dear Dr. Freud." *Cultural Anthropology* 29(2): 312–343.

Briggs, Charles L., and Clara Mantini-Briggs. 2003. *Stories in the Time of Cholera: Racial Profiling during a Medical Nightmare*. Berkeley: University of California Press.

———. 2005. "Hegemonía comunicativa y salud emancipadora: Un contradicción inédita (El Ejemplo del Dengue)." In *Informe Alternativo sobre la Salud en América*

Latina, edited by Observatorio Latinoamericano de Salud, Centro de Estudios y Asesoría en Salud. Quito: Global Health Watch/CEAS.

———. 2009. "Confronting Health Disparities: Latin American Social Medicine in Venezuela." *American Journal of Public Health* 99(3): 549–555.

Briggs, Charles L., Norbelys Gómez, Tirso Gómez, Clara Mantini-Briggs, Conrado Moraleda Izco, and Enrique Moraleda Izco. 2015. *Una enfermedad monstruo: Indígenas derribando el cerco de la discriminación en salud*. Buenos Aires: Lugar Editorial.

Briggs, Charles L., and Daniel C. Hallin. 2007. "Biocommunicability: The Neoliberal Subject and Its Contradictions in News Coverage of Health Issues." *Social Text* 25(4): 43–66.

———. 2016. *Making Health Public: How News Coverage Is Remaking Media, Medicine, and Contemporary Life*. London: Routledge.

Brown, Phil. 1997. "Popular Epidemiology Revisited." *Current Sociology* 45(3): 137–156.

Butler, Judith. 1993. *Bodies That Matter*. New York: Routledge.

———.1997. *Excitable Speech: A Politics of the Performative*. New York: Routledge.

———. 2004. *Precarious Life: The Powers of Mourning and Violence*. London: Verso.

Cañizález, Andrés. 2010. "Medios, gobernabilidad democrática y políticas públicas. La presidencia mediática: Hugo Chávez (1999–2009)." Unpublished dissertation, Department of Political Science, Universidad Simón Bolívar, Caracas, Venezuela.

Castro, Arachu, and Merrill Singer, eds. 2004. *Unhealthy Health Policy: A Critical Anthropological Examination*. Walnut Creek, CA: Altamira.

Chakrabarty, Dipesh. 2000. *Provincializing Europe*. Princeton, NJ: Princeton University Press.

Chávez Frías, Hugo. 2002. "Discurso ante la FAO," 16 October 2002. http://www.embavenefao.org/Doc/DiscursoantelaFAOHugoChavez16deoctubrede2002.pdf, accessed 6 August 2015.

Chen, Mel Y. 2012. *Animacies: Biopolitics, Racial Mattering, and Queer Affect*. Durham, NC: Duke University Press.

Cheng, Anne Anin. 2000. *Melancholy of Race: Psychoanalysis, Assimilation, and Hidden Grief*. Cary, NC: Oxford University Press.

Cicourel, Aaron V. 1982. "Interviews, Surveys, and the Problem of Ecological Validity." *American Sociologist* 17(1): 11–20.

———. 1992. "The Interpenetration of Communicative Contexts: Examples from Medical Encounters." In *Rethinking Context: Language as an Interactive Phenomenon*, edited by Alessandro Duranti and Charles Goodwin, 291–310. Cambridge: Cambridge University Press.

Clarke, Adele E., Janet K. Shim, Laura Mamo, Jennifer Ruth Fosket, and Jennifer R. Fishman. 2003. "Biomedicalization: Technoscientific Transformations of Health, Illness, and U.S. Biomedicine." *American Sociological Review* 68(2): 161–194.

Clifford, James. 1997. *Routes: Travel and Translation in the Late Twentieth Century*. Cambridge, MA: Harvard University Press.

———. 2013. *Returns: Becoming Indigenous in the Twenty-First Century*. Cambridge, MA: Harvard University Press.

Collier, Stephen J., Andrew Lakoff, and Paul Rabinow. 2004. "Biosecurity: Towards an Anthropology of the Contemporary." *Anthropology Today* 20(5): 3–7.

Conrad, Peter. 1992. "Medicalization and Social Control." *Annual Review of Sociology* 18: 209–232.

Coronil, Fernando. 1997. *The Magical State: Nature, Money, and Modernity in Venezuela*. Chicago: University of Chicago Press.

Couldry, Nick. 2012. *Media, Society and World: Social Theory and Digital Media Practice*. Cambridge: Polity.

Couldry, Nick and Andreas Hepp. 2013. "Conceptualizing Mediatization: Contexts, Traditions, Argument." *Communication Theory* 23(3): 191–202.

Crapanzano, Vincent. 1973. *The Hamadsha: A Study in Moroccan Ethnospychiatry*. Berkeley: University of California Press.

Cueto, Marcos. 1997. *El regreso de las epidémias: Salud y sociedad en el Perú del siglo XX*. Lima: Instituto de Estudios Peruanos.

Danz, Shari M. 2000. "A Nonpublic Forum or a Brutal Bureaucracy? Advocates' Claims of Access to Welfare Center Waiting Rooms." *New York University Law Review* 75(4): 1004–1044.

Das, Veena. 1985. "Anthropological Knowledge and Collective Violence: The Riots in Delhi, November 1984." *Anthropology Today* 1(3): 4–6.

———. 1995. "Suffering, Legitimacy and Healing: The Bhopal Case." *In Critical Events: An Anthropological Perspective on Contemporary India*, 137–174. Delhi: Oxford.

———. 2007. *Life and Words: Violence and the Descent into the Ordinary*. Berkeley: University of California Press.

———. 2015. *Affliction: Health, Disease, Poverty*. New York: Fordham University and Oxford University Press.

Das, Veena, and Ranendra K. Das. 2006. "Pharmaceuticals in Urban Ecologies: The Register of the Local." In *Global Pharmaceuticals: Ethics, Markets, Practices*, edited by Adriana Petryna, Andrew Lakoff, and Arthur Kleinman, 171–205. Durham, NC: Duke University Press.

Davidson, Brad. 2001. "Questions in Cross-Linguistic Medical Encounters: The Role of the Hospital Interpreter." *Anthropological Quarterly* 74(4): 170–178.

de Certeau, Michel. 1984. *The Practice of Everyday Life*. Berkeley: University of California Press.

de la Cadena, Marisol. 2010. "Indigenous Cosmopolitics in the Andes: Conceptual Reflections beyond 'Politics.'" *Cultural Anthropology* 25(2): 334–370.

de la Cadena, Marisol, and Orin Starn, eds. 2007. *Indigenous Experience Today*. Oxford: Berg.

Descola, Philippe. 1996 (1986). *In the Society of Nature: A Native Ecology in Amazonia*. Translated by Nora Scott. Cambridge: Cambridge University Press.

———. 2009. "Human Natures." *Social Anthropology/Anthropologie Sociale* 17(2): 145–157.

Dirección de Salud Indígena (DSI), Ministerio del Poder Popular para la Salud. n.d. *Medicina Tradicional Warao*. DVD. Caracas: Dirección de Salud Indígena, Ministerio del Poder Popular para la Salud.

Du Bois, W. E. B. (1903) 1990. *The Souls of Black Folk.* Chicago: A. C. McClurg.

Dumit, Joseph. 2012. *Drugs for Life: How Pharmaceutical Companies Define Our Health.* Durham, NC: Duke University Press.

Dutta, Mohan J. 2008. *Communicating Health: A Culture Centered Approach.* Cambridge, UK: Polity.

Dutta, Mohan J., and Ambar Basu. 2011. "Culture, Communication, and Health: A Guiding Framework." In *The Routledge Handbook of Health Communication,* edited by Teresa L. Thompson, Roxanne Parrott, and Jon F. Nussbaum, 320–334. New York: Routledge.

Dutta, Mohan J., and Uttaran Dutta. 2013. "Voices of the Poor from the Margins of Bengal: Structural Inequities and Health." *Qualitative Health Research* 23(1): 14–25.

Ellison, Ralph. 1972. *Invisible Man.* New York: Vintage.

Epstein, Steven. 1996. *Impure Science: AIDS, Activism, and the Politics of Knowledge.* Berkeley: University of California Press.

Escalante, Bernada, and Librado Moraleda. 1992a. *Narraciones warao: Origen, cultura, historia.* Caracas: Instituto Caribe de Antropología y Sociología, Fundación La Salle.

———. 1992b. *Warao a rejetuma.* Caracas: Instituto Caribe de Antropología y Sociología, Fundación La Salle.

Evans-Pritchard, E. E. 1958. *Witchcraft, Oracles and Magic among the Azande.* Oxford: Clarendon.

Fanon, Frantz. 1963. *Wretched of the Earth.* Trans. Richard Philcox. New York: Grove.

———. 1967. *Black Skin, White Masks.* New York: Grove.

Farmer, Paul. 1992. *AIDS and Accusation: Haiti and the Geography of Blame.* Berkeley: University of California Press.

———. 1999. *Infections and Inequalities: The Modern Plagues.* Berkeley: University of California Press.

———. 2003. *Pathologies of Power: Health, Human Rights, and the New War on the Poor.* Berkeley: University of California Press.

Fassin, Didier. 2012. *Humanitarian Reason: A Moral History of the Present.* Translated by Rachel Gomme. Berkeley: University of California Press.

Feinsilver, Julie M. 1993. *Healing the Masses: Cuban Health Politics at Home and Abroad.* Berkeley: University of California Press.

Feld, Steven. (1982) 2012. *Sound and Sentiment: Birds, Weeping, Poetics, and Song in Kaluli Expression,* 3rd ed. Durham, NC: Duke University Press.

———. 1990. "Wept Thoughts: The Voicing of Kaluli Memories." *Oral Tradition* 5: 241–266.

Feldman, Allen. 1991. *Formations of Violence: The Narrative of the Body and Political Terror in Northern Ireland.* Chicago: University of Chicago Press.

Fernandes, Sujatha. 2010. *Who Can Stop the Drums? Urban Social Movements in Chávez's Venezuela.* Durham, NC: Duke University Press.

Ferrándiz, Francisco. 2004. *Escenarios del cuerpo: Espiritismo y sociedad en Venezuela.* Bilbao, Spain: Universidad de Deusto.

Fisher, Daniel. 2013. "Intimacy and Self-Abstraction: Radio as New Media in Aboriginal Australia." *Culture, Theory and Critique* 54(3): 372–393.

Freud, Sigmund. (1900) 1965. *The Interpretation of Dreams.* Translated by James Strachey. New York: Basic.

———. (1905) 1960. *Jokes and Their Relation to the Unconscious.* Translated by James Strachey. New York: Norton.

———. (1917) 1957. "Mourning and Melancholia." In *The Standard Edition of the Complete Psychological Works of Sigmund Freud*, translated by James Strachey, 14: 243–258. London: Hogarth.

Garcia, Angela. 2010. *The Pastoral Clinic: Addiction and Dispossession along the Rio Grande.* Berkeley: University of California Press.

Garro, Linda C., and Cheryl Mattingly. 2000a. "Narrative as Construct and Construction." In *Narrative and the Cultural Construction of Illness and Healing*, edited by Cheryl Mattingly and Linda C. Garro, 1–49. Berkeley: University of California Press.

———. 2000b. "Narrative Turns." In *Narrative and the Cultural Construction of Illness and Healing*, edited by Cheryl Mattingly and Linda Garro, 259–269. Berkeley: University of California Press.

Geertz, Clifford. 1973. *The Interpretation of Cultures: Selected Essays.* New York: Basic.

Geissler, P. W. 2013. "Public Secrets in Public Health: Knowing Not to Know While Making Scientific Knowledge." *American Ethnologist* 40(1): 13–34.

Getrich, Christina, et al. 2007. "An Ethnography of Clinic 'Noise' in a Community-Based, Promotora-Centered Mental Health Intervention." *Social Science and Medicine* 65(2): 319–330.

Gieryn, Thomas F. 1983. "Boundary-Work and the Demarcation of Science from Non-science: Strains and Interests in Professional Ideologies of Scientists." *American Sociological Review* 48(6): 781–795.

Gilbert, Amy T., Brett W. Petersen, Sergio Recuenco, Michale Niezgoda, Jorge Gómez, V. Alberto Laguna-Torres, and Charles Rupprecht. 2012. "Evidence of Rabies Virus Exposure among Humans in the Peruvian Amazon." *American Journal of Tropical Medicine and Hygiene* 87(2): 206–215.

Ginsburg, Faye. 2008. "Rethinking the Digital Age." In *The Media and Social Theory*, edited by David Hesmondhalgh and Jason Toynbee, 127–144. New York: Routledge.

Goffman, Erving. 1981. *Forms of Talk.* Philadelphia: University of Pennsylvania Press.

Goldstein, Ruth Elizabeth. 2014. "Consent and Its Discontents: On the Traffic in Words and Women." *Latin American Policy* 5(2): 236–250.

———. 2015. "The Triangular Traffic in Women, Plants, and Gold: Along the Interoceanic Road in Brazil, Peru, and Bolivia." Ph.D. dissertation, Medical Anthropology, University of California, Berkeley.

Good, Byron J. 1994. *Medicine, Rationality, and Experience: An Anthropological Perspective. Cambridge*: Cambridge University Press.

Good, Byron J., and Mary-Jo DelVecchio Good. 2000. " 'Fiction' and 'Historicity' in Doctors' Stories: Social and Narrative Dimensions of Learning Medicine." In *Narrative and the Cultural Construction of Illness and Healing*, edited by Cheryl Mattingly and Linda C. Garro, 50–69. Berkeley: University of California Press.

Gordis, Leon. 2004. *Epidemiology*, 3rd ed. Philadelphia: Elsevier Saunders.

Gordon, Avery. 1997. *Ghostly Matters: Haunting and the Sociological Imagination*. Minneapolis: University of Minnesota Press.

Gordon, Deborah R. 1988. "Tenacious Assumptions in Western Medicine." In *Biomedicine Examined*, edited by Margaret Lock and Deborah Gordon, 19–56. Dordrecht: Kluwer.

Gröger, Udo, and Lutz Wiegrebe. 2006. "Classification of Human Breathing Sounds by the Common Vampire Bat, *Desmodus Rotundus*." *BMC Biology* 4: 18.

Gupta, Akhil. 2012. *Red Tape: Bureaucracy, Structural Violence, and Poverty in India*. Durham, NC: Duke University Press.

Hall, Stuart, Chas Critcher, Tony Jefferson, John N. Clarke, and Brian Robert. 1978. *Policing the Crisis: Mugging, the State, and Law and Order*. New York: Holmes and Meier.

Hallin, Daniel C., and Charles L. Briggs. 2010. "Health Reporting as Political Reporting: Biocommunicability and the Public Sphere." *Journalism: Theory, Practice, and Criticism* 11(2): 149–165.

Harper, Richard. 1998. *Inside the IMF: An Ethnography of Documents, Technology, and Organizational Action*. San Diego: Academic Press.

Harvey, T. S. 2008. "Where There Is No Patient: An Anthropological Treatment of a Biomedical Category." *Culture, Medicine, and Psychiatry* 32(4): 577–606.

Hayden, Cori. 2010. "The Proper Copy: The Insides and Outsides of Domains Made Public." *Journal of Cultural Economy* 3(1): 85–102.

Healy, David M. 2004. *Let Them Eat Prozac: The Unhealthy Relationship between the Pharmaceutical Industry and Depression*. New York: New York University Press.

Heimer, Carol A. 2006. "Conceiving Children: How Documents Support Case versus Biographic Analyses." In *Documents: Artifacts of Modern Knowledge*, edited by Annelise Riles, 95–126. Ann Arbor: University of Michigan Press.

Heinen, H. Dieter. 2009. *The Kanobo Cult of the Warao Amerindians of the Central Orinoco Delta: The Nahanamu Sago Ritual*. Munich: Lit Verlag.

Hepp, Andreas. 2012. *Cultures of Mediatization*. Cambridge: Polity.

Heritage, John, and Douglas W. Maynard, eds. 2006. *Communication in Medical Care: Interaction between Primary Care Physicians and Patients*. Cambridge: Cambridge University Press.

Hertz, Robert. 1960. *Death and the Right Hand*, translated by Rodney and Claudia Needham. Glencoe, IL: Free Press.

Hill, Jane H. 2008. *The Everyday Language of White Racism*. Chichester, U.K.: Wiley-Blackwell.

Hirschkind, Charles. 2006. *The Ethical Soundscape: Cassette Sermons and Islamic Counterpublics*. New York: Columbia University Press.

———. 2008. "Cultures of Death: Media, Religion, Bioethics." *Social Text* 26(3): 39–58.

Hjavard, Sigurd. 2013. *The Mediatization of Culture and Society*. London: Routledge.

Horton, Sarah. 2014. "Debating 'Medical Citizenship': Policies Shaping Undocumented Immigrants' Learned Avoidance of the U.S. Health Care System." In

Hidden Lives and Human Rights in the United States, edited by Lois Ann Lorentzen, vol. 2, 297–319. Santa Barbara: Praeger.

Hull, Matthew W. 2012. *Government of Paper: The Materiality of Bureaucracy in Urban Pakistan*. Berkeley: University of California Press.

Hunt, Nancy Rose. 1999. *A Colonial Lexicon: Of Birth Work, Medicalization, and Mobility in the Congo*. Durham, NC: Duke University Press.

Hutchins, Edwin. 1995. *Cognition in the Wild*. Cambridge, MA: MIT Press.

Hymes, Dell H. 1981. *"In Vain I Tried to Tell You": Essays in Native American Ethnopoetics*. Philadelphia: University of Pennsylvania Press.

Instituto Nacional de Estadística. 2003. *XII Censo de población y vivienda. Población y pueblos indígenas: anexo estadístico*. Caracas: Ministerio de Planificación y desarrollo/ Instituto Nacional de Estadística.

Irvine, Judith T. 1996. "Shadow Conversations: The Indeterminacy of Participant Roles." In *The Natural History of Discourse*, edited by Michael Silverstein and Greg Urban, 131–159. Chicago: University of Chicago Press.

Jackson, Alan C. 2000. "Rabies." *Canadian Journal of Neurological Sciences* 27: 278–283.

Jaén, Maria Helena. 2001. *El sistema de salud venezolano: Desafíos*. Caracas: Ediciones IESA.

Jakobson, Roman. 1957. *Shifters, Verbal Categories, and the Russian Verb*. Cambridge, MA: Harvard University Russian Language Project.

———. 1960. "Closing Statement: Linguistics and Poetics." In *Style in Language*, edited by Thomas A. Sebeok, 350–377. Cambridge, MA: MIT Press.

———. 1971. "Signe zéro." In *Selected Writings of Roman Jakobson*, vol. 2, *Word and Language*, edited by S. Rudy, 211–219. The Hague: Mouton.

Jensen, Jakob D., et al. 2010. "Making Sense of Cancer News Coverage Trends: A Comparison of Three Comprehensive Content Analyses." *Journal of Health Communication* 15(2): 136–151.

Joffe, Hélène, and Georgina Haarhoff. 2002. "Representations of Far-Flung Illnesses: The Case of Ebola in Britain." *Social Science and Medicine* 54: 955–969.

Keane, Webb. 2013. "Ontologies, Anthropologists, and Ethical Life." *HAU: Journal of Ethnographic Theory* 3(1): 186–191.

Kleinman, Arthur. 1988. *The Illness Narratives: Suffering, Healing and the Human Condition*. New York: Basic Books.

Kohn, Eduardo. 2007. "How Dogs Dream: Amazonian Natures and the Politics of Transspecies Engagement." *American Ethnologist* 34(1): 3–24.

Kohn, Eduardo. 2013. *How Forests Think: Toward an Anthropology Beyond the Human*. Berkeley: University of California Press.

Kopytoff, Igor. 1986. "The Cultural Biography of Things: Commoditization as Process." In *The Social Life of Things*, edited by Arjun Appadurai, 64–91. Cambridge: Cambridge University Press.

Krieger, Nancy. 2011. *Epidemiology and the People's Health: Theory and Context*. Oxford: Oxford University Press.

Kristeva, Julia. 1989. *Black Sun: Depression and Melancholia*. Translated by Leon S. Roudiez. New York: Columbia University Press.

Labov, William, and Joshua Waletzy. 1967. "Narrative Analysis." In *Essays on the Verbal and Visual Arts*, edited by June Helm, 12–44. Seattle: University of Washington Press.

Laclau, Ernesto, and Chantal Mouffe. 1985. *Hegemony and Socialist Strategy*. London: Verso.

Lakoff, Andrew. 2008, "The Generic Biothreat, or, How We Became Unprepared." *Cultural Anthropology* 23(3): 399–428.

Lakoff, Andrew, and Stephen J. Collier, eds. 2008. *Biosecurity Interventions: Global Health and Security in Question*. New York: Columbia University Press.

Laplanche, Jean. (1992) 1999. *Essays on Otherness*. Translated by John Fletcher. London: Routledge.

Latour, Bruno. 1987. *Science in Action*. Cambridge, MA: Harvard University Press.

———. 1988. *The Pasteurization of France*. Cambridge, MA: Harvard University Press.

———. 1993. *We Have Never Been Modern*. Translated by Catherine Porter. Cambridge, MA: Harvard University Press.

———. 1999. "Circulating Reference." *Pandora's Hope: Essays on the Reality of Science Studies*. Cambridge, MA: Harvard University Press.

Laurell, Asa Christina. 2003. "What Does Latin American Social Medicine Do When It Governs: The Case of the Mexico City Government." *American Journal of Public Health* 93(12): 2028–2031.

Leavitt, Judith Walzer. 1996. *Typhoid Mary: Captive to the Public's Health*. Boston: Beacon.

Levinson, Stephen C. 1988. "Putting Linguistics on a Proper Footing: Explorations in Goffman's Participation Framework." In *Goffman: Exploring the Interaction Order*, edited by Paul Drew and Anthony J. Wootton, 161–227. Oxford: Polity.

Linares, Omar. 1986. *Murciélagos de Venezuela*. Caracas: Cuadernos de Lagoven.

Lindenbaum, Shirley. 2001. "Kuru, Prions, and Human Affairs: Thinking about Epidemics." *Annual Review of Anthropology* 30: 363–385.

Lloyd, G. E. R. 2012. *Being, Humanity, and Understanding*. Oxford: Oxford University Press.

López, Leslie. 2005. "De Facto Disentitlement in an Information Economy: Enrollment Issues in Medicaid Managed Care." *Medical Anthropology Quarterly* 19(1): 26–46.

Lundby, Kurt. 2009. *Mediatization: Concept, Changes, Consequences*. New York: Peter Lang.

Lupton, Deborah. 1994a. "Toward the Development of a Critical Health Communication Praxis." *Health Communication* 6(1): 55–67.

———. 1994b. *Moral Threats and Dangerous Desires: AIDS in the News Media*. London: Falmer.

Mann, Jonathan M., Sofia Gruskin, Michael A. Grodin, and George J. Annas, eds. 1999. *Health and Human Rights: A Reader*. New York: Routledge.

Martín Barbero, Jesús. 1987. *De los medios a las mediaciones: Comunicación, cultura y hegemonía*. Mexico: Ediciones G. Gili.

Marx, Karl. (1939) 1973. *Grundrisse: Introduction to the Critique of Political Economy*. New York: Vintage.

Mattingly, Cheryl. 1998. *Healing Dramas and Clinical Plots: The Narrative Structure of Experience*. Cambridge: Cambridge University Press.

Menéndez, Eduardo L. 1981. *Poder, estratificación y salud: Análisis de las condiciones sociales y económicas de la enfermedad en Yucatán.* Mexico: La Casa Chata.

———. 2005. Intencionalidad, experiencia y función: La articulación de los saberes médicos. *Revista de Antropología Social* 14: 33–69.

———. 2009. *De sujetos, saberes y estructuras: Introducción al enfoque relacional en el estudio de la salud colectiva.* Buenos Aires: Lugar Editorial.

Menéndez, Eduardo L., and Renée B. Di Pardo. 1996. *De algunos alcoholismos y algunos saberes: Atención primaria y proceso de alcoholización.* Mexico City: CIESAS.

———. 2010. *Miedos, riesgos e inseguridades: El papel de los medios, de los profesionales y de los intelectuales en la construcción de la salud como catástrofe.* Mexico City: CIESAS.

Minkler, Meredith, and Nina Wallerstein, eds. 2008. *Community-Based Participatory Research for Health: From Process to Outcomes,* 2nd ed. San Francisco: Jossey-Bass.

Mishler, Elliot. 1984. *The Discourse of Medicine: Dialectics of Medical Interviews.* Norwood, NJ: Ablex.

———. 1986. *Research Interviewing: Context and Narrative.* Cambridge, MA: Harvard University Press.

Mol, Annemarie. 2008. *The Logic of Care: Health and the Problem of Patient Choice.* London: Routledge.

Monserrat, Rubén Ayalón. 2005. "Barrio Adentro: Combatir la exclusión profundizando la democracia." *Revista Venezolana de Economía y Ciencias Sociales* 11(3): 219–244.

Montoya, Michael. 2011. *Making the Mexican Diabetic: Race, Science, and the Genetics of Inequality.* Berkeley: University of California Press.

Moraleda, Librado. 1979. *Mawaraotuma, karata teribukitane naminaki: Primer libro de lectura Warao.* Caracas: Ministerio de Educación, Oficina Ministerial de Asuntos Fronterizos Indígenas.

Moraleda, Librado, and Basilio López. 1982. *Ka jobaji ekuya kujuki: Viajemos por nuestra tierra.* Caracas: Ministerio de Educación, Dirección de Asuntos Indígenas.

Morgan, Lynn M. 1993. *Community Participation in Health: The Politics of Primary Care in Costa Rica.* Cambridge: Cambridge University Press.

Muntaner, Carles, et al. 2006. "Venezuela's Barrio Adentro: An Alternative to Neoliberalism in Health Care." *International Journal of Health Services* 36(4): 803–811.

Nasio, Juan-David. 2004. *The Book of Love and Pain: Thinking at the Limit with Freud and Lacan.* Translated by David Pettigrew and François Raffoul. Albany: State University of New York Press.

Nations, Marilyn, and Christina Monte. 1996. "'I'm Not Dog, No!' Cries of Resistance against Cholera Control Campaigns." *Social Science and Medicine* 43(6): 1007–1024.

Nelson, Diane. 1999. *A Finger in the Wound: Body Politics in Quincentennial Guatemala.* Berkeley: University of California Press.

———. 2009. *Reckoning: The Ends of War in Guatemala.* Durham, NC: Duke University Press.

Nichter, Mark. 2008. *Global Health: Why Cultural Perceptions, Social Representations, and Biopolitics Matter.* Tucson: University of Arizona Press.

Nichter, Mark, and Vinay Kamat. 1998. "Pharmacies, Self-Medication and Pharmaceutical Marketing in Bombay India." *Social Science and Medicine* 47(6): 779–794.

Olsen, Dale A. 1996. *Music of the Warao of Venezuela: Song People of the Rain Forest.* Gainesville: University Press of Florida.

Organización Panamericana de la Salud (OPS). 2006. *Barrio Adentro: Derecho a la salud e inserción social en Venezuela.* Caracas: Organización Panamericana de la Salud.

Osborn, Henry. 1958. "Textos folkloricos en Guarao." *Boletin Indigenísta Venezolano* 3–5: 163–170; 6: 157–173.

———. 1960. "Textos folklóricos guarao." *Antropológica* 9: 21–38; 10: 71–80.

———. 1964. "Adivinanzas Warao." *Boletin Indigenista Venezolano* 9(1–4): 37–58.

———. 1967. "Warao III: Verbs and Suffixes." *International Journal of American Linguistics* 3: 46–64.

Parsons, Talcott. 1951. *The Social System.* London: Routledge.

Peirce, Charles Sanders. 1932. *Collected Papers of Charles Sanders Peirce.* Vol. 2, *Elements of Logic.* Edited by C. Hartshorne and P. Weiss. Cambridge, MA: Harvard University Press.

———. (1940) 1955. *Philosophical Writings of Charles Sanders Peirce.* Edited by Justus Buchler. New York: Dover.

Petryna, Adriana. 2002. *Life Exposed: Biological Citizens after Chernobyl.* Princeton, NJ: Princeton University Press.

Plotkin, Stanley A. "Rabies." *Clinical Infectious Diseases* 30 (2000): 4–12.

Pollak-Eltz, Angelina. 1972. *María Lionza: Mito y culto venezolano.* Caracas: Universidad Católica "Andres Bello," Instituto de Investigaciones Históricas.

Poovey, Mary. 1998. *A History of the Modern Fact: Problems of Knowledge in the Sciences of Wealth and Society.* Chicago: University of Chicago Press.

Povinelli, Elizabeth. 2006. *The Empire of Love: Toward a Theory of Intimacy, Genealogy, and Carnality.* Durham, NC: Duke University Press.

Ramos, Alcida. 2012. "The Politics of Perspectivism." *Annual Review of Anthropology* 41: 481–494.

Redfield, Peter. 2013a. "Commentary: Eyes Wide Shut in Transnational Science and Aid." *American Ethnologist* 40(1): 33–37.

———. 2013b. *Life in Crisis: The Ethical Journey of Doctors without Borders.* Berkeley: University of California Press.

Ricoeur, Paul. 1980. "Narrative Time." In *On Narrative,* edited by W. J. F. Mitchell, 165–186. Chicago: University of Chicago Press.

Riles, Annelise. 1998. "Infinity within the Brackets." *American Ethnologist* 25(3): 378–398.

———. 2000. *The Network Inside Out.* Ann Arbor: University of Michigan Press.

Riles, Annelise, ed. 2006. *Documents: Artifacts of Modern Knowledge.* Ann Arbor: University of Michigan Press.

Rose, Nikolas. 2006. *The Politics of Life Itself: Biomedicine, Power, and Subjectivity in the Twenty-First Century.* Princeton, NJ: Princeton University Press.

Rosenberg, Charles E. 1992. *Explaining Epidemics and Other Studies in the History of Medicine.* Cambridge: Cambridge University Press.

Roth, Walter. 1915. "An Inquiry into the Animism and Folklore-Lore of the Guiana Indians." *Thirtieth Annual Report of the Bureau of American Ethnology*. Washington, DC: Government Printing Office.

Sacks, Oliver. 1985. *The Man Who Mistook His Wife for a Hat and Other Clinical Tales*. New York: Perennial.

Salas de Lecuna, Yolanda. 1985. *El cuento folklórico en Venezuela: Antología, clasificación y estudio*. Caracas: Academic Nacional de la Historia.

Salazar, Juan Francisco, and Amalia Córdova. 2008. "Imperfect Media and the Poetics of Indigenous Video in Latin America." In *Global Indigenous Media*, edited by Pamela Wilson and Michelle Stewart, 39–57. Durham, NC: Duke University Press.

Samet, Robert Nathan. 2012. "Crime, Journalism, and Fearful Citizenship in Caracas, Venezuela." Unpublished PhD diss., Department of Anthropology, Stanford University, Palo Alto, California.

Sangaramoorthy, Thurka. 2014. *Treating AIDS: Politics of Difference, Paradox of Prevention*. New Brunswick, NJ: Rutgers University Press.

Scheper-Hughes, Nancy. 1992. *Death without Weeping: The Violence of Everyday Life in Brazil*. Berkeley: University of California Press.

———. 2002. "Commodity Fetishism in Organs Trafficking." In *Commodifying Bodies*, edited by Nancy Scheper-Hughes and Loïc Wacquant, 31–62. London: Sage.

Schiller, Naomi. 2013. "Reckoning with Press Freedom: Community Media, Liberalism, and the Processual State in Caracas, Venezuela." *American Ethnologist* 40(3): 540–554.

Schneider, M. C., P. C. Romijn, W. Uieda, H. Tamayo, D. F. da Silva, A. Belotto, J. B. da Silva, and L. F. Leanes. 2009. "Rabies Transmitted by Vampire Bats to Humans: An Emerging Zoonotic Disease in Latin America?" *Revista Panamericana de Salud Pública* 25: 260–269.

Schoch-Spana, Monica. 2004. "Bioterrorism: U.S. Public Health and a Secular Apocalypse." *Anthropology Today* 20(5): 8–13.

Seale, Clive. 2002. *Media and Health*. Thousand Oaks, CA: Sage.

Sekoff, Jed. 1999. "The Undead: Necromancy and the Inner World." In *The Dead Mother: The Work of André Green*, edited by Gregorio Kohon, 109–127. London: Routledge.

Seremetakis, C. Nadia. 1991. *The Last Word: Women, Death, and Divination in Inner Mani*. Chicago: University of Chicago Press.

Servicio de Apoyo Local, A. C. (SOCSAL). 1998. "Registro sociodemográfico warao de Punta Pescador." Photocopy.

Shuman, Amy. 2005. *Other People's Stories: Entitlement Claims and the Critique of Empathy*. Urbana: University of Illinois Press.

Singer, Merrill. 2009. *Introduction to Syndemics: A Critical Systems Approach to Public and Community Health*. San Francisco: Jossey-Bass.

Singer, Merrill, and Scott Clair. 2003. "Syndemics and Public Health: Reconceptualizing Disease in Bio-Social Context." *Medical Anthropology Quarterly* 17(4): 423–441.

Slater, Candace. 1994. *Dance of the Dolphin: Transformation and Disenchantment in the Amazonian Imagination*. Chicago: University of Chicago Press.

Smedley, Brian D., Adrienne Y. Stith, and Alan Nelson, eds. 2002. *Unequal Treatment: Confronting Racial and Ethnic Disparities in Health Care*. Washington, DC: National Academies Press.

Smith, Linda Tuhiwai. 1999. *Decolonizing Methodologies: Research and Indigenous Peoples*. London: Zed.

———. 2008. "Decolonizing Methodologies: Research and Indigenous Peoples." In *Handbook of Critical and Indigenous Methodologies*, edited by Norman K. Denzin, Yvonna S. Lincoln, and Linda Tuhiwai Smith. Los Angeles: Sage.

Star, Susan Leigh, and James Griesemer. 1989. "Institutional Ecology, 'Translations,' and Boundary Objects: Amateurs and Professionals in Berkeley's Museum of Vertebrate Zoology, 1907–39." *Social Studies of Science* 19(3): 387–420.

Stengers, Isabelle. 2005. "The Cosmopolitical Proposal." In *Making Things Public: Atmospheres of Democracy*, edited by Bruno Latour and Peter Weibel, 994–1003. Cambridge, MA: MIT Press.

Stevenson, Lisa. 2014. *Life Beside Itself: Imagining Care in the Canadian Artic*. Berkeley: University of California Press.

Stewart, Kathleen. 2007. *Ordinary Affects*. Durham, NC: Duke University Press.

Strathern, Marilyn. 1999. *Property, Substances and Effect: Anthropological Essays on Persons and Things*. London: Athlone.

———. 2006. "Bullet-Proofing: A Tale from the United Kingdom." In *Documents: Artifacts of Modern Knowledge*, edited by Annelise Riles, 181–205. Ann Arbor: University of Michigan Press.

Sundberg, Johan. 1974. "Articulatory Interpretation of the 'Singing Formant.'" *Journal of the Acoustic Society of America* 55: 838–844.

Tannen, Deborah, and Cynthia Wallat. 1983. "Doctor/Mother/Child Communication: Linguistic Analysis of a Pediatric Interaction." In *The Social Organization of Doctor-Patient Communication*, edited by Sue Fisher and Alexandra Dundas Todd, 203–219. Washington, DC: Center for Applied Linguistics.

Taussig, Michael. (1980) 1992. "Reification and the Consciousness of the Patient." In *The Nervous System*, 83–109. New York: Routledge.

———. 1987. *Shamanism, Colonialism, and the Wild Man: A Study in Terror and Healing*. Chicago: University of Chicago Press.

———. 1993. *Mimesis and Alterity: A Particular History of the Senses*. New York: Routledge.

———. 1999. *Defacement: Public Secrecy and the Labor of the Negative*. Palo Alto, CA: Stanford University Press.

Taylor, Diana. 2003. *The Archive and the Repertoire: Performing Cultural Memory in the Americas*. Durham, NC: Duke University Press.

Ticktin, Miriam. 2011. *Casualties of Care: Immigration and the Politics of Humanitarianism in France*. Berkeley: University of California Press.

Treichler, Paula A. 1999. *How to Have Theory in an Epidemic: Cultural Chronicles of AIDS*. Durham, NC: Duke University Press.

Trostle, James A. 1998. "Medical Compliance as an Ideology." *Social Science and Medicine* 27(12): 1299–1308.

———. 2005. *Epidemiology and Culture*. Cambridge: Cambridge University Press.

Tsing, Anna. 2005. *Friction: An Ethnography of Global Connection*. Berkeley: University of California Press.

Turner, Terence S. 2009. "The Crisis of Late Structuralism: Perspectivism and Animism: Rethinking Culture, Nature, Spirit, and Bodiliness." *Tipití: Journal of the Society for the Anthropology of Lowland South America* 7(1): 1–40.

Ungar, Sheldon. 1998. "Hot Crises and Media Reassurance: A Comparison of Emerging Diseases and Ebola Zaire." *British Journal of Sociology* 49(1): 36–56.

Urban, Greg. 1988. "Ritual Wailing in Amerindian Brazil." *American Anthropologist* 90(2): 385–400.

Urciuoli, Bonnie. 1996. *Exposing Prejudice: Puerto Rican Experiences of Language, Race and Class*. Boulder, CO: Westview.

Urry, John. 2007. *Mobilities*. Cambridge: Polity.

Vaughan, Megan. 1991. *Curing Their Ills: Colonial Power and African Illness*. Stanford: Stanford University Press.

Villalba, Julian A., Yushi Liu, Mauyuri K. Alvarez, et al. 2013. "Low Child Survival Index in a Multi-dimensionally Poor Amerindian Population in Venezuela." *PLoS ONE* 8(12): 1–13. http://dx.doi.org/10.1371/journal.pone.0085638.

Viveiros de Castro, Eduardo. 1998. "Cosmological Deixis and Amerindian Perspectivism." *Journal of the Royal Anthropological Institute* 4(3): 469–488.

———. 2004. "Exchanging Perspectives: The Transformation of Objects into Subjects in Amerindian Ontologies." *Common Knowledge* 10(3): 463–484.

Vološinov, V. N. 1973 (1930). *Marxism and the Philosophy of Language*. Translated by Ladislav Metejka and I. R. Titunik. New York: Seminar Press.

Wacquant, Loïc. 2002. "From Slavery to Mass Incarceration: Rethinking the 'Race Question' in the US." *New Left Review* 13: 41–60.

Wagner, Roy. 1984. "Ritual as Communication: Order, Meaning, and Secrecy in Melanesian Initiation Rites." *Annual Review of Anthropology* 13: 143–155.

Waitzkin, Howard. 1991. *The Politics of Medical Encounters: How Patients and Doctors Deal with Social Problems*. New Haven, CT: Yale University Press.

———. 2005. "The Contribution of Salvador Allende to Epidemiology." *International Journal of Epidemiology* 34(4): 739–741.

———. 2011. *Medicine and Public Health at the End of Empire*. Boulder, CO: Paradigm.

Waitzkin, Howard, Cecilia Iriat, Alfredo Estrada, and Silvia Lamadrid. 2001. "Social Medicine in Latin America: Productivity and Dangers Facing the Major National Groups." *Lancet* 358: 315–323.

Wald, Patricia. 2008. *Contagious: Cultures, Carriers, and the Outbreak Narrative*. Durham, NC: Duke University Press.

Walsh, Catherine. 2010a. "Development as Buen Vivir: Institutional Arrangements and (De)Colonial Entanglements." *Development* 53(1): 15–21.

———. 2010b. "Fundamentos para una interculturalidad crítica. In *Construyendo interculturalidad crítica*, by Jorge Viaña, Luis Tapia, and Catherine Walsh. La Paz, Bolivia: Instituto Internacional de Integración del Convenio Andrés Bello.

Wasik, Bill, and Monica Murphy. 2012. *Rabid: A Cultural History of the World's Most Diabolical Virus*. New York: Viking.

Weber, Max. 1978. *Economy and Society.* Berkeley: University of California Press.

Weisbrot, Mark, and Tara Ruttenberg. 2010. "Television in Venezuela: Who Dominates the Media?" *MR Zine*, December 13, http://mrzine.monthlyreview.org/2010 /wr131210.html.

Wilbert, Johannes. 1980. "Genesis and Demography of a Warao Subtribe: The Winikina." In *Demographic and Biological Studies of the Warao Indians*, edited by Johannes Wilbert and Miguel Layrisse, 13–47. Los Angeles: UCLA Latin American Center.

———. 1987. *Tobacco and Shamanism in South America.* New Haven, CT: Yale University Press.

———. 1993. *Mystic Endowment: Religious Ethnography of the Warao Indians.* Cambridge, MA: Harvard University Center for the Study of World Religions.

Wilbert, Werner. 1996. *Fitoterápia Warao: Una teoría pnéumica de la salud, la enfermedad y la terápia.* Caracas: Instituto Caribe de Antropología y Sociología.

Wilbert, Werner, and Cecilia Ayala Lafée-Wilbert. 2007. "Los Warao." In *Salud Indígena en Venezuela*, edited by Germán Freire and Aimé Tillett, 331–396. Caracas: Gobierno Bolivariano de Venezuela, Ministerio del Poder Popular para la Salud.

Wilson, Pamela, and Michelle Stewart, eds. 2008. *Global Indigenous Media: Cultures, Poetics, and Politics.* Durham, NC: Duke University Press.

Woolard, Kathryn. 1989. "Sentences in the Language Prison: The Rhetorical Structuring of an American Language Policy Debate." *American Ethnologist* 16(2): 268–278.

World Health Organization. 2010. "Rabies Vaccines: WHO Position Paper." *Weekly Epidemiological Record* 85: 309–320.

———. 2014. "Rabies." Fact Sheet No. 99. Last modified September 2014. http://www .who.int/mediacentre/factsheets/fs099/en/, accessed 1 January 2015.

Zentella, Ana Celia. 2002. "Latin@ Languages and Identities." In *Latinos: Remaking America*, edited by Marcelo M. Suárez-Orozco and Mariela M. Páez, 321–338. Berkeley: University of California Press.

Zoller, Heather M., and Mohan J. Dutta, eds. 2008. *Emerging Perspectives in Health Communication: Meaning, Culture, and Power.* New York: Routledge.

INDEX

Benjamin, Walter, 168, 170, 172
Bernstein, Alissa, 200
Beverley, John, 166
Biehl, João, 9, 268
biocommunicability, 24, 230–32, 250, 252, 258;
    and health/communicative inequities, 241,
    266, 270–71, 272, 285n4
biomediatization, 23–25, 47–48, 125, 138, 224,
    225–44, 260, 285n4, 286n7; of cholera
    epidemic, 25, 247; criminalization of
    popular participation in, 244; defined, 24;
    and epidemiology, 234, 270; and health/
    communicative inequities, 235, 243, 269;
    internet and social media, 23, 129, 155,
    227, 228, 260, 270; of rabies epidemic, 24,
    123–24; and racial stereotypes, 242; and
    symbolic violence, 242
biomedicalization, 241, 253, 266
biosecurity, 266–67
Blackwell, Maylei, 265–66
blame, 4, 6, 13, 89, 92, 93, 98, 133, 135, 147, 165,
    226, 261
blood, 23, 93, 114, 120, 121, 142, 186, 191, 193,
    194, 195, 196, 237, 282n16; menstrual, 104,
    105, 282n11
body, 6, 95, 125, 134, 140, 159, 164, 168, 169, 181,
    182, 185, 186, 192, 193, 196, 197, 206, 207, 220,
    229, 242, 256–57, 261, 264, 279n6, 282n2;
    biomedical constructions of, 192; dead
    bodies, 20, 173, 179, 180, 184, 206, 207, 216,
    241, 260, 261; and hygiene, 248, 250; and
    indexical calibration, 184–87, 202, 203; and
    laments, 207, 208, 210, 219; and narratives,
    34, 161, 168, 169, 186, 197
Bolivia, 23, 200, 272; constitution, xix, 23, 75,
    144, 251, 265
Bolivarian revolution, 2, 137, 140, 144, 253, 262
bongueros (itinerant merchants), 31, 71
boundary objects, 21, 194, 206, 207, 241;
    defined, 182; diagnosis as, 181; narratives as,
    206; and social inequity, 183
boundary-work, 9, 200, 240, 242, 243, 267
Bourdieu, Pierre, 183, 256
Bowker, Geoffrey, 182, 202, 206, 223, 229
Brazil, 72, 142, 219, 284n1
Breilh, Jaime, 9, 171, 254–55, 265, 272
Brown, Phil, 167, 272
Brudzinski sign, 120, 283n15

bureaucratic disentitlement, 7
Buenaventura, Carmen (El Nacional health
    reporter), 137–54, 172, 176, 187, 188, 232,
    235, 237
buen vivir (good living), 23, 265
Butler, Judith, 209, 221–22

Cáceres, Ricardo (resident physician, Nabasa-
    nuka Clinic), 18, 33, 34, 36, 43, 45, 80,
    92–93, 106, 107, 112, 114, 120, 121, 122, 139,
    143, 185, 199, 271; and autopsies, 188; and
    indexical calibration, 186–87; and participa-
    tion frameworks, 187–88; perception by
    residents of Nabasanuka, 81; perception of
    healers, 164; view of parents, 186
Cadena, Marisol de la, 22, 195
Campero, Avelino (Bamutanoko healer who
    treated Elbia Torres Rivas), 65, 100–102, 212
cancer, 54, 79, 194, 246
Cañizález, Miguel, 285n2
canoes, 2, 10, 30, 62, 65, 67, 100, 216
Capuchin priests and boarding school, 77, 84, 152
Caracas, xix, 13, 15, 25, 26, 47, 83, 129, 130, 137,
    138, 144, 149, 150, 152, 251; biomediatiza-
    tion in, 232–33, 235–39, 241, 242, 244–53;
    as center of biomedical calculation, 112,
    114, 120, 121, 123, 124, 125, 136, 139, 143, 175,
    161, 163, 264; journalists in, 138, 141, 142,
    189; and Mission Barrio Adentro, 251–52;
    and social inequality, 140, 153, 175, 177, 226
carceral apparatus, 249–50
care, 180, 196, 246; and Bolivarian revolu-
    tion, 2–3, 20; coproduction of care and
    communication, 5, 6, 7, 9, 17; in epidemic,
    1, 4, 9, 31–67; and health/communicative
    inequities, 9–10, 263, 268, 272; and health/
    communicative labor, 268; and humanitari-
    anism, 263, 264–65; inadequacies of, 41; and
    knowledge production, 21–22, 179–204, 255;
    labor of, 5, 6, 7, 18, 262–63, 268; lay contribu-
    tions to, 31–67, 268, 271; logic of, 5; and nar-
    ration, 18–20; palliative, 14, 65; of racialized
    populations, 6–7, 268; relational distribution
    of, 262–63; specialized, 11, 36, 37–40, 44,
    57–59, 267; temporalities of, 171
Carrasquero, Matilse (mother of Adalia and
    Ángel Gabriel), 34–36, 112, 150
cartoon, 53, 169, 242

Coronil, Fernando, 282n2
cosmopolitics, 22, 195, 207
criminalization, 143, 148–49, 161, 186, 189, 202, 277, 266
criollo (non-indigenous), 31, 38, 40, 44, 63, 190, 221–22, 242, 246; bad medicine, 95, 101, 103, 105–6, 109
critical epidemiology, 9, 20, 21, 171, 254, 255, 265
Cuba, biomediatization in, 233
Cuban epidemiologists, xvii, xxi, 12, 118, 119, 142, 280n3, 280n4, 281n6
Cuban physicians in Venezuela, xix, xx, 2, 251, 252, 267, 286n8. *See also* Mission Barrio Adentro
cultural logics, 1, 15, 135, 146, 147, 150, 152, 172, 188, 231–32, 242; and epidemiological apparatus, 250; and Latinos, 270
cultural production, 241–42
culture, incarcerated by, 161, 202, 248
crabs, 231–32

Danz, Shari, 7
Das, Veena, 23, 167, 170, 256–57
Davidson, Brad, 8, 164
death, 171, 172, 177, 186, 208, 226, 239, 250, 261, 262; of animals, 190, 195; in cholera epidemic, 247–48; enumeration of, 199, 205, 235, 237–38; and hospital practices, 281n7; and lament, 206–24; narratives and, 183, 185, 188; normal, 2, 15, 111, 116, 132, 146, 183, 198, 238, 246, 247, 255, 256, 260; social, 173, 193, 261
de Certeau, Michel, 160
decolonial, 208, 248, 257, 265–66
decolonization, 265, 266, 273
dehydration, 2, 247
dengue fever, 120, 137, 253
denuncia, 130, 131, 133, 135, 136, 138, 144, 146, 236–37
Derrida, Jacques, 201
Department of Homeland Security, 266
Descola, Philippe, 191–92, 193
diabetes, 269, 270
diagnosis, xvii, xviii, 14, 15, 24, 84, 89, 96, 186, 192, 205, 271; and autopsies, 81, 143; as boundary object, 183, 203; and circulation, 13, 27, 182; empirical, 180; and epidemiology, 109, 123, 125–26; failure of, 3, 5, 11, 21–22, 77,

92, 94, 130, 165, 173, 180, 184, 203, 232, 237; and health/communicative inequities, 8; and narratives, 17, 20; as performance, 261; and political liability, 182, 198; presumptive diagnosis of rabies, 71–73, 140, 142, 149, 154, 180, 260; self-diagnosis, 168, 268; and symbolic authority, 181–83
dialogue, 3, 169, 197, 204, 261, 263, 269
Diario VEA (national newspaper aligned with government), 144, 228, 232, 233, 236
diarrhea, 88, 111, 119, 120, 121, 134, 145, 146, 152, 153, 172, 175, 182, 183, 198, 234–35, 237, 241, 246
dipyrone (fever, pain, and spasm reducing medication), 92
DirectTV, 53, 141, 242, 257
disability, 263, 272
discrimination, xx, xxi, 16, 59, 93, 106, 153, 180, 221, 242, 244, 246, 255
divination, xvi, 103
distortion, and health journalism, 7, 229
doctor-patient interaction, 6, 8, 18, 163, 251, 252, 256, 267
documents, 45, 116–17, 118–19, 131; aesthetics, of, 200; epidemiological, 114, 176, 199; and iconic transparency, 196; and political resistance, 239; team's report, 15, 138, 140, 146, 186, 190, 202, 237
dogs, 183, 261
Domínguez, Ronaldo (nurse from Tucupita), 10, 116–17, 123–24
double consciousness, 242
dreams, xiv, 22, 45, 56
Dr. Luís Beltrán Zabaleta Hospital (new facility in Nabasanuka), 79
Dr. Manuel Núñez Tovar Hospital (in Maturín), 36, 38–39, 112
Du Bois, W. E. B., 222, 242
Dutta, Mohan, 8, 163, 165, 167, 168, 257, 263–64, 269, 272–73
dysphagia (difficulty swallowing), xiii, 34, 43, 68, 94, 102, 112, 119

Ebola hemorrhagic fever, 1–2, 228, 229, 261; and health/communicative inequities, 270
Ecuador, 73, 272
Ecuadorian constitution, 23, 265
El Cocal, xiii–xvi, 102, 103, 107

Ellison, Ralph, 262

El Nacional (national opposition newspaper), 127, 128, 129, 136–54, 223, 224, 228, 235, 236; Carmen Buenaventura, 137–54; and official control of health knowledge, 240; as opposition newspaper, 15, 241

El Universal (national opposition newspaper), 140–41, 142, 143, 144, 147, 228, 236

empire, 15, 123, 146–47

encephalitis (inflammation of the brain), 71, 119

enterovirus, 119, 175, 255

entitlement, 197; defined, 184

ethnomethodology, 163

empathy, 3, 124, 125, 184, 264

engaged anthropology, 21

enregisterment, defined, 183–84

environmental degradation, 142, 171, 195, 246

environmental samples, 186

epidemiological apparatus, 246–50, 258, 260, 262, 268

epidemiological investigation, 21; of diarrheas, 121; and participation frameworks, 188; by RHS, 13; by team, 13

epidemiologists, xvii, xix, xxi, 2, 3, 5, 8, 18, 22, 24, 83, 94, 100, 109–26, 165, 167, 186, 187, 188, 190, 198, 254–55, 261, 267, 272; and affect, 124–25; assistant regional, 111, 119–22, 125, 234–35; chronotopes of, 185–86, 222; Cuban, 12, 118–19, 142, 199; of Monagas state, 112, 113; municipal, 111, 115–16, 123; national, 15, 139, 247; and politics, 125–26, 130–33, 182; regional, 12, 110–13, 183–84, 186, 199, 237, 247; reports by, 176, 197, 199, 201; of RHS, 21, 109–26; visit to Mukoboina, 13, 94, 165, 197, 246, 269. *See also* Escalante, Diego; Godoy, Froilán; López, Benjamín; Othegui, Yolanda

epidemiology, 121, 183–84; and biomediatization, 23, 129–30, 134–35, 146, 172–73, 188, 228, 229, 234, 235, 270; critical, 9, 171; of cholera epidemic, 247; and health/communicative inequities, 19, 165, 171–72, 175, 269; and health/communicative justice, 268; and iconic transparency, 199; and multilingualism, 256; and narrative, 169, 171–72, 197; and normalcy, 111, 112, 255; nurses perform, 116–18; popular, 167; social, 9

Epstein, Steven, 286n6

equality, 251

erasure, 108, 202–4, 223

Erinnerungen (memories), 209, 210

errors, 21, 22, 233

Erwartungen (expectations), 209

Escalante, Diego (Cuban epidemiologist), 12, 118–19, 142, 199

Estrella, Basilio (wisidatu from Guayo), 53, 206

ethical soundscapes, 220

ethics, 22, 192, 220, 281n7

Eurocentrism, 221, 257

evidence, xvii, xviii, 3, 17, 19, 71, 73, 104, 112, 116, 121, 165, 180, 273; evidence-based, 165, 263, 273; and genre, 197, 203; lack of evidence, 154; for mercury hypothesis, 114, 115; myth as, 203; and official monopoly of health knowledge, 236–50, 271

experts, 233, 257, 269

failure to diagnose epidemic, 21, 94, 106–8

Fanon, Frantz, 58, 222

Farmer, Paul, 167, 248, 256, 261, 279n3

Fassin, Didier, 264

Fe y Algería Radio, 141, 281n10

fear, 93, 96, 100, 101, 148, 169, 212, 231, 245

Feinsilver, Julie, 251

Feld, Steven, 215

Feldman, Allen, 184

Fernández, José, 130–31

Ferrándiz, Francisco, 282n12

fetishization, 265

fever, xiii, xiv, xv, 10, 32, 33, 34, 36, 37, 38, 40, 41, 43, 44, 52, 53, 54, 60, 63, 64, 65, 67, 68, 82, 85, 91, 92, 93, 94, 96, 99, 100, 112, 119, 120, 134, 136, 152, 171, 235; and medications, 57, 80, 86–88, 89, 102, 106

Figueroa, María Luz (indigenous deputy congressional representative), 145

Florín, Adalia (patient from Mukoboina), 34–36, 107, 112–13, 114, 115–16

Florín, Ángel Gabriel (patient from Mukoboina), 34, 35, 36, 41, 43, 86, 87, 112, 184, 185, 188, 280n4

Florín, Graciano (father of Adalia and Ángel Gabriel), 34–36, 41, 107, 112

Fogón Comunitario (Community Hearth), 30, 96, 115, 116, 151

framing, 181, 238; of news stories, 236, 237, 241, 270
Freud, Sigmund, 20, 208, 210, 211, 212, 218, 222, 284n3, 284n2
funerals, 15, 45, 53, 64, 65, 225
futures, 186, 212, 221, 226; and care and communication, 177; and diagnosis, 177; and narratives, 171–72

Gandhi, Indira, 256
García, Hector (*New York Times* reporter), 138, 140, 141, 154
Garay, Jesús (patient from El Cocal), xiii–xiv, xv, 13, 102, 103, 261
Garay, Lizandro (patient from El Cocal), xiii, xiv–xvi, 13, 103, 105, 106, 108, 261
Garay Mata, Dario (father of Jesús and Lizandro), xiii, xv
Garcia, Angela, 284n2
gardening, 30, 60, 62, 77, 85, 214; as theme in laments, 210, 214, 216
Garro, Linda, 19, 160, 161
Geertz, Clifford, 176, 221
Geissler, P.W., 280n9
gender, xix, 47, 185, 193, 216, 254, 261, 263, 264, 272; and healing, 95
genre, 20, 22, 196–97, 198, 268
geographies of blame, 261
Gieryn, Thomas F., 9, 240
Gilbert, Amy, 72, 73, 194, 195
Ginsburg, Faye, 241
global health, 2, 3, 4, 243, 264–65, 273
Globovisión (opposition TV station), 141
Godoy, Froilán (regional epidemiologist), 113–14, 121, 123, 124, 134–35, 183–84, 186, 199, 237
Goffman, Erving, 181, 187, 219–21, 284n2
gold mining, 185, 283n10
Gómez, Jacinta (Elbia's grandmother), 64, 216
Gómez, Norbelys (nurse/EMT and team member), xix, 5, 13, 14, 15, 16, 25, 31, 64, 137, 138, 189, 226; and health/communicative justice, 271; and journalists, 139–42, 153, 243, 244; at Muaina meeting, 205; and state reprisals, 243; trip to Caracas, 223
Gómez, Tirso (healer and team member), xix, 5, 13, 25, 31, 65, 95, 138, 153, 189; as healer, 22; and health/communicative justice, 271; and journalists, 139–42, 243, 244; at Muaina meeting, 205; and multispecies relations, 190–95; and state reprisals, 16, 243; trip to Caracas, 223
Good, Byron, 7, 18–19, 160, 162, 163–64
Gordon, Deborah, 192
government contractors, xvi, 99, 102, 103, 106, 109, 171, 194, 210, 212
Grandmothers of the Plaza de Mayo, 239
graphic ideologies, 199–201
Griesemer, James, 21
grievability, 221–22, 224, 260–61
Guatemala, 260, 262
Guayo. *See* San Francisco de Guayo
Gupta, Akhil, 200
Guyana, 95, 117, 147
Guzmán Antonio, Roberto (prosecutor), 143, 186

H1N1 (swine flu), 127, 285n4
Haarhoff, Georgina, 229
Haiti, 167, 256, 269
Hallin, Daniel, 229, 258, 280n11, 286n2, 286n7
hallucinations, 10, 53, 56, 71, 194
handicraft production, 30, 32
Harper, Richard, 200
Harvey, T. S., 6, 164
haunting, 286n8
headache, xv, 54, 57, 71, 80, 82, 83, 89, 94, 101, 119
healers, xiv, xv, 3, 25, 36, 47, 94–106, 282n7; accused of killing patients, 132, 133, 135, 239; Avelino Campero, 100–102, 106, 212; *bahanarotu*, 95; Francisco Pérez, 98–100, 179, 225; and gender, 105; and health/communicative inequities, 108, 183, 197–98, 257, 258, 267; *hoarotu*, 32, 56; Inocencio Torres, 96–98; Paulino Zapata, 102–6; perception of, 164; physicians' antipathy towards, 92–93; and symbolic authority, 182, 183; *wisidatu*, 32, 49, 82, 85, 95, 96–98, 102–6, 172, 205, 226, 282n8; *yarokotarotu*, 41, 53, 88–89, 95, 105, 145, 180, 282n10
health committee, 11, 235, 252, 253, 269, 286n8
health communication, 6, 8, 228, 230, 253; critical perspectives in, 8, 165, 167, 257, 263–64, 269, 272–73

mediatization, 240, 249. *See also* biomediatization

medical anthropology, 228, 261

medical education, 7, 19, 162, 163, 164, 182, 183

medical interns, 82–83, 143, 185, 282n5; Leoncio D'Ambrosio, 82–83; Roselia Narváez, 82–83, 170

medicalization, 5, 172, 229, 240, 266

medical logics, 229

medical technologies, 38, 58, 59, 63, 180, 182, 188, 190

medical versus media opposition. *See* communication: as analytic construct

médico rural (recently graduated physician working in underserved population), 79, 82, 94, 188

Medina, Vicente, 237, 284n3

melancholia, 209, 222, 284n2

memory, 212; and laments, 214; and biomediatization, 226

Menéndez, Eduardo, 5, 19, 168, 243, 254, 262–63, 268

menstruation, 104, 105

mercury, 23, 71, 112, 113, 114, 115–16, 117, 119, 120, 174, 182, 184, 255, 283n10

mermaid (*la madre del aqua*), 105

metrics, 269

Millán, Emeri Mata (former Delta Amacuro governor), 248

mimesis, 196

mining, 116, 142, 147, 283n10

Ministry of Popular Power for Health (MPPS), 15, 79, 108, 121, 137–39, 154, 161, 201, 223, 260; and control of health knowledge, 139, 151, 186, 189, 201; deny presumptive diagnosis, 260; and health/communicative inequities, 269. *See also* Martinelli, Mariela; Regional Health Service; Serrano, Rafael

Ministry of Popular Power for Indigenous Peoples (MPPPI), 139, 145, 150, 152, 232, 236, 238

Minkler, Meredith, 167, 272

Mishler, Elliot, 8, 163, 167, 284n2

missions and missionaries, 49, 77, 78, 221, 249

Mission Barrio Adentro, 12, 118, 175, 199, 251–53, 256, 267, 269, 280n7, 286n7, 286n8

mobility, of knowledge, 25, 26, 175, 180–81, 182, 198, 200, 203–4, 206, 266

modernity, 249, 265

Mol, Annemarie, 5, 168

Monagas State, 113

Mondragón, Julio (former RHS director), 132, 142

monikata nome nakakitane (dispute mediation process), 47, 99

Montoro, Micaela (governor), 125, 130, 136, 142, 145, 147, 187, 189–90, 259

Moraleda, Alonzo (Nabasanuka nurse), 89–94, 120, 130, 131, 133, 161, 226, 233

Moraleda, Aureliano (Nabasanuka nurse), 89–94

Moraleda, Conrado (team member), xix, 3, 4, 25, 114, 120, 121, 125, 133, 137, 138, 139, 143, 152, 153, 237, 242; and autopsies, 185; and biomediatization, 225–27; as challenging stereotypes, 189; and February 2008 meeting, 13, 120, 125, 131, 170, 200, 226, 233, 236, 239; and health/communicative justice, 242, 271; and journalists, 139–42, 236, 243, 244, 247–48; "kidnapping," 234–35; meeting with national epidemiologist, 15; organizing team 13; perception of media, 226, 242; as president of Health Committee, 11, 137, 235; threats against, 16, 243–44

Moraleda, Enrique (team member), xix, 3, 4, 25, 47–48, 59, 137, 138, 139–42, 143, 145, 152, 153, 223; challenges health/communicative inequities, 237; challenges stereotypes, 189; and colonialism, 171, 222; engagement in politics, 137, 248; and health/communicative justice, 271; and journalists, 139–42, 243, 244; media reception, 242; media strategy, 227; at Muaina meeting, 206; organizing team, 13; on racism, 221; threats against, 16, 243–44; and team's report, 198, 202

Moraleda, Jesús (Nabasanuka nurse), 54, 89–94

Moraleda, Librado (deceased indigenous leader), 3, 46, 50, 54, 87, 138, 153, 221, 248, 281n8

Morales, Santa (mother of Yanilka), 37–40, 75, 285

morbidity, 248

Morgan, Lynn, 272

morgue, 40,

Morichito, 102, 282n14

mortality, 248

mosquito nets, 139, 141, 142, 150

mourning, 205–24; contradictory nature of, 209; and epidemiology, 20; and hyper-cathexis, 209; vis-á-vis melancholia, 222; and poetics, 209, 210–19, 221–23; temporal-ity of, 209; work of, 20, 21, 26, 108, 167, 205–24. *See also* laments

Movement toward Socialism Party (MAS), 248

Muaina, 13, 46–60, 64, 71, 83, 87–89, 102, 150, 203, 210, 216, 220; and biomediatization, 225–27; description of, 46; government contractors in, 99–100, 102, 210; laments in, 205–6; meeting in, 99, 183, 205–6, 225

Mukoboina, 2, 10–12, 30–45, 71, 80, 81, 85, 90, 93, 144, 165, 269; cemetery, 73, 150; com-mission in, 199–202; community meeting, 31; description of, 30; as epidemic ground zero, 31, 124, 185, 197; and epidemiologists, 113–19, 165, 175, 197; healer of, 96–98; in news coverage, 150, 153; nurses visit, 117; and participation frameworks, 187

multilingualism, 152, 175, 176, 267, 284n4

multiple ontologies, 23

multispecies relationship, 5, 22–23, 182, 190–95

myth, 22, 194; of bats, 22, 191–93; of *hoarani* water spirits, 104, 105

nabarao (water spirits), 104, 105, 106, 282n17

Nabasanuka, 50, 87, 93, 133, 281n1; description of, 77; visit by vice minister, 133, 235

Nabasanuka clinic, 10, 12, 30, 32, 33, 36, 43, 44, 56, 57, 60, 77–81, 85, 89–94; history of, 77; nurses of, 89–94, 106; two-way radio, 81, 90, 198

nahanamu (ceremony), 95

narratives, 159–78; of care and communication, 177; circulation of, 173–74; defined, 184; events of narration and narrated events, 169; failure of, 173; and global health, 177; and health/communicative inequities, 268; and heteroglossia, 169; and labor, 168; and laments, 221; and mobility, 206–7; practices, 161; and research, 206; social lives of, 160–73; and symbolic authority, 183; and temporality, 170–72, 185; and violence, 260

Narváez, Roselia (medical intern in Nabasa-nuka), 82–83, 170

Nasio, Juan-David, 218

National Dengue Fever Program, 153, 253

National Institute of Hygiene, 112, 114, 123

National Office of Health Committees, 252

naturalism, 192

natureculture, 192, 265

nehimanoko (menstrual house), 43, 105

Nelson, Diane, 110, 262

neoliberalism, 9, 273

neurological abnormalities, 68, 71, 83, 120, 194, 281n12

Newcastle virus, 195

news coverage. *See* media

New York Times, 10, 15, 140, 154, 228, 279n2

noncompliance, 247, 271

nonknowledge, 21, 22, 181, 263, 280n9; defined, 181; and indexical calibration, 187

normalcy, 115, 116, 118, 121, 125, 183, 198, 238, 246, 247, 255, 260

Notidiario, 120, 127, 128–36, 142, 148, 176, 197, 228, 237; coverage of February 2008 meeting, 130, 234–35; coverage of cholera epidemic, 247; coverage of rabies epidemic, 120, 130–36, 142–43, 149, 226, 227, 234; as definer of public sphere in Delta Amacuro, 242; of diarrheal investigation, 133–35, 235; health reporting, 129, 228; journalistic prac-tices, 135, 147, 152, 192; Leo Romero, 129–36; Oscar Marcano, 129–30, 135; and regional government, 241

nurses, xv, 10, 16, 25, 37, 82, 84–94, 102, 116–18, 234, 267, 282n6; Alonzo Moraleda, 89–94, 120, 130; Antonio Peña, 116–17; Aureliano Moraleda, 89–94; and biomediatization, 270; defined, 281n3; and diagnosis, 91, 94; and healers, 92–93; Ildebrando Zapata, 102; and indexical calibration, 186; Jesús Moraleda, 89–94; José Perez, 84–87; Mirna Pizarro, 87–89; and multilingualism, 176; of Nabasanaku clinic, 89–94; Ronaldo Domínguez, 116–17, 124; and symbolic authority, 183

nursing stations, 74, 84–89, 94, 263, 279n7

object relations theory, 208

Office of Indigenous Health, 137

oil production, 242, 251, 282n2

Oliver, Paul (AP reporter), 141–42, 144, 154

Olsen, Dale, 282n9, 282n14
ontological perspectives, 204, 268; and indexical calibration, 186–87; and multilingualism, 176
ontological relations, 190–95
ontological turn in anthropology, 22
ontologies: and narratives, 174, 177; and symbolic authority, 182
opposition, political, 137, 149, 232–33; and health policy, 250–52
optimism, 244
oración (type of healing and bad medicine), 95, 97–98, 100–102
Organic Law of Ingenious Peoples, 144
organ transplantation, 163
Orinanoko, 234
Orinoco River, xviii, 10, 29, 32, 43, 173
Osborn, Dale, 285n4
Othegui, Yolanda (municipal epidemiologist), 115, 118, 123–24, 185
overhearers, 207

Padre Barral Municipality, 98, 226
pain, 10, 31, 37, 40, 45, 67, 88, 93, 106, 140, 144, 219; and acoustic materiality, 220; and grief, 209–10, 219; some narratives as increasing, 160, 172, 173; as symptom, xiv, 14, 44, 56, 65, 68, 83, 89, 94, 100, 101, 119, 120
palliative care, 14, 65, 93, 94, 180
palm heart factories, 46, 60, 248
Pan American Health Organization, 72, 112
paresthesia (itching or tingling sensation), 10, 53, 54, 68, 71, 83, 89
Parsons, Talcott, 6, 164
participation framework, 181, 187–95, 196, 203, 204, 284n2; and circulation, 190
pasts, 186, 212, 216, 221, 226, 249; and narrative, 171–72
pathologization, 168, 272
patient advocate, 38, 44, 45
patriarchy, 47, 193
Pedernales clinic, 247
pediatricians, 112, 115, 129, 199
Peirce, Charles S., 181–82, 184, 195–96
performativity, 200, 239, 261; and archives, 239–40; of biomediatization, 240; and listening, 220; and narratives, 177; and participation frameworks, 190; and science, 239

Peña, Antonio (nurse from Tucupita), 116–17, 185
penicillin, 89
Pérez, Francisco (healer of Heukukabanoko), 98–100, 225
Pérez, Rafael (opposition politician), 133
Pérez, Rómulo (national epidemiologist), 139. *See also* epidemiologists
Pérez, José (Siawani nurse), 33, 34, 84–87, 89, 94, 106, 116
Peru, 72, 73, 142, 194, 229, 281n13, 284n1
personal narratives. *See* narratives
perspectivism, 192, 193, 194
pharmaceuticals, 8, 9, 24, 254, 273
pharmaceutical industry, 7, 8, 23, 286n6
photographs, 14, 15, 25–26, 79, 196, 197, 202, 239; in cholera epidemic, 229–30, 248; of Elbia Torres Rivas and family, 65, 138, 139, 142, 223–24; and mourning, 138, 223–24; in newspaper coverage, 131, 133, 134, 140, 141, 142, 150, 152, 229; in scientific documents, 196; and the work of memory, 223–24
physicians, xix, 1, 2, 111, 163, 238, 270, 273; and biomediatization, 7, 128, 134, 136, 153–54, 187, 188, 227, 228, 233, 237; and care, 180; and doctor-patient interaction, 6, 7, 8, 18–19, 163–64, 175, 251–52, 256, 257; and documentation, 7, 94, 201, 268; as epidemiologists, 115, 126, 184; and healers, 43, 92–93, 98, 102, 104, 106, 108, 164, 182; and health/communicative inequities, 4, 81, 92, 94, 168, 172, 268, 271, 272; and institutional hierarchies, 83, 89, 94, 263; and multilingualism, 38, 164, 175, 198, 267; and Nabasanuka clinic, 10, 77, 78, 79, 82; and narratives, 18–19, 161, 162, 164, 172, 175, 183, 196–97, 271; and nurses, 79, 89, 90, 93, 94; perceptions of, 36, 43, 44, 45, 81–82, 164, 175; relational definition, 6, 153, 170, 269; and stereotypes, 4, 133, 153–54, 164, 175, 233, 242, 249, 268; and symbolic capital, 181–84, 267; in urban hospitals, 36, 38, 44, 57, 58, 59, 63, 93, 112, 120. *See also* Cáceres, Ricardo; clinical medicine; diagnosis; medical interns; *médico rural*; Mission Barrio Adentro
Pineda, Alfredo (RHS zoonosis director), 121–22

rationality, 9, 18, 24, 170, 175, 248, 249, 254, 257

rattle, xv, 53, 93, 95, 96, 100, 102, 106, 180, 190, 196

reality testing, 211, 212, 216; defined, 209; and scale, 221

Redfield, Peter, 264

regimes of care, 263

regional epidemiologists, 12, 110–13, 114, 119–22; and chronotopes, 185. *See also* Godoy, Froilán

Regional Health Service (RHS), 3, 12, 84, 92, 129, 131, 138, 142; and biomediatization, 5, 129–36, 142–43, 233–36, 237; and cholera epidemic, 165, 232, 247–49; and Conrado Moraleda, 4, 12, 170, 200, 234–35; criticisms of, 13, 82–83, 121, 138, 139–40, 141; and epidemiological apparatus, 246–50; and health inequities, 175, 183, 197, 224, 226; controlling health communication, 16, 186, 198, 182–83, 198–99, 200–201, 232, 234–35, 237; and political power, 110, 112, 125, 184; Ricardo Cáceres, 81, 92. *See also* Ministry of Popular Power for Health; Rendón, Guillermo

Regional Office of Indigenous Affairs, 247

registers, 183–84, 196, 231, 256, 260, 267

relational definitions, 136, 192, 262–63; of biomedicine and indigenous medicine, 194, 254; of indigenous/nonindigenous, 170, 175, 246, 254; and narratives, 161, 169–70, 177; and perspectivism, 22, 192; of physicians and patients, 6, 7, 170, 175, 263, 268, 269

relational distribution of care and communication, 263

Rendón, Guillermo (RHS director), 114, 123, 133, 135, 237, 258–59; and epidemiology, 118, 123, 200, 235; and indexical calibration, 186; and news coverage, 134, 136, 138, 142, 143, 145, 237; and participation frameworks, 186, 189; political influence, 125; and visit of vice minister, 133, 235

resilience, 153, 246

resistance, 164, 171, 239, 247, 267, 271

respiratory problems, xxi, 79, 113, 119, 120, 237, 246

response cries, 219–20

Ricoeur, Paul, 170

rights: human rights, 163, 271; and research, 166; violations, 235, 259, 268, 269, 272

Riles, Annelise, 200, 201, 280n9

Rigoberta Menchu, 166

Rivas, Anita (mother of Elbia Torres Rivas), 60–67, 100, 223; laments for Elbia Rivas Torres, 212–18, 219

Rivas, Romeliano (brother of Elbia Torres Rivas), 213

Rivas, Tomás (radio journalist and member of Legislative Council), 130

Rivero, Inez (mother of Jesús and Lizandro), xiii–xvi, 102, 103

Rodríguez, Daniel (former regional epidemiologist), 247

Rodríguez, Lourdes (MPPPI representative), 150–52, 153, 172, 187, 188, 232

Romero, Leo (*Notidiario* journalist), 129–31, 133–36, 197

Rose, Nikolas, 9, 286n7

Rosenberg, Charles, 2, 172

Roth, Walter, 105, 282n15

rumors, 143, 186, 188, 196, 201, 227, 283n5; spread by health officials, 118, 131–33, 172, 226, 239, 283n5

Rupprecht, Charles, 142

saberes medicos (contrastive forms of medical knowledge), 254

Sakoinoko, 75, 119, 120, 121

Salazar, Armando (MAS leader and former governor), 248

Salazar, Pedro (mayor of Antonio Díaz Municipality and gubernatorial candidate), 125, 145, 148, 189, 241

salivation, xv, 23, 32, 34, 43, 63, 68, 71, 80, 83, 112, 117, 119, 120, 134

Samet, Robert, 232

San Diego Union-Tribune, 270

San Francisco de Guayo 49, 52, 53, 56, 77, 98, 100

Sangaramoorthy, Thurka, 268

sanitary engineer, 114–15, 142, 185

sanitary infrastructure, 145, 152, 246

Santa Rosa de Guayo, 13, 75, 98, 150, 152, 190, 238

Sapir, Edward, 201

scales, 47, 221, 237, 251, 256, 264, 269, 270, 273

Scheper-Hughes, Nancy, 163

Schneider, M. C., 72,
Schoch-Spana, Monica, 266
school boat drivers, 48, 99
science-technology-society (STS), 8, 21, 152,
   162, 181, 196, 200, 203, 224, 227, 228, 264
Seale, Clive, 8, 227, 228, 257
seizures, xiv, xv, 80, 83, 117, 134, 194
self-diagnosis, 168, 268
self-medication, 233, 268
septicemia, 120, 283n16
Seremetakis, Nadia, 220
Serrano, Rafael (MPPS minister), 137, 155,
   200–201, 231–32, 237; and biomediatization,
   146–47, 155; and indexical calibration, 186;
   and MPPS control of health knowledge, 189,
   200–201
settlement, defined, 279n6
sexual abuse, 63, 185
sexuality, 104, 105, 195, 256, 261, 263, 272
sexualization, 253
sexually transmitted infections, 7, 83
shaman, as racialized figure, 231, 241, 265
Siawani, xix, 33, 34, 49, 56, 75, 80, 83, 84–87,
   94, 105, 106, 116, 120, 210
signe zero, 201
silence, 4, 65, 93, 107, 123, 166, 167, 172, 180,
   198, 234, 235, 256, 257, 259, 267
Singer, Merrill, 246, 269
singer's formant, suppression of, 220
Slater, Candace, 104
sleep, xiii, xiv, xv, 45, 56, 59, 60, 62, 63, 71, 191,
   194, 195
sloths, 190, 195
smallpox, 248
Smith, Linda Tuhiwai, 208, 265–66
social class, 231, 263, 272
social conflicts, 180, 184
social death, 20, 25, 160, 173, 222, 261
social epidemiology, 9, 255–56
socialist revolution, xix, xx, 2, 5, 57, 137, 140,
   144, 145, 184, 202, 221, 234–35, 250, 262;
   and health communication, 250–53; and
   health/communicative inequities, 250–51;
   and media, 232–33, 240
social justice, 5, 138, 235, 241, 258. See also
   health/communicative justice
social movements, 252. See also indigenous
   social movement

social right to health, xx, 75, 161, 233, 251
social suffering, 264
solidarity, 184, 251
Sosa, Wilfredo (sanitary engineer), 114–15,
   142, 185
soursop (Annona muricata), 53
space, 22, 165, 169, 172, 182, 185, 186, 188, 193, 253;
   acoustic, 220; clinical, 77–79, 194; epidemiological, 124, 126; and health/communicative
   inequities, 187, 269; and laments, 207, 215–16;
   and narratives, 185, 196, 257
Spain, 260
spirit possession, 194, 282n12
squatter's settlement, 44–45, 63, 64
Star, Susan Leigh, 21, 182, 202, 206, 223, 229
statistics, 131, 142, 162, 262, 273; and biomediatization, 145, 146, 238–39; epidemiological,
   110–13; erasure of, 249; and health inequities, 238
stereotypes, 133, 139, 153–54, 164,189, 233,
   242, 249, 268; and biomediatization, 227,
   228, 235–36; epidemiological apparatus,
   250; of indigenous Warao ethic group, 4,
   131, 174–75, 183, 224, 228, 231–32, 250; and
   linguistic inequities, 267; and symbolic
   authority, 183
stethoscope, 190, 283n14
Stevenson, Lisa, 26
Stewart, Kathleen, 224
stigmatization, 250, 261, 271; and biocommunicability, 270–71; and biomediatization, 242;
   and health/communicative inequities, 268;
   and language, 176. See also stereotypes
Strategic Plan for Epidemiological Intervention, 134
Stengers, Isabel, 16, 22, 207, 209, 280n8
Stories in the Time of Cholera, xix, 279n4
Strathern, Marilyn, 200, 280n9
structural bases of health inequities, 1, 6, 13, 82,
   152, 163, 260, 261
Sundberg, Johan, 220
superstition, 21, 186, 202, 204, 232, 236, 265
symbol, defined, 181
symbolic authority, 181–84, 196, 202, 203;
   and genre, 197; and linguistic difference,
   267
symbolic capital, 181–87, 196, 256; defined, 183
syndemics, 246